FIFTH EDITION

Zoltan's Vision, Perception, and Cognition

Evaluation and Treatment of the Adult With Acquired Brain Injury

FIFTH EDITION

Zoltan's Vision, Perception, and Cognition

Evaluation and Treatment of the Adult With Acquired Brain Injury

Tatiana A. Kaminsky, PhD, OTR/L
University of Puget Sound
Tacoma, Washington

Janet M. Powell, PhD, OTR/L, FAOTA
Associate Professor Emerita
University of Washington
Seattle, Washington

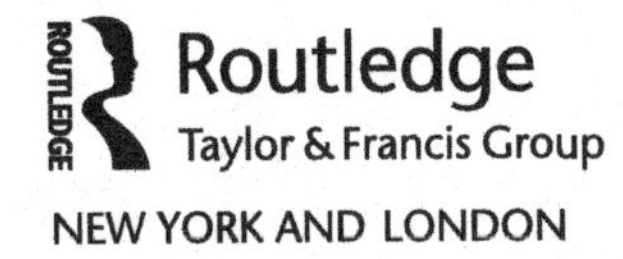

NEW YORK AND LONDON

Zoltan's Vision, Perception, and Cognition: Evaluation and Treatment of the Adult With Acquired Brain Injury, Fifth Edition includes ancillary materials specifically available for faculty use. Included is an *Instructor's Manual.* Please visit www.routledge.com/9781617110818 to obtain access.

First published in 2023 by SLACK Incorporated

Published 2024 by Routledge
605 Third Avenue, New York, NY 10017

and by Routledge
4 Park Square, Milton Park, Abingdon, Oxon OX14 4RN

Routledge is an imprint of the Taylor & Francis Group, an informa business

Dr. Tatiana A. Kaminsky *and* Dr. Janet M. Powell *reported no financial or proprietary interest in the materials presented herein.*

Cover: Tinhouse Design

Library of Congress Cataloging-in-Publication Data
Names: Kaminsky, Tatiana A., author. | Powell, Janet, author. | Zoltan, Barbara. Vision, perception, and cognition.
Title: Zoltan's vision, perception, and cognition : evaluation and treatment of the adult with acquired brain injury / Tatiana A. Kaminsky, Janet M. Powell.
Other titles: Vision, perception, and cognition
Description: Fifth edition. | Thorofare, NJ : SLACK Incorporated, [2023] | Preceded by Vision, perception, and cognition / Barbara Zoltan. 4th ed. Thorofare, NJ : SLACK Inc., c2007. | Includes bibliographical references and index.
Identifiers: LCCN 2023002322 (print) | ISBN 9781617110818 (hardcover)
Subjects: MESH: Brain Injuries--rehabilitation | Cerebrovascular Disorders--rehabilitation | Vision Disorders--diagnosis | Vision Disorders--therapy | Cognition Disorders--diagnosis | Cognition Disorders--therapy
Classification: LCC RC387.5 (print) | NLM WL 354 | DDC 617.4/81044--dc23/eng/20230313
LC record available at https://lccn.loc.gov/2023002322

ISBN: 9781617110818 (hbk)
ISBN: 9781003526896 (ebk)

DOI: 10.4324/9781003526896

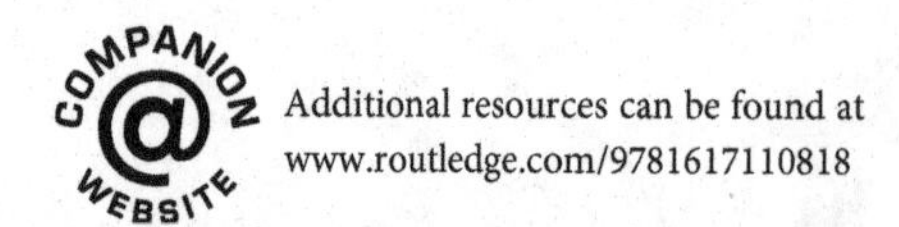

Additional resources can be found at
www.routledge.com/9781617110818

Dedication

To Mark, Ace, and Josephine for your never-ending love and patience.

—Tatiana A. Kaminsky, PhD, OTR/L

To Chris, Anne, and Colleen for your encouragement and support at every turn, and to Nancy Torgerson, OD, FCOVD, for 30 years of unparalleled interdisciplinary collaboration.

—Janet M. Powell, PhD, OTR/L, FAOTA

Contents

Zoltan's Vision, Perception, and Cognition: Evaluation and Treatment of the Adult With Acquired Brain Injury, Fifth Edition includes ancillary materials specifically available for faculty use. Included is an *Instructor's Manual.* Please visit http://www.routledge.com/9781617110818 to obtain access.

Acknowledgments

We are especially grateful to Nancy Torgerson, OD, FCOVD, and Jacqueline Daniels, MA, CCC-SLP, CBIS, for their consultation and insights into interprofessional work with adults with acquired brain injury. In addition, we would like to acknowledge the work by the occupational therapy pioneers who have come before us in the rehabilitation of adults with visual, perceptual, and cognitive disorders after acquired brain injury, with special thanks to Barbara Zoltan, MA, OT, whose previous texts have served as the foundation for this edition. We extend our thanks to Brien Cummings at SLACK Incorporated for his encouragement and eternal patience with us throughout this process. Finally, we would like to thank our clients, colleagues, and students for stimulating and supporting our lifelong learning.

About the Authors

Tatiana A. Kaminsky, PhD, OTR/L, received her Bachelor of Science in occupational therapy from the University of Wisconsin–Madison in Madison, Wisconsin, and her Master of Science in rehabilitation medicine and Doctor of Philosophy in nursing science from the University of Washington, Seattle, Washington. She has been a clinician for more than 25 years providing services to adults, especially those with neurological disorders, in a wide variety of inpatient and outpatient settings. She has also worked as a low vision therapist in a hospital outpatient setting and a low vision clinic where she partnered with optometrists. Her current clinical work focuses on home- and community-based care. Dr. Kaminsky taught full time in the School of Occupational Therapy at the University of Puget Sound in Tacoma, Washington, from 2005 until 2021 and continues to teach in an adjunct capacity. The courses she has taught have primarily focused on neuroscience and the treatment of adults with neurological disorders. Her research has focused on people with visual and/or cognitive deficits. She is especially interested in examining the use of everyday technology for adults with cognitive deficits after acquired brain injury.

Janet M. Powell, PhD, OTR/L, FAOTA, is an associate professor emerita and former Master of Occupational Therapy program director in the Division of Occupational Therapy at the University of Washington in Seattle, Washington. She holds three degrees from the University of Washington: a Bachelor of Science in occupational therapy; a Master of Science in rehabilitation medicine; and an interdisciplinary Doctor of Philosophy degree in rehabilitation medicine, psychology, biostatistics, and education. Dr. Powell's research and teaching expertise is in adult neurological rehabilitation. She has been supported by a number of federal grants to better understand the lives of people who have sustained traumatic brain injury and to investigate telephone-based, problem-solving interventions for survivors of traumatic brain injury and their family and friend caregivers. Her research has also included studies of the assessment of saccadic eye movements in adults. Dr. Powell has authored numerous journal articles, chapters in occupational therapy and optometry textbooks, and consumer resources. She has copresented nationally with an optometrist/physiatrist team on assessing and treating visual impairments in adults with acquired brain injury. Before becoming a full-time faculty member in 2001, she provided occupational therapy services to children and adults with neurological disorders in a variety of clinical settings for more than 20 years.

CHAPTER 1

Key Perspectives

The contents of this book represent a combined 60 years of clinical, research, and/or teaching experience as occupational therapists specializing in adult neurological rehabilitation—26 years for Tatiana A. Kaminsky and 34 for Janet M. Powell. These experiences have been highly influential in the decisions we have made in writing this book (e.g., the topics we have included, how we have presented the information, and our thoughts on the role of occupational therapy in this area of practice). In this chapter, we share some additional details about each of our backgrounds to help the reader better understand those decisions, explain how our experiences have shaped our thinking on the role of occupational therapy practitioners in the treatment of vision and cognitive impairments after acquired brain injury (ABI), and give a brief overview of the chapters that follow.

Our Backgrounds

Tatiana A. Kaminsky, PhD, OTR/L

Since graduating with my Bachelor of Science degree in occupational therapy in 1995, I have always worked with adults. In the beginning of my clinical career, I worked as a generalist, treating people with a wide variety of diagnoses, although those with neurological conditions were the most frequent clients on my caseload. In recent years, my clinical practice has focused exclusively on working with adults with neurological disorders, most commonly people recovering from cerebrovascular accident or traumatic brain injury (TBI). I have also worked in just about every clinical setting. I started my career in inpatient rehabilitation. Since then, I have worked in skilled nursing facilities; acute care hospitals, including the intensive care unit; transitional care units; outpatient clinics; and, most recently, home and community settings. I have always appreciated that my varied experience helps me understand the continuum of care and what our client populations often look like at different stages of recovery.

Kaminsky, T. A., & Powell, J. M.
Zoltan's Vision, Perception, and Cognition: Evaluation and Treatment of the Adult With Acquired Brain Injury, Fifth Edition (pp. 1-9).

My entry into working with people with visual disorders had a clear starting point. It began in 1997 when I took the first of what would be many courses about working with people with visual impairment. Two of those courses were taught by Mary Warren, PhD, OTR/L, SCLV, FAOTA. The first was in 1999, and the second was in 2001. The latter was a course Dr. Warren taught with the late Dr. Josephine Moore, PhD, OTR, FAOTA, who was a neuroanatomist in addition to being an occupational therapist. That course was the one that inspired my passion and interest in the neurological basis of vision. I was able to apply the concepts from these courses directly in my clinical practice, most notably through my work at the Lions Low Vision Clinic in Bellevue, Washington (which, sadly, has since shut down). I worked there once per week for almost 2 years. I worked in close partnership with optometrists who would conduct vision evaluations and then make referrals to me. I then helped people learn to use low vision devices and other strategies to facilitate their independence and safety with their occupational performance.

It is more difficult for me to pinpoint the exact moment when my interest in cognition started. I have gradually increased my knowledge in this area of practice over the years by reading a lot of research and taking courses, including in 2008 when I took the first of what would be several workshops with Joan Toglia, PhD, OTR/L, FAOTA, about the multicontext approach. However, I do remember feeling dissatisfied with my knowledge in cognitive rehabilitation, especially early in my career. I worked steadily to improve my understanding of cognition and its influence on occupational performance, work that continues today.

Much as I loved (and still love) being a clinician, my dream was always to teach. So, in 2001, I started my postprofessional education at the University of Washington (UW), Seattle, Washington, first earning a Master of Science degree in 2003 and then my Doctor of Philosophy degree in 2008. My research during this time period focused on people with neurological disorders (Parkinson's disease was the focus of my master's thesis) and low vision. For my dissertation, I studied physical and social environmental influences on the occupational functioning of people with diabetic retinopathy. Before my graduation, in 2005, I started teaching full time at the University of Puget Sound in Tacoma, Washington, where I was hired partly because of my expertise in working with people with visual disorders. One of the goals of my teaching is to make sure that every student I teach knows how to screen vision, especially for people with neurological conditions (because vision is so frequently disrupted with a brain injury), and how to work with people with visual disorders while staying within their scope of practice (see more details of that viewpoint later). In 2021, for a variety of reasons, I left full-time teaching at the University of Puget Sound, although I continue to work with students in an advisory capacity and as an adjunct instructor.

My teaching shifted over the 16 years I taught full time from more foundational courses to classes that focus on neurological conditions. I taught neuroscience to entry-level students, in addition to teaching courses focusing on the evaluation and treatment of adults, especially adults with neurological conditions. The change in my teaching continued to drive my exploration of cognitive rehabilitation, and I have been thrilled with the major changes in our profession in recent years to a more defined focus on functional cognition. I have worked with numerous colleagues in the past, including occupational therapy practitioners, who do not understand the incredibly important perspective occupational therapy brings to the rehabilitation of people with cognitive deficits. I have even been told that cognition is not something occupational therapy practitioners should work on because it is covered by other disciplines, including speech-language pathologists and neuropsychologists. I have always found that to be a confusing viewpoint. Cognitive functioning is such an integral part of people's ability to complete occupation that to not address cognition feels as irrational to me as not addressing functional mobility would be.

One of the challenges I have faced in my clinical practice, and in my teaching, is in the evaluation of people with cognitive deficits. Cognition is often difficult to quantify and is very complex. Looking at individual impairments never felt like it captured the whole complex picture of how people were struggling or succeeding. Becoming certified to use the Assessment of Motor and Process Skills (AMPS) in 2015 has helped. The AMPS is a very powerful and occupationally based tool that can help clinicians identify the way in which the clients' deficits are impacting occupational performance. In addition to my AMPS certification, having access to increasing numbers of functionally based assessment tools that are being developed by occupational scientists helps, as do the conversations the profession is having about functional cognition. This evolution in our discipline helps to define the unique role the occupational therapist has in cognitive rehabilitation. In recent years, my area of research has been more focused on how occupational therapy practitioners can use everyday technology (e.g., smartphones, tablets, laptops) in cognitive rehabilitation. With the increasingly widespread use of technology in all areas of occupation, not addressing its use with our client populations does them a disservice.

Janet M. Powell, PhD, OTR/L, FAOTA

My interest in vision and cognition and the interrelationship between the two started in 1992 when I attended a workshop by Mary Warren, MS, OTR (her credentials at that time) on the assessment and treatment of visual impairments after ABI. I had wondered about the role of vision in the perceptual functioning of children with cerebral palsy as a new therapist working in pediatrics in the early 1970s, but I was not able to find anyone who could answer my questions and had put them aside. It was not until I heard Mary Warren speak that my curiosity returned. The workshop covered the same content that Warren presented in the two seminal articles published in the *American Journal of Occupational Therapy* a few months later, including her framework describing the previously overlooked role of foundational visual skills in perception and cognition. At the time, I had been working in adult neurorehabilitation for 5 years, and the ideas she presented resonated with me as a possible missing piece of optimal treatment services for clients with stroke and TBI.

Warren's ideas were made even more relevant to me by some vision and cognitive difficulties I was personally experiencing at that time. I had reached the age when I needed glasses to read. Hoping to avoid the logistical and esthetic issues of wearing glasses, I asked my vision provider about other options. He suggested I try monovision in which I would wear a contact in one eye for near vision and leave the other eye uncorrected for distance vision. The vision provider assured me that this worked well for many people, and I embraced the possibility. At first, things went well. In almost all instances, I was able to see clearly. The only situation in which I experienced difficulty was with watching a movie in a theater, which I solved by removing the contact beforehand. I did occasionally experience a sensation of "pulling" in one eye, especially when reading, and had a few instances when my depth perception was clearly off. Those ranged from the slightly embarrassing when I missed a straw when reaching for it to the potentially life-threatening when I stopped much too close on the freeway to a pickup truck carrying a load of lumber extending out from the truck bed. I also experienced some minor visual distortions such as thinking I had left my purse on the top of the car when I was actually seeing some objects in the distance. However, I continued to think that the advantages of not wearing glasses offset the disadvantages of these experiences and vowed to be more careful in situations that might prove dangerous.

Then, I started having some cognitive issues. It started with difficulty with time; at first, I was not sure what day of the week it was, which progressed to not being sure of the month, and eventually I was not even sure what season it was. Next, I started having difficulty counting change even though I had routinely paid for purchases with cash for years. When I was unable to figure out what combination of coins to give the grocery store cashier for a purchase of so many dollars and 37 cents, I realized that I had reached the limit of what I was willing to accept regarding the impact of monovision on my daily occupations. I went back to the vision provider, who prescribed bifocals with clear glass in the upper lenses. Within a few days of wearing the glasses instead of the one contact, my cognitive symptoms completely disappeared.

Connecting my personal experiences with the information on vision dysfunction provided in Warren's workshop made me wonder if any vision issues that my clients with ABI might be having could also be impacting their cognitive function. This made it seem even more worthwhile to provide better vision services, and I decided to pursue setting up a neurovision program at the outpatient rehabilitation facility where I was working. Over the next few months, I identified a local developmental optometrist, Nancy Torgerson, OD, FCOVD, whose approach fit with what I was looking for (i.e., an emphasis on individualized client-centered treatment based on functional goals and a willingness to start treatment with less expensive, less time-consuming options and only progress to more intensive and costly therapy if the lower-level interventions did not work) and who was interested in collaborating with me. The two of us met with the clinic's physiatrists to obtain their approval. We educated them on the role of foundational vision in perception and cognition and how the optometrist could help those issues. We stressed that we would take a scientific approach, gathering data on referrals and outcomes as the basis for deciding if the program was successful. Dr. Torgerson and I collaborated on developing a vision screen and referral criteria, trained the other clinicians, and launched the program.

Two years later, after seeing many clients benefit from the vision services that were now being provided routinely, I became interested in doing research in this area. Realizing that I needed advanced training, I entered a Master of Science program at UW 15 years after graduating with my Bachelor of Science degree in occupational therapy. My Master of Science degree led to a Doctor of Philosophy degree, which led to a full-time faculty position in the UW Division of Occupational Therapy in 2001 with joint responsibilities for teaching in the Master of Occupational Therapy program and research. The courses I took in the UW Psychology Department on the science of vision and cognition during my graduate studies have been another key influence in shaping my thinking.

Two comments made during my faculty position interviews continue to stand out for me as examples of where the field was 20 years ago. After sharing my background and vision-related research goals, the most senior occupational therapy faculty member asked, "Why would an occupational therapist be interested in vision?" The physiatrist overseeing the brain injury program stated with full conviction, "Patients with brain injury have perceptual problems, not vision issues." Fortunately, with additional education and experience, their thinking changed. The physiatrist became a strong advocate for vision services for people with ABI and a valued collaborator in presenting on vision issues after ABI to physiatrists and other rehabilitation clinicians.

My experiences as a researcher in the first 10 years of my faculty appointment before taking on the Master of Occupational Therapy program director role have greatly influenced my perspective on the role of research evidence in clinical decision making. As a faculty member at a research-intensive university with expectations for conducting externally funded research, I learned firsthand the large amount of funding required to conduct high-quality studies; the challenges of obtaining funding for any research, especially when the research questions of interest to you do not fit with the priorities of funding agencies; and the logistical challenges of conducting research within complex clinical systems and with people dealing with the aftermath of ABI. During those 10 years, I was funded on multiple large-scale randomized controlled trials examining interventions for people with TBI and stroke as well as caregivers of people with TBI. I was also able to conduct some smaller-scale vision-related studies. However, because of the challenges that I encountered, none of those were the ones I considered the highest priority (e.g., examining the use of prisms to treat diplopia and of providing appropriate glasses early on in recovery and comparing optometric and ophthalmologic approaches). These experiences made me appreciate the difficulties, the field of rehabilitation, in general, and occupational therapy and optometry, more specifically, have in generating sufficient high-quality evidence as a basis for clinical decision making. As a result, I am careful not to interpret "lack of evidence" or "negative" results from lower-quality studies as "evidence against."

My experiences as an investigator on multiple randomized controlled trials also clarified for me that a statistically significant difference between the intervention and the control group is just that—a mathematical difference indicating that "on average" one group performed better than the other on the study outcome measures. I saw firsthand that a finding in favor of the intervention group does not indicate that the treatment worked well for everyone in that group or that nobody in the control group got better without the treatment. I learned that statistically significant findings cannot and should not be generalized to everyone and that we need to continue to value clinician experience, in addition to research findings and client perspectives, as one of the three key prongs of evidence-based practice as originally described by Sackett and colleagues (1996).

As an occupational therapist who graduated with my entry-level degree in the early 1970s, the first 20 years of my clinical practice were strongly based in a bottom-up assessment and treatment approach with a clear delineation between remediation and compensation. My focus in providing occupational therapy services during that time was to identify as precisely as possible what deficits were impairing each client's function and then work to improve those underlying abilities. There was some possibility of using compensatory methods to help people improve their everyday functioning. However, at least in the settings I was working in, this was seen as a much less desirable approach than remediation and did not garner nearly as much time or attention.

My clinical reasoning started to change in 1993 when I took a certification course in the AMPS. After incorporating the AMPS into my clinical practice, I saw the advantages of a top-down assessment approach in which I could identify how each individual's particular subset of impairments interacted to support or hinder their performance of everyday tasks through observing their occupational performance. Each time I gave the AMPS, I found that I learned something important that had not been evident from my bottom-up approach and began incorporating the AMPS as a routine piece of my evaluations.

The AMPS also gave me a new way of thinking and talking about cognition from an occupational therapy perspective through the concepts and vocabulary of the AMPS process skills (subsequently incorporated as part of the observable performance skills in the *Occupational Therapy Practice Framework: Domain and Process, Fourth Edition* [American Occupational Therapy Association {AOTA}, 2020]). My approach to cognitive assessment and treatment, as well as my thinking about remediation and compensation, changed further with an in-depth study of the work of Joan Toglia, PhD, OTR/L, FAOTA. Through reading her publications and attending workshops she presented (including the one referenced previously by Dr. Kaminsky), I learned how occupational therapy practitioners could use strategy training to address cognitive dysfunction after ABI along with a new understanding of remediation and compensation as more of a continuum than two separate approaches.

At this time, I am struck by how much more knowledge we have as occupational therapy practitioners than when I was a new therapist almost 50 years ago and, yet, how much more there is to discover and learn. My hope is that someday we will know precisely what combination of approaches and therapeutic techniques would serve best to improve the occupational performance and quality of life of each of our clients in a fully individualized, client-centered approach.

The Role of Occupational Therapy in Vision Assessment and Treatment for Individuals With Acquired Brain Injury

As the reader will see in the subsequent chapters in this book, we believe that occupational therapy practitioners have an ethical and legal obligation to collaborate with qualified vision providers in identifying and treating vision impairments after ABI. This is not an opinion that is shared by all occupational therapy practitioners or all vision providers, and we thought it would be useful to explain to the reader how we came to this opinion. Ours is not a theoretical position but rather one based on firsthand experience working in the field.

From an ethical perspective, we consider this collaboration essential in upholding several of the principles and associated standards of conduct for occupational therapy practitioners outlined in the *Occupational Therapy Code of Ethics* (AOTA, 2015). These principles include beneficence, nonmaleficence, and fidelity. The principles of beneficence and nonmaleficence relate to promoting good while preventing and removing harm. The standards of conduct for these two principles include providing appropriate client-specific evaluations and interventions that are within the practitioner's level of competence and scope of practice and referring to other providers to meet client needs. Risks of harm should be avoided even when there is not malicious or harmful intent, with the goals of occupational therapy services balanced with potential risks for harm. The principle of fidelity relates to treating others with respect, fairness, discretion, and integrity, with the standards for conduct including promoting collaboration with other professionals as part of providing quality care.

Our clinical experiences over the years have demonstrated to us time and time again that occupational therapy practitioners who attempt to assess and treat vision impairments after ABI on their own without a qualified vision provider are at great risk for doing harm rather than good. At the same time, we have experienced firsthand the positive outcomes associated with care from a qualified provider. As such, we see collaborating with professionals who have the expertise needed to do good rather than harm as an essential component of this specialized area of practice. A few examples are as follows:

- After referral from the outpatient occupational therapist, a client with TBI was found by a rehabilitation optometrist to still have a contact in one eye several months postinjury. The contact had been missed by providers in the emergency department, intensive care unit, acute neurology floor, and inpatient rehabilitation. Fortunately, the optometrist was able to remove the contact without damaging the client's cornea.
- A client with severe diplopia after a cerebellar stroke was referred by the outpatient occupational therapy practitioner to a rehabilitation optometrist who found that the diplopia was a result of the client wearing an old pair of glasses in an attempt to correct for her astigmatism because the ataxia from her stroke prevented her from using her contacts. The diplopia resolved completely in a few days with a new glasses prescription.
- A client several years poststroke who wanted to read but had been told that poststroke cognitive impairments were limiting her ability to comprehend text was seen in a teaching clinic. Based on the results of a vision screen conducted by the student occupational therapist, the client was referred to a rehabilitation optometrist who diagnosed the client with oculomotor dysfunction. After the prescription of prism glasses, the client's complaints of fatigue and headache resolved, and she was able to read again.

- In multiple clients with visual symptoms after ABI, including diplopia in some instances, their symptoms resolved with simply a new or updated glasses prescription. This was often a different prescription for each eye, which would not be the case if the recommendation from the occupational therapy practitioner had been that the client purchase over-the-counter reading glasses.
- Multiple clients had findings that were similar on the occupational therapy vision screen but whose diagnoses and recommended treatments from the rehabilitation optometrist were quite different.

We also are acutely aware of the possibility of an undiagnosed brain tumor, glaucoma, or other medical condition being responsible for visual symptoms that look like the visual symptoms commonly seen after stroke or TBI. Many of these medical conditions have the potential to cause serious harm if not identified and treated in a timely fashion. Other conditions, such as cataracts, can typically be treated successfully if identified. However, none of these medical conditions can be identified by the vision screens performed by occupational therapy practitioners.

We appreciate the frustration of occupational therapy practitioners working in settings where access to qualified vision providers and services is limited. However, in keeping with the ethical principles of autonomy and justice and to ensure, from a legal perspective, that we are operating within our scope of practice, we do not believe that the solution is taking on responsibilities for evaluation and treatment that we do not have the training to do well. Rather, we suggest that occupational therapy practitioners take an active role in advocating for changes to the systems that limit access to these essential services while looking for innovative ways to establish collaborative relationships with providers in their communities.

The Role of Occupational Therapy in Cognitive Assessment and Treatment for Individuals With Acquired Brain Injury

As stated earlier, we believe that it is important for occupational therapy practitioners to work within our scope of practice. At times, that means taking steps to avoid evaluating and treating in a way that goes beyond our training. At other times, that means ensuring that we evaluate and treat clients in a fully holistic manner, even when there are areas of overlap with other disciplines. Occupational therapy is one of several disciplines that considers the cognitive functioning of people with ABI. Speech-language pathologists and neuropsychologists are members of the team who will also address cognition (see Chapter 2). The role of occupational therapy in cognitive rehabilitation has not been fully understood, both within and outside the profession. As a result, it is likely that readers work with or will work with colleagues who do not realize that cognitive rehabilitation is well within the occupational therapy domain (AOTA, 2020). To fully engage in occupation requires a variety of skills, including cognitive processing skills. Those who have cognitive impairment after ABI are at high risk of experiencing disruption in their occupations. Occupational therapy practitioners who do not address cognition with their clients will not be as successful in helping their clients with "[a]chieving health, well-being, and participation in life through engagement in occupation" (AOTA, 2020, p. 5). Indeed, inadequately addressing cognition can lead to lower rates of return to work (Wolf et al., 2009) and independence (Toglia, 2018) for our client populations. As a result, cognitive rehabilitation is an essential part of occupational therapy practice (AOTA, 2019).

One of the skills all occupational therapy practitioners have relates to advocacy, both for our clients and for our profession (AOTA, 2020). All occupational therapy practitioners have likely had vast experience in educating people about occupational therapy, both what it is and what it is not. Educating about the role of occupational therapy in cognitive rehabilitation provides another opportunity to advocate for our client populations and our profession. Our work with cognition does not need to be in competition with what other members of the team are doing. Instead, it can enhance the overarching rehabilitation process. We see the client's functioning through a unique occupational lens and can contribute information that helps all members of the team better understand the client's strengths and challenges. The use of sound occupationally based evaluation tools, including our own skilled observation of occupational performance, will help to better articulate this lens. Similarly, occupational therapy practitioners who maintain focus on occupational outcomes in treatment with clients will best ensure that we are working within our scope of practice.

The way that we approached the cognitive rehabilitation chapters in this book looks different from many other texts addressing this area of practice. Rather than focusing on the treatment of individual impairments (e.g., attention or memory deficits), we discuss general treatment strategies that can be used for clients with a variety of cognitive deficits. We made that choice for several reasons. First, it is consistent with a top-down approach in occupational therapy practice and the direction our profession has been moving, especially in recent years. Second, cognitive skills interact with and influence each other. It is extremely rare for a client to have only one type of cognitive deficit, so rather than considering individual skills, we address cognitive functioning as a whole, including with a focus on learning potential. A third reason is a personal one that stems directly from our experience with students. Several years ago, Dr. Kaminsky was teaching her students about cognitive rehabilitation. As was typical at the time, she had organized the class sessions based on the types of impairment. At one point, one of her students remarked that the intervention approaches for memory seemed to be the same as the ones for attention. That one remark changed the way that Dr. Kaminsky approached her teaching in this area. She has found that teaching students about the "big picture" of cognitive rehabilitation has enabled them to understand this area of practice in a much more holistic way and that they are better able to focus on the client's occupational performance rather than getting overly caught up in the impairments.

Book Overview

This book provides comprehensive coverage of occupational therapy perspectives on vision and cognitive evaluation and treatment after ABI. It is intended to be an accessible, foundational textbook for students in entry-level occupational therapy and occupational therapy assistant programs, while also serving as a resource for those clinicians already in practice who wish to expand their knowledge in this area. We begin with a discussion of teams and health care teams in general and, more specifically, the members of the specialized neurorehabilitation teams that address vision and cognitive dysfunction after ABI. The next chapter presents an overview of how the visual system works, followed by a chapter describing the assessment and treatment of visual dysfunction after ABI from occupational therapy perspectives. The next two chapters focus on visual perception and inattention. The following four chapters provide an overview of the cognitive system, including the types of cognitive skills and their neurological basis, and describe the assessment and treatment of cognitive dysfunction after ABI from an occupational therapy perspective. The final chapter describes the use of technology in supporting everyday function for those with visual and/or cognitive impairments after ABI.

A collection of instructional resources for faculty to use in conjunction with the *Fifth Edition* is available at www.efacultylounge.com. These resources are a sample of the materials we have created over the years for use in our comprehensive adult neurorehabilitation courses for entry-level occupational therapy students at our respective universities. They include complete descriptions of case-based learning and lab activities, written exam questions, and a practical exam. There are also brief descriptions of websites, videos, and documentary films that we have found useful in helping students understand this content.

References

American Occupational Therapy Association. (2015). Occupational therapy code of ethics (2015). *American Journal of Occupational Therapy, 69*(Suppl. 3), 6913410030. https://doi.org/10.5014/ajot.2015.696S03

American Occupational Therapy Association. (2019). Cognition, cognitive rehabilitation, and occupational performance. *American Journal of Occupational Therapy, 73*, 7312410010. https://doi.org/10.5014/ajot.2019.73S201

American Occupational Therapy Association. (2020). Occupational therapy practice framework: Domain and process (4th ed.). *American Journal of Occupational Therapy, 74*(Suppl. 2), 7412410010. https://doi.org/10.5014/ajot.2020.74S2001

Sackett, D. L., Rosenberg, W. M., Gray, J. A., Haynes, R. B., & Richardson, W. S. (1996). Evidence-based medicine: What it is and what it isn't. *British Medical Journal, 312*, 71-72. https://doi.org/10.1136/bmj.312.7-23.71

Toglia, J. (2018). The dynamic interactional model and the multicontext approach. In N. Katz & J. Toglia (Eds.), *Cognition, occupation, and participation across the lifespan* (4th ed., pp. 355-385). AOTA Press.

Wolf, T. J., Baum, C., & Connor, L. T. (2009). Changing face of stroke: Implications for occupational therapy practice. *American Journal of Occupational Therapy, 63*, 621-625. https://doi.org/10.5014/ajot.63.5.621

CHAPTER 2

The Team Approach

Acquired brain injury (ABI) typically results in multiple physical, cognitive, emotional, behavioral, and psychosocial difficulties that are often interrelated in complicated and confusing ways. It is widely understood that no one discipline has the knowledge and skill set to evaluate and treat the complex and wide-ranging array of symptoms typically observed in neurorehabilitation (Karol, 2014). Rather, effective neurorehabilitation care for a client after ABI takes a coordinated team effort with providers from multiple disciplines working together in a cooperative and collaborative fashion to identify the different deficits that are present and how those deficits are impacting the client's functioning. However, who makes up a neurorehabilitation team, the responsibilities of each team member, and how the members of a team work together vary widely. In this chapter, we discuss how teams are defined, including the different types of health care teams; the characteristics of effective teams; strategies teams use to manage challenges; the makeup of general rehabilitation teams; and the structure of neurorehabilitation vision and cognitive-perceptual teams.

Defining Teams

A team is defined as a group of two or more people who work together toward a common aim, purpose, goal, or objective (Payne, 2000). In health care, the common purpose of formal and informal teams is centered around providing high-quality care (Mitchell et al., 2012). The expertise of the different team members typically varies in ways that complement each other so that each person contributes something important to the shared outcome. Teams develop processes over time for communicating about, collaborating on, and consolidating their different knowledge bases in order to make decisions and determine actions. Team members may share common

Kaminsky, T. A., & Powell, J. M.
Zoltan's Vision, Perception, and Cognition: Evaluation and Treatment of the Adult With Acquired Brain Injury, Fifth Edition (pp. 11-32).

values and a common approach. There is often a feeling of membership and loyalty to the team among the team members, with an understanding that more is being achieved collectively by the team than could be accomplished individually.

Types of Health Care Teams

Health care teams are often described as being multidisciplinary, interdisciplinary, or transdisciplinary. These terms reflect variations in the degree of collaboration, the amount of professional autonomy, and the extent of adherence to discipline identity within these different team structures (D'Amour et al., 2005; Malec, 2013; Payne, 2000).

In a multidisciplinary team, individual team members remain in their traditional roles to address the treatment goals that are within their expertise. There may be a shared overall discharge goal, but most decision making, including short- and long-term goal setting, is done by each team member separately without intentional adjustment to or consideration of the work of the other team members. Each team member has limited formal interaction with other providers, with communication often taking place through the medical record rather than in person at scheduled structured meetings. Although multidisciplinary teams are often considered inferior to more collaborative team structures, Malec (2013) noted that this type of team can be the most appropriate approach in neurorehabilitation when a client has a small number of specific problems. For example, a person with good emotional adjustment and self-awareness after traumatic brain injury (TBI) whose symptoms are limited to mild memory impairment and minor balance issues could be treated in a multidisciplinary fashion by occupational therapy, speech-language pathology, or neuropsychology for the memory impairment and physical therapy for gait.

In an interdisciplinary team, team members still use their disciplinary-specific expertise in addressing treatment goals. However, there is greater coordination and cooperation than in a multidisciplinary approach. Team members come together to collaborate on shared treatment planning and coordination of services. Team communication is planned and structured through mechanisms such as the daily "rounding" or "huddles" that typically occur in a hospital setting or scheduled case/team conferences in other inpatient or outpatient settings. Each team member is aware of the goals and treatment approaches of the other providers on the team. Team members may adapt their interactions with the client to reinforce the work of the other disciplines when appropriate. This type of approach is viewed as being particularly important when there are multiple problems that can interact with and compound each other (Malec, 2013). As a result, most intensive neurorehabilitation programs use an interdisciplinary team approach (Malec, 2013).

Transdisciplinary teams are also made up of members from different disciplines who provide treatment in a coordinated fashion. What differs in a transdisciplinary team is that members adopt each other's roles, sometimes on a temporary basis and sometimes more permanently. Information, knowledge, and skills are transferred from one discipline to another (Payne, 2000) so that team members can provide interventions that are typically viewed as being outside of their own discipline. In neurorehabilitation, a transdisciplinary approach is most often used in residential day treatment programs with clients with severe cognitive impairments and impaired self-awareness (Malec, 2013). For example, a client with severe anger management issues would likely benefit more from treatment if all team members took the same approach to managing outbursts under the direction of the psychologist. The deliberate blurring of traditional role delineations that occurs in transdisciplinary teams is sometimes referred to as *role release*. This type of team structure requires a great deal of mutual trust and coordination among team members and frequent team communication.

There is increasing use of the term *interprofessional* in referring to coordinated health care teams that were previously characterized as interdisciplinary. The term interprofessional is also widely used to describe educational opportunities in which students learn how to work more collaboratively with providers from other disciplines by engaging in shared learning experiences. The shift in terminology from interdisciplinary to interprofessional is intended to shift the focus from the body of specialized theories, knowledge, and skills that belongs to each discipline to the group of individuals who apply their specialized knowledge in the interest of others in their professional roles. Thus, interprofessional is a somewhat broader term because it emphasizes the functions and activities of the people who make up different professional groups on a team, whereas interdisciplinary focuses more narrowly on the knowledge and skills of various disciplines (Payne, 2000). The term interprofessional also serves to highlight that each profession has their own unique educational, entrance, and membership requirements that are typically regulated by a professional association (Greenwood, 1957) along with their own code of ethics and professional culture. Despite these underlying distinctions, interdisciplinary and interprofessional are often used interchangeably. Another term that is starting to be used more frequently in health care for interdisciplinary and interprofessional teams is *collaborative practice.*

Characteristics of Effective Teams

A group of people may be labeled a *team* with the expectation that they will work together but not have the attitudes, skills, or processes needed to move from a discipline-specific perspective to collaborative work. The characteristics of effective teams along with how to recognize if a team is not functioning well are summarized in Table 2-1. Developing relationships in which team members act as collaborative partners in working toward shared goals starts with understanding and valuing the perspectives and contributions of the other team members. Based on that knowledge, an effective team develops clear expectations for each team member's role and responsibilities and how each team member will be accountable to the others (Mitchell et al., 2012; Rothberg, 1981). An open discussion of scope of practice issues in areas of care in which one or more disciplines have overlapping interests and proficiencies is critical. When team members know that they can rely on the expertise, contributions, and participation of other team members to do what is needed to address the client's needs and meet shared goals, they are more likely to feel comfortable relying on the other members of the team, and the team is more likely to function in an interdependent fashion.

Having this type of respect and trust among the team members is one of the key elements of an effective team (D'Amour et al., 2005; Mitchell et al., 2012). However, a high level of respect and trust can be challenging to develop because health care providers have typically been socialized in their professional education to adopt a strong professional identity and culture (Hall, 2005). Students learn discipline-specific theoretical perspectives, problem-solving approaches, decision-making styles, and practice frameworks as well as discipline-specific values, attitudes, customs, and behaviors. As a result, each discipline represented on a team brings its own view of the client, what treatment should be offered, how the treatment should be delivered, and the desired outcomes of that treatment. Students in each discipline often learn about other disciplines only in terms of how the other disciplines relate to what they will be doing in their new professional roles. As a result, team members may see their own discipline as "the most central, the most important, and the most correct" (Rothberg, 1981, p. 409). Students also learn the language and jargon specific to their discipline. Not having a fully shared language can make it more difficult for treatment team members from different disciplines to fully and accurately understand each other. These discipline-focused perspectives can lead to varying degrees of distrust of other disciplines and result in an approach that is more competitive than collaborative.

Table 2-1

Characteristics of Effective Teams

CHARACTERISTIC	WHAT THIS LOOKS LIKE	SIGNS OF TROUBLE
Clear purpose	The vision, mission, goals, and tasks of the team have been clearly defined and accepted by everyone.	Different team members have different responses if asked about the team vision, mission, goals, and tasks, or do not know.
Informality	The atmosphere for team meetings or discussions is informal, comfortable, and relaxed.	The atmosphere in team meetings is tense and/or one or more team members seem bored.
Broad participation	There is a lot of discussion with everyone encouraged to participate. Clear progress is made toward identified goals.	Team members appear on the surface to be involved, but there is not much tangible output or progress toward goals.
Active listening	Team members use listening techniques such as questioning, paraphrasing, and summarizing.	Team members talk but do not listen to each other well. Techniques to clarify and ensure understanding of other's perspectives are rarely used.
Civilized disagreement	When there is disagreement, the team is comfortable with this.	Conflict is avoided, smoothed over, or suppressed. Differences are aired in private without the people most directly involved.
Consensus decisions	Team members strive for substantial, but not necessarily unanimous, agreement through open discussion and assessment of everyone's ideas.	The team relies primarily on formal voting with a tendency toward easy compromise. The information being gathered is not actually used in making decisions.
Open communication and trust	Team members freely express their opinions on the tasks and processes of the team.	Team members do not feel comfortable saying what they really think.
Clear roles and work assignments	There are clear expectations about each team member's role. Assignments are clearly made, accepted, and carried out.	Team members are unsure what they should be doing and do not always follow through.

(continued)

Table 2-1 (continued)

Characteristics of Effective Teams

CHARACTERISTIC	WHAT THIS LOOKS LIKE	SIGNS OF TROUBLE
Shared leadership	Although the team has a formal leader, leadership functions shift from time to time depending on the circumstances, the needs of the group, and the skills of the members. The formal leader models the appropriate behavior and helps establish positive norms.	One person maintains leadership of the group at all times, even when another is better situated to handle a situation that has arisen.
Strong external relations	The team actively develops key outside relationships, mobilizing resources, and building credibility with important people in other parts of the organization.	People outside the team do not know what is going on or are not supportive.
Diversity of style	The team has a broad spectrum of team player styles including members who emphasize attention to task, goal setting, focus on process, and questions about how the team is functioning.	Members all have similar team player styles (having varied expertise is typically not enough).
On-going self-assessment	Periodically, the team stops to examine how well it is functioning, assess both processes and products, and identify what may be interfering with its effectiveness.	The team does not regularly assess progress toward goals and evaluate team process.

Adapted from Parker, G. M. (2008). *Team players and teamwork: New strategies for developing successful collaboration* (2nd ed.). Jossey-Bass.

Effective communication is one key way of developing respect and trust and overcoming these inherent barriers to collaborative teamwork. The importance of ongoing communication among team members can be seen in the Centers for Medicare & Medicaid Services (CMS; 2017) requirement that the members of interdisciplinary teams in inpatient rehabilitation facilities meet in person at least once per week (Figure 2-1). If a team member cannot attend one of the scheduled meetings, another provider from that discipline with current knowledge of the patient must go in their place. (In this book, we use the term *patient* when referring specifically to individuals receiving services in a hospital setting and *client* for all other instances.) The team meetings must include an assessment of how well the patient is progressing toward the goals of the inpatient rehabilitation stay, identification of any issues that are negatively impacting progress toward the goals, and revision of the treatment plan and/or goals as needed.

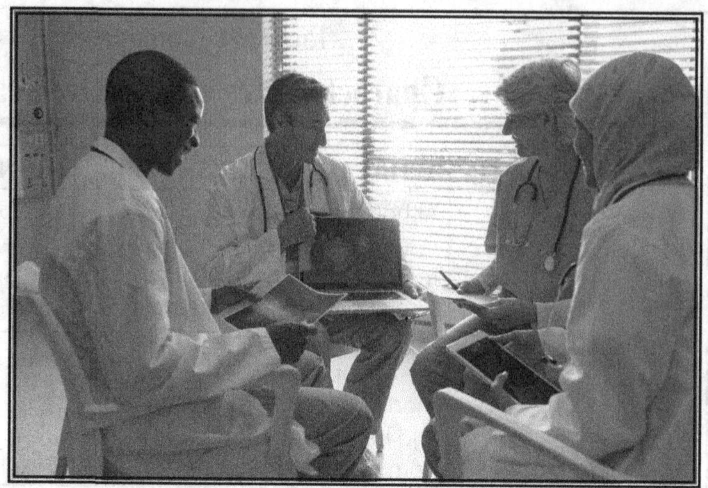

Figure 2-1. The team on which the occupational therapy practitioner works will include colleagues from a variety of professions. Some common team members include physicians, nurses, psychologists, case managers, physical therapy practitioners, and speech-language pathologists. Clients and caregivers are also important members of health care teams, although their ability to fully participate will be influenced by a number of factors. No matter who is on the team, regular communication is essential. (Wavebreakmedia/shutterstock.com)

It is not enough, however, to have a meeting structure in place in which communication is focused on client care needs. In order to build a collaborative team in which the perspectives of the various team members are well integrated and team members respect and trust each other, teams must also prioritize communication about the team process itself (i.e., what they are doing and how they are doing it). They must discuss what they have in common, their relationships, their interdependence, and the power differentials and dynamics within the team (D'Amour et al., 2005). Team members who work effectively in a collaborative fashion typically develop and refine their shared goals over time along with shared values and shared philosophies for how care should be given. They also develop processes for sharing decision making and treatment and discharge planning. This often requires negotiation and compromise along with good conflict resolution skills.

Managing Challenges

At any level of team development, there can be challenges that arise from how power among the team members is recognized and used. Challenges stemming from status and power dynamics can be difficult to recognize and, even when recognized by one or more team members, often difficult to address openly. The most effective balance of power varies depending on the team. Although power is often based on people's functions and titles, teams in which power is determined by knowledge and experience often operate at a more collaborative level. In teams with the highest level of collaboration, power is often shared among the team members, with each team member recognizing and valuing the power of the other members.

Taylor (2020) stresses that all collaborative relationships, even those in which there is a great deal of similarity in backgrounds and beliefs, must be approached in an intentional manner to ensure that people are working effectively. This can be done by (a) asking collaborators about their beliefs, values, and preferred approaches; (b) clearly describing your own beliefs, values, and preferred approaches; (c) recognizing the weaknesses along with the strengths of your orientation to practice; (d) clearly describing your client impressions and goals while being willing to learn and receive input from others; (e) monitoring collaborative relationships for potential issues; (f) promptly addressing any issues that arise; and (g) using conflict resolution techniques to resolve differences and prevent long-term negative consequences. When team members have a major difference in opinion regarding a client's care, they should make an intentional, conscious decision about whether or not to let the client know (Taylor, 2020). This decision should be based on the best interests of the client. In some instances, it is not appropriate to inform the client (e.g., when it would cause confusion or damage the reputation of one of the team members). On the other hand, when it would be useful for the client or family to hear both perspectives in order to make their own decision about how to proceed, team members may have an ethical responsibility to share both sides.

Rehabilitation Team Members

How is it decided who makes up a rehabilitation treatment team? Although each client's needs and goals are instrumental in making a decision, governmental policies, including those related to reimbursement, also play a key role. For example, CMS (2017) only considers care received in an inpatient rehabilitation facility (IRF) as reasonable and necessary (and, therefore, reimbursable) if the patient has nursing, medical management, and rehabilitation needs that are so complex that an interdisciplinary team approach is needed. The CMS guidelines specify that these treatment teams must be led by a rehabilitation physician responsible for coordinating care and making final decisions. The team must include, at minimum, a registered nurse with specialized training or experience in rehabilitation, a social worker or case manager (or both), and a licensed or certified practitioner from each of the disciplines treating the patient. One of the therapists on the team must be either an occupational or physical therapist.

IRF treatment team membership is also influenced by a policy that is often referred to as the *3-hour rule*. This policy defines the CMS requirement for an intensive rehabilitation program by the amount of therapy a patient receives. The 3-hour rule was first proposed in 1978 by a committee established by the American Academy of Physical Medicine and Rehabilitation in response to a request by the Health Care Financing Administration to establish admission criteria for IRFs that would distinguish them from medical-surgical units. The committee recommended three criteria for IRF admission: (a) the patient is medically stable, (b) there is a reasonable expectation that the patient will experience significant functional improvement in a reasonable amount of time, and (c) the patient will be able to tolerate and participate in 3 hours of daily (i.e., 5 days/week) therapy (Braddom, 2005; Reinstein, 2014). The requirement for participation in at least 3 hours of therapy each day for at least 5 days/week remains an industry standard, although, in certain instances, it is now allowable for the 15 hours of therapy to be spread over a 7-day period. At the time that the 3-hour rule was adopted, only occupational and physical therapy minutes could contribute toward the required therapy time. As a result, occupational and physical therapy services typically split the time with patients receiving 1.5 hours of each of these therapies per day. Shortly after the implementation of the 3-hour rule, the American Speech-Language-Hearing Association began lobbying for the inclusion of speech-language pathology services in the required therapy time (Intagliata & Hollander, 1987). At the time of this writing, speech-language pathology and prosthetic/orthotics services can also be counted toward the 3 hours of therapy per day, resulting in more variation in the core treatment team. Recreational therapists are currently advocating for the inclusion of their services, which will further shift how the 3-hour rule is implemented if those efforts are successful.

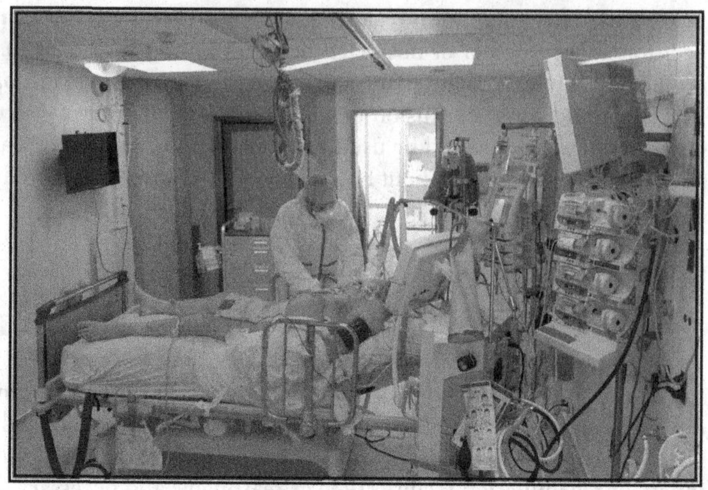

Figure 2-2. In the intensive care unit, the focus of the team is on medical management of the patient. Therapy services are involved but to a lesser extent than in other settings. (Alexandros Michailidis/shutterstock.com)

Neurorehabilitation Teams

As discussed previously, the disciplines represented in neurorehabilitation teams vary depending on the needs and goals of each client over the course of their recovery and the setting where the services are provided (Ivanhoe et al., 2013). There can also be variation by facility within the same level of care depending on factors such as treatment philosophy and organizational constraints (D'Amour et al., 2005). In general, the most common health care professionals providing services to individuals with stroke or TBI throughout the continuum of care (in alphabetical order) are neuropsychologists, occupational therapists and occupational therapy assistants, physical therapists and physical therapist assistants, physicians, recreational therapists, rehabilitation counselors, rehabilitation nurses, social workers, speech-language pathologists, and vocational counselors (Miller et al., 2010). Psychologists are also often included in treatment teams. In the more acute stages, as in the intensive care unit, the focus of the treatment team is typically on medical management by physicians and nurses with lesser involvement from the various rehabilitation therapy disciplines (Ivanhoe et al., 2013; Miller et al., 2010; Figure 2-2). As a person progresses from the intensive care unit to acute care, inpatient rehabilitation, and outpatient care, there is typically a gradual decrease in nursing staffing and an increase in the amount and number of therapy services provided (Figure 2-3). There is also a shift in the specialty of the physicians involved, with neurologists often playing a key role in the early stages of treatment for ABI along with orthopedists if there are co-occurring musculoskeletal injuries. Medical care then typically shifts to physiatrists (i.e., physical medicine and rehabilitation physicians) if rehabilitation services are indicated. Early on, dieticians, respiratory therapists, and pharmacists may be involved in the health care team to varying extents depending on the patient's needs, whereas later on driving specialists, vocational counselors, and other community reintegration specialists may play a role (Ivanhoe et al., 2013). Additional personnel, including behavior attendants, certified nursing assistants, and rehabilitation aides and technicians, who provide key aspects of care, but do not have the same level of decision-making responsibilities, may or may not be formally recognized as part of the team, depending on the facility.

Although various health care professions often describe their care provision as "client or patient centered," the extent to which clients and their families are fully included in the workings of the health care team varies considerably. In some settings, clients and families are seen as integral members of the team, whereas in others their role is much more peripheral. The role of clients in the neurorehabilitation health care teams is often compromised by cognitive, communication, and/or emotional difficulties stemming from the brain injury. As a result, family members are

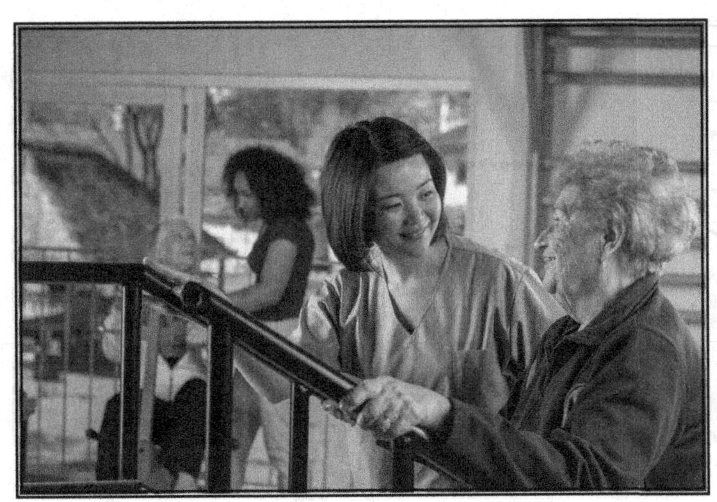

Figure 2-3. In settings such as inpatient rehabilitation units and outpatient clinics, the members of the team who represent therapy services (e.g., occupational therapy, physical therapy, speech-language pathology, recreational therapy) play major roles in the treatment of the clients. (GagliardiPhotography/shutterstock.com)

often viewed as important sources of information to the team about the premorbid life and abilities of the individual with a brain injury (Belanger et al., 2009) and may serve as a proxy to the client in goal setting, treatment, and discharge decisions. Family members typically take on an even bigger role when caregiving is needed after discharge to the community. In some instances, family members are not interested in or available to participate as a member of the team or may not have the skills needed to do so effectively. Further complexity is added if family members have needs or concerns of their own that require support and/or referral from the health care team. This can result in dual roles for those individuals as a family member/caregiver on one team and a client on another, potentially overlapping, team.

Neurorehabilitation Vision and Cognitive-Perceptual Teams

It is common for providers on neurorehabilitation teams to target the same or closely related deficits from different discipline-specific perspectives (Karol, 2014). In the following section, we describe how this can be observed in vision and cognitive-perceptual treatment teams.

Neurorehabilitation Vision Teams

In 2016, the American Congress of Rehabilitation Medicine Stroke Interdisciplinary Special Interest Group (Roberts et al., 2016) presented a conceptual model to describe how different health care professionals could work collaboratively in a rehabilitation setting to assess and manage vision dysfunction. As noted in Figure 2-4, this model makes a distinction between impairments in visual function and impairments in functional vision and between providers who are vision specialists and those who are nonspecialists. *Vision function* refers to the workings of the eye and the associated structures in the visual system. Vision function is assessed and treated by specialized vision providers, such as ophthalmologists and optometrists. *Functional vision* refers to the use of vision in everyday life and the impact of vision problems on activities of daily living (ADLs), instrumental activities of daily living (IADLs), work, and leisure as well as a person's physical, cognitive, emotional, and social function. According to this model, functional vision falls within the

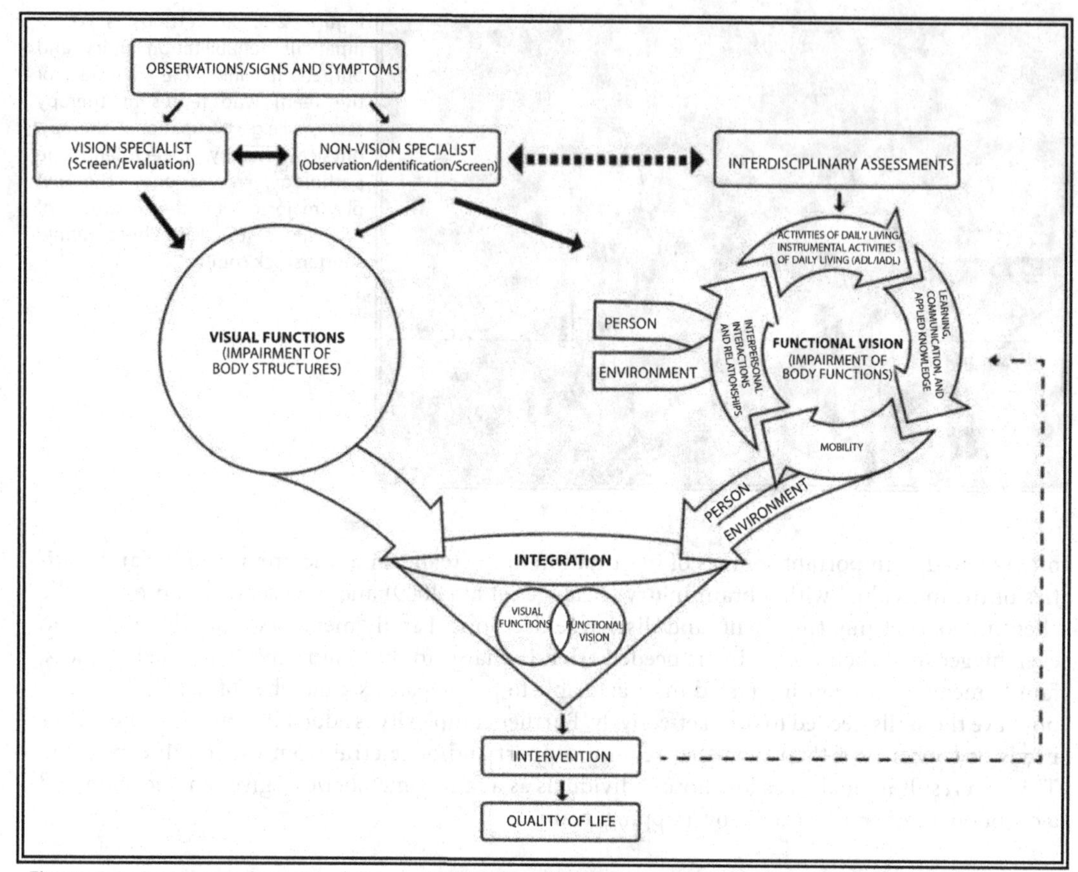

Figure 2-4. A conceptual model of vision rehabilitation. (Reproduced with permission from Roberts, P. S., Rizzo, J., Hreha, K., Wertheimer, J., Kaldenberg, J., Hironaka, D., Riggs, R., & Colenbrander, C. [2016]. A conceptual model for vision rehabilitation. *Journal of Rehabilitation Research and Development, 53*, 693-704. https://doi.org/10.1682/JRRD.2015.06.0113)

domain of all of the other members of the rehabilitation team whose primary training and expertise are in areas other than vision. The role of these nonvision specialists is to observe the impact of vision on function within their areas of expertise, to screen for potential vision problems, and/or to refer to vision specialists as appropriate.

In many rehabilitation settings, the occupational therapist is the nonvision specialist who takes on the primary responsibility for the identification of functional vision problems and subsequent referral to a vision specialist as well as the role of liaison between the vision specialist and the rest of the treatment team (Berrymann & Rasavage, 2011). Depending on the treatment approach for a particular setting, the occupational therapy practitioner may also work under the supervision of an optometrist or ophthalmologist in assisting with vision therapy (Suter, 2017). As explained in more detail in Chapter 4, the occupational therapy practitioner is more often involved with teaching a person how to compensate for vision deficits through new ways of performing everyday tasks or environmental modifications.

There is much greater variation in who fulfills the role of the vision specialist. As noted previously, this is most commonly either an ophthalmologist or an optometrist, but could also be a provider within either of those fields with a subspecialty in the treatment of vision dysfunction that results from neurological insult or injury. Furthermore, there are specialized vision providers within optometry who assess and treat both vision function and functional vision. Understanding

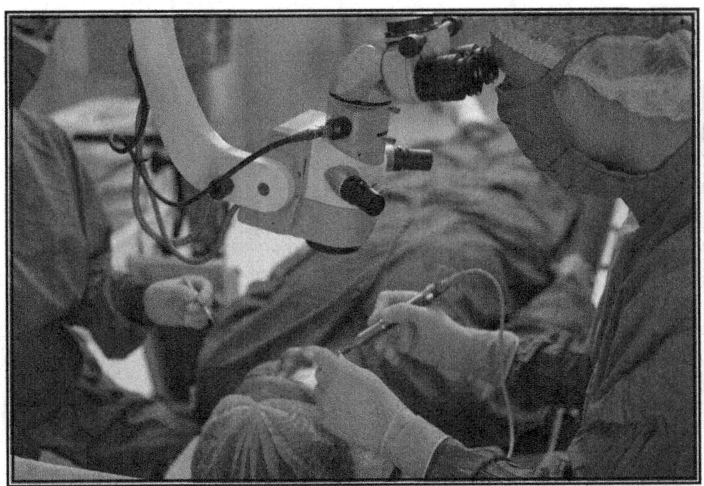

Figure 2-5. Ophthalmologists are medical doctors who diagnose and treat eye conditions, including surgical intervention. One example is surgery to treat diplopia (double vision) caused by misalignment of one or both eyes after TBI. (Dragon Images/shutterstock.com)

more about the background and training of these various vision providers and when or why one versus another might be included in a treatment team helps with understanding how neurorehabilitation vision care teams form and operate.

Ophthalmologists are medical (MD) or osteopathic (DO) doctors who are licensed to practice medicine and perform surgery (American Academy of Ophthalmology, 2020), diagnose and treat diseases of the eye, perform eye surgery, and prescribe eyeglasses and contact lenses (Figure 2-5). The educational background of ophthalmologists includes 4 years of undergraduate studies, 4 years of medical school, and 3 years of ophthalmology residency. Ophthalmologists may elect to complete 1 or 2 additional years of fellowship training in a subspecialty area. These subspecialties are based on a particular part of the eye (e.g., cornea, retina), disease or condition (e.g., glaucoma, pediatric strabismus), or treatment (e.g., plastic or refractive surgery).

The ophthalmology subspecialists who work most often with clients with ABI are neuro-ophthalmologists. Neuro-ophthalmologists focus on the diagnosis and treatment of neurologically based dysfunction of the vision system (Suter, 2017) using a combination of neurological, ophthalmologic, and medical perspectives (North American Neuro-Ophthalmology Society, 2018). Some neuro-ophthalmologists perform surgeries for eye misalignment (strabismus) after ABI (Suter, 2017), whereas others refer those cases to a neurosurgeon. Neuro-ophthalmologists are more likely than general ophthalmologists to use additional nonsurgical or pharmacological intervention approaches, such as tints for glasses (Suter, 2017). Some ophthalmologists work with orthoptists who are trained by ophthalmologists to treat problems with the two eyes working together (i.e., eye teaming) that result from strabismus (Suter, 2017).

Optometrists, who are sometimes referred to as *optometric physicians*, are primary eye care providers with a Doctor of Optometry (OD) degree. For many years, the primary focus of optometry was the prescription of lenses (glasses and contacts) to correct for conditions such as myopia, hyperopia, presbyopia, and astigmatism (Figure 2-6). More recently, the practice of optometry has expanded to include the diagnosis and nonsurgical management of eye conditions, such as infection and inflammation, and common eye diseases, such as glaucoma and macular degeneration. Optometrists in the United States are now licensed to prescribe all topical eye medications, such as eye drops for glaucoma, and most oral medications. They may provide pre- and postoperative care in a comanagement model with an ophthalmologist. In a few states, optometrists are also licensed to perform some types of eye surgery. Optometrists complete 4 years of education at an accredited Doctor of Optometry program, most typically after obtaining a bachelor's degree (American Optometric Association, n.d.). Graduates must pass the National Board of Examiners in Optometry examinations to be licensed to practice.

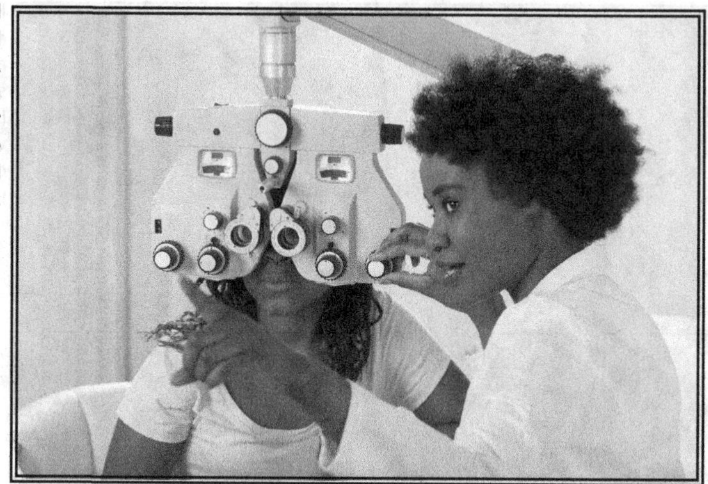

Figure 2-6. Optometrists are licensed to prescribe corrective lenses and topical medication for eye conditions. They also work in partnership with ophthalmologists to administer pre- and postsurgical care. In some locations, optometrists are licensed to perform selected eye surgeries. (Andrey_Popov/shutterstock.com)

Optometrists may choose to complete a postprofessional residency to gain advanced competency in a particular area (Association of Schools and Colleges of Optometry, 2019). The two optometric residencies most relevant to ABI are vision therapy and rehabilitation and brain injury vision rehabilitation. Residencies in vision therapy and rehabilitation focus on treating eye movement, accommodative, and binocular dysfunction; reductions in visual acuity and visual fields; and visual processing. Residencies in brain injury vision rehabilitation focus on the assessment and management of clients with a brain injury and neurological disease from an interdisciplinary perspective.

There are also optometric fellowships and board certification options. The American Academy of Optometry (n.d.) and the American Board of Optometry (2019) both offer general optometry fellowships. Successful completion is indicated by the credentials FAAO (Fellow of the American Academy of Optometry) or diplomate of the American Board of Optometry. The College of Optometrists in Vision Development (n.d.) offers board certification in vision development, vision therapy, and vision rehabilitation. A board-certified optometrist is designated by the credential FCOVD (Fellow of the College of Optometrists in Vision Development). The Neuro-Optometric Rehabilitation Association (n.d.) offers a fellowship with the aim of promoting and recognizing the highest level of clinical competence and knowledge in neuro-optometric rehabilitation. Recognition as a Fellow of the Neuro-Optometric Rehabilitation Association requires publication in the field in addition to coursework and an examination. As of 2021, 21 providers have been awarded Fellow of the Neuro-Optometric Rehabilitation Association status.

There are several terms used to describe optometrists who specialize in the treatment of clients with ABI. These practitioners may be referred to as developmental, behavioral, neuro-, rehabilitative, or neurorehabilitative optometrists. Optometrists working with children who have learning issues typically use the term *developmental* or *behavioral*, whereas those working with clients with ABI lean toward the neurorehabilitative terminology (N. Torgerson & L. Press, personal communication, July 2, 2021). In many instances, these providers have completed advanced training, such as residencies or fellowships, as described earlier.

The focus of neurorehabilitative optometrists is broader than that of general optometrists. There is typically a greater emphasis on evaluating visual function (i.e., the use of vision in everyday tasks) in addition to basic visual skills. There is also a greater emphasis on the rehabilitative treatment of acquired loss of visual acuity, strabismus, diplopia, binocular dysfunction, vergence and/or accommodation disorders, and oculomotor dysfunction (Figure 2-7). These providers also assess and treat deficits in visual processing (Suter, 2017).

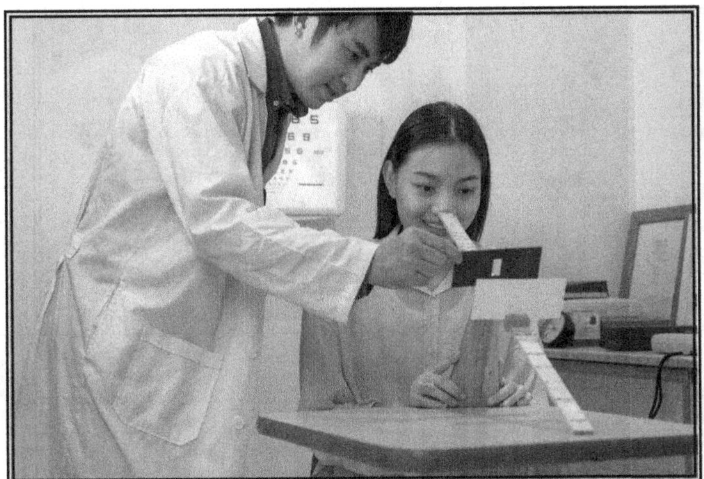

Figure 2-7. Some optometrists complete advanced training in remediation/rehabilitation services for clients with vision disorders that occur as a result of brain injury. These professionals use a variety of treatments, including vision therapy. (chomplearn/shutterstock.com)

The approaches used by neurorehabilitative optometrists to treat the various types of visual system dysfunction after ABI include optical devices and optometric vision therapy (Simpson-Jones & Hunt, 2019). One of the optical devices used is standard lenses (eyeglasses) to improve a person's ability to see clearly. In some instances, tints are added to the lenses. Other optical devices are more specialized. These devices include sectoral occlusion and several types of prisms. With sectoral occlusion, a specific sector (i.e., part) of the visual field is partially or fully blocked. This is often done by placing tape on eyeglasses, either with or without prescription lenses. Specialized prisms used by neurorehabilitative optometrists include microprisms that change how the light and, therefore, the image on the retina, is coming into one or both eyes by a very small amount; yoked prisms that shift images in the same direction and amount in both eyes; and prisms that shift the image coming into an eye that is turning outward or inward so that it aligns with the image from the other eye. Depending on the type and purpose of the prism, they are either permanently ground into or temporarily applied to eyeglass lenses.

The overall goal of optometric vision therapy is to improve the speed, flexibility, endurance, and accuracy of the visual system, including eye tracking, eye focusing, and eye teaming (i.e., the eyes working together). Because vision therapy addresses all basic visual skills, it can lay the foundation for the rest of rehabilitative care. Vision therapy techniques include oculomotor training, with or without the use of the optical devices described previously (Simpson-Jones & Hunt, 2019). Optical devices may also be used in isolation.

Historically, vision therapy research has focused on case studies, retrospective case series, and retrospective chart reviews. Even though research in this area is still fairly limited, there is a growing body of evidence for the effectiveness of vision therapy interventions after ABI (Simpson-Jones & Hunt, 2019). Although the sample sizes remain small, recent studies have used more rigorous prospective experimental designs to examine the effect of various treatment protocols, including home-, clinic-, or laboratory-based oculomotor training alone or with prisms on outcomes such as foundational visual function (e.g., fixation, saccades, accommodation) and reading speed and accuracy. These study designs include single-subject methodology (Schaadt et al., 2014), pre-post comparisons (Conrad et al., 2017), experimental and placebo crossover (Thiagarajan & Ciuffreda, 2013, 2014a, 2014c; Thiagarajan et al., 2014) with longer-term follow-up (Thiagarajan & Ciuffreda, 2014b), and small-scale randomized controlled trials (Berryman et al., 2020).

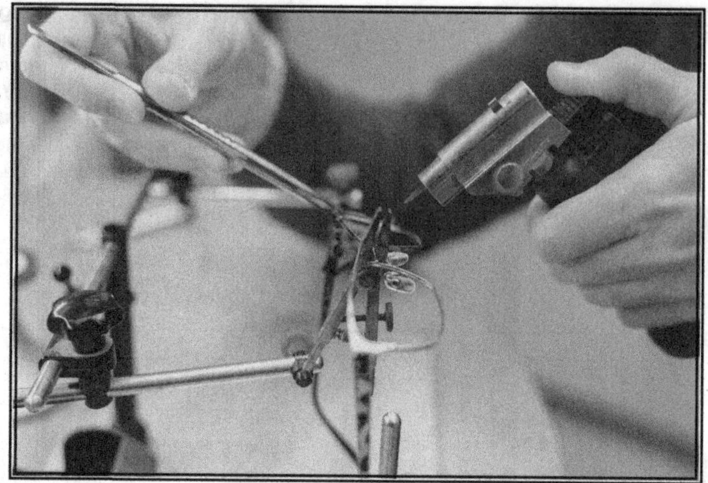

Figure 2-8. Opticians work from prescriptions received from optometrists or ophthalmologists to fit and adjust eyeglasses, contact lenses, and other optical aids. (MarkoBeg/shutterstock.com)

Opticians are providers of glasses or other eyewear. They are trained to fit eyeglass lenses and frames, contact lenses, and other devices to correct eyesight. They work from a prescription written by an ophthalmologist or optometrist and do not evaluate or diagnose eye or visual function (Figure 2-8). There are several avenues to becoming an optician. Some individuals arrange for on-the-job training after high school graduation. Others complete a 1-year certificate or a 2-year community college training program (U.S. Bureau of Labor Statistics, 2021).

Optometrists and/or ophthalmologists may serve as consultants to or integral members of the primary treatment team as specialists of the eye and visual system. The degree to which they are integrated into the overall care of the client depends on many factors including the client's needs, the program philosophy, facility constraints, scope of practice issues, and licensure laws. There is a relatively long-standing history of involvement of neuro-ophthalmology as a consultant to the primary rehabilitation treatment team. Over the past 40 years, there have been multiple calls in the literature to add optometrists to the ABI rehabilitation team. Early proponents included neuropsychologist Rosamond Gianutsos and optometrists Allen Cohen and Robert Perlin (Cohen & Rein, 1992; Cohen & Soden, 1981; Gianutsos & Ramsey, 1988; Gianutsos et al., 1988, 1989). They were joined in the early 1990s by several occupational therapists who advocated more specifically for collaborations between optometry and occupational therapy in the care of persons with ABI (e.g., Bouska & Gallaway, 1991; Maley et al., 1991; Schlageter et al., 1993; Schlageter & Shaw, 1991; Schnell, 1992). More recently, optometrist Mitchell Scheiman (2011) described the benefits of a synergistic relationship between optometry and occupational therapy in which each discipline respects the other's areas of expertise in developing collaborative relationships.

Following are two examples of collaboration between occupational therapy and neurorehabilitative optometry in addressing visual dysfunction in people with ABI.

First, imagine Anand, a 56-year-old man who is being seen for occupational therapy after a stroke. The stroke did not result in any cognitive or physical dysfunction. The occupational therapy practitioner does not see any signs of hemi-inattention in her evaluation but identifies a possible left visual field cut and decreased near visual acuity on the vision screen. She refers him to the neurorehabilitative optometrist for further evaluation. The optometrist confirms the presence of a field cut stemming from the stroke and decreased near visual acuity as a result of normal aging. She also confirms the absence of hemi-inattention and determines that neither prisms nor visual therapy are indicated for this client. The optometrist issues an updated eyeglasses prescription and refers him back for occupational therapy to compensate for the field cut (N. Torgerson, personal communication, July 2, 2021). Anand identifies two main long-term goals: (a) to return to his position as a purchasing agent at a large manufacturing company and (b) to be able to walk through unfamiliar environments without bumping into objects on the left. The occupational therapy practitioner instructs Anand in the use of anchoring and scanning techniques (see Chapter 4) for working on the computer, reading, and walking and how to adjust his computer workstation for optimal viewing without neck strain.

Next, consider Avery, a 33-year-old non-binary individual who sustained a TBI and complex lower limb fracture as a result of a bicycle accident. On the initial evaluation, the occupational therapist finds that Avery is having difficulties performing everyday household tasks and is unable to work because of issues with memory, attention, and executive function. On the vision screen portion of the evaluation, Avery reports that they are reading more slowly than before their accident and that their eyes are getting tired more often. Avery says that they seem to be having difficulty focusing their eyes, seem clumsier than usual when reaching for objects, and are getting carsick for the first time in their life. The occupational therapist identifies possible decreased near visual acuity on the vision screen and refers Avery to the neurorehabilitative optometrist for further evaluation.

The optometrist confirms that Avery has decreased near visual acuity as well as occasional diplopia (double vision) that impacts their depth perception when reaching for objects. She diagnoses Avery with convergence insufficiency (eyes not aiming together when looking at close objects as needed to support binocular vision) and intermittent exotropia (one eye occasionally turning out). The optometrist prescribes vision therapy to be provided in her office by her staff to improve (a) the stability of the binocular and accommodative systems so that the eyes are working together (eye teaming) and moving appropriately for task demands and (b) the integration of the central and peripheral visual systems. The treatment plan also includes the temporary use of prescription eyeglasses for near work, with tint provided if needed, to decrease the focusing strain as well as specialized microprisms and sectoral occlusion on Avery's eyeglasses to reduce the motion sickness they are currently experiencing (N. Torgerson & L. Press, personal communication, July 2, 2021). The overall functional goals for the optometric vision treatment are for Avery to be able to (a) read without special lighting or other compensatory strategies for 1 hour at a time without getting a headache or their eyes feeling tired, (b) reach and grasp objects without hesitation 100% of the time while performing familiar household tasks, and (c) drive or ride in a car for up to 1 hour without motion sickness.

In the meantime, the occupational therapy practitioner instructs Avery and their family on how to use contrast, magnification, and lighting to make it easier to read for pleasure and while performing everyday tasks and how to modify the environment to reduce irritating visual stimulation (see Chapter 4). The occupational therapy practitioner also works with Avery's speech-language pathologist and physical therapist on how to effectively incorporate contrast and magnification into printed material used in therapy activities and home exercise instructions while avoiding visual overload.

To date, formal collaborations of rehabilitation clinicians with optometry and full inclusion of optometrists on neurorehabilitation teams have been limited. The decreased access of clients and clinicians to optometrists results in part from barriers to optometrists gaining approval to see patients in hospital settings. This often stems from concerns from physicians regarding allowing nonmedical providers access. As a result, there are only a small number of optometrists in the United States with hospital privileges. The restrictions in workplace interaction along with the unfamiliarity of many rehabilitation clinicians with the optometry literature contribute to limited knowledge of the optometry field within many rehabilitation settings. These factors may explain why Schaadt and colleagues (2014), whose backgrounds are in clinical neuropsychology, described their study intervention to improve binocularity after TBI as novel despite being similar to vision therapy treatment techniques used by optometrists for many years (e.g., Berne, 1990; Ciuffreda et al., 2009; Scheiman & Galloway, 2001) and the intervention in the study published by Thiagarajan and Ciuffreda (2013) the previous year.

For clinicians interested in establishing a new or expanding an existing interdisciplinary team to include optometry, we suggest starting by interviewing potential optometry colleagues to identify those who use an individualized, functional, goal-driven treatment approach. In bringing an optometrist into an existing team, we have found it helpful to use a low-key, education-oriented focus combined with a systematic approach to gathering and analyzing objective data on referral patterns and client outcomes (Powell & Torgerson, 2011).

The Vision Clinic at Craig Hospital in Denver, Colorado, provides an example of how an interdisciplinary vision team functions (Ripley et al., 2010). The clinic is structured as an ancillary, or support, service to the primary care provided in an acute rehabilitation program for people with TBI. The clinic only sees patients in whom a potential vision problem has been identified. The identification of appropriate patients typically starts with a screening conducted by the occupational therapy practitioner that includes visual acuity, eye alignment, fixations, eye movements, and visual field screening (confrontation method; see Chapter 4). To be considered an appropriate candidate for referral, patients need to have sufficient awareness and emotional control to be able to participate in a full vision examination. It is also common to wait until any initial eye-related surgical treatment (e.g., surgical repair of the orbit) has been completed. However, patients do not need to be able to travel off-site to access the Vision Clinic services. Portable equipment allows for examination at bedside or in other rooms on the rehabilitation unit to increase access and reduce costs.

The occupational therapist who conducted the screening typically accompanies patients to their initial Vision Clinic visit to present the findings from the vision screen to the primary vision provider on the team. At this site, an optometrist is typically in the primary vision provider role (Cilo et al., 2010). The vision provider performs a full examination, including a record review, visual history, and observations followed by assessment of visual acuity, ocular alignment, fixations and eye movements, reflexes, visual fields, papillary reflexes, ocular health (including eye pressure), and refraction (see Cilo et al., 2010 for additional vision examination details). The examination is similar to the one used by other optometrists specializing in the care of people with a brain injury, including the staff at the Optometry Polytrauma Inpatient Clinic, Veterans Affairs Palo Alto Health Care System (Goodrich et al., 2007).

After the examination, the vision provider discusses any treatment recommendations with the occupational therapist. The occupational therapist is responsible for communicating the plan of care to the rest of the rehabilitation team to facilitate integration with other rehabilitation services in which vision will likely play a key role in the assessment and treatment, including physical therapy, speech-language pathology, recreation therapy, and neuropsychology. Nursing is responsible for performing any medication orders, whereas behavioral attendants assist with exercises outside of therapy sessions. Family members also assist with exercises outside of therapy and help the patient understand the importance of vision treatment to help with adherence. The vision provider at the Vision Clinic may also refer the patient to other vision specialists, including general ophthalmology, neuro-ophthalmology, and oculoplastic surgery (e.g., for reconstruction of the eyelids, orbit, tear system, and face) who serve as consultants to the primary vision team.

Neurorehabilitation Cognitive-Perceptual Treatment Teams

The makeup of the core cognitive-perceptual team in adult neurorehabilitation differs from the core vision team and also varies depending on whether the primary focus is on cognition or visual-perceptual issues. Many neurorehabilitation teams include a clinical neuropsychologist

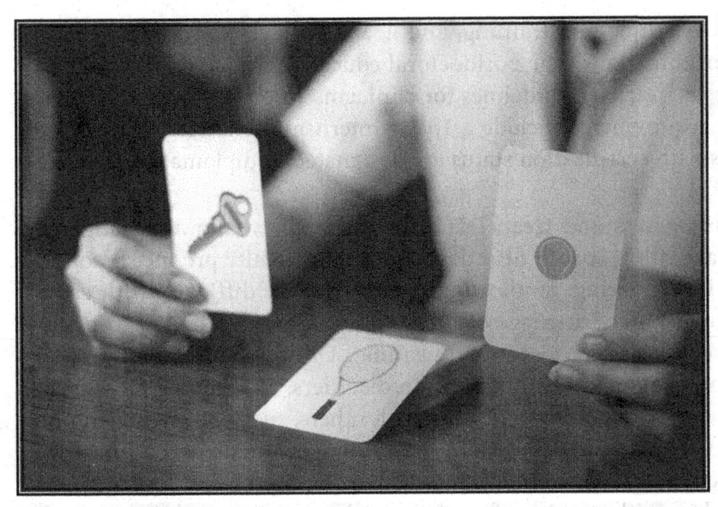

Figure 2-9. Neuropsychological testing is often performed with tabletop activities. One example of a common subtest is the ability to name and categorize objects. (Atthapon Raksthaput/shutterstock.com)

who will likely be involved to some extent in the assessment of perceptual dysfunction and a key team member in the assessment and/or treatment of cognitive-related impairments. It is also highly likely that a speech-language pathologist will be involved in the assessment and treatment of cognitive impairments. In some cases, a neurorehabilitative optometrist is also involved in assessing and treating deficits in visual processing (Suter, 2017). Understanding more about the fields of clinical neuropsychology and speech-language pathology will help in clarifying the roles of the various team members.

Clinical neuropsychology is a specialty area of practice within the field of clinical psychology. Clinical neuropsychologists work with individuals with suspected or known involvement of the central nervous system to understand the relationship between the functioning of the brain and an individual's cognitive, emotional, and behavioral function (American Psychological Association, 2008; Hannay et al., 1998). Their clinical expertise includes the administration and interpretation of standardized assessments of cognition, attention, learning and memory, problem solving, sensorimotor, and psychological function. The assessments used by neuropsychologists are typically well developed with strong psychometric properties. They are most often performed sitting at a table (Figure 2-9), although behavioral observations also contribute to a neuropsychologist's findings. The role of the clinical neuropsychologist in providing treatment can vary. They are often involved with counseling clients and their families on the adjustment to disability and injury and using psychotherapy approaches to manage emotional conditions, such as depression and anxiety. In some settings, clinical neuropsychologists provide direct individual- or group-based interventions for remediation and compensation of cognitive functions, whereas in others they refer to other professionals for treatment (American Board of Professional Psychology, 2022).

The American Psychological Association first recognized clinical neuropsychology as a specialty area of practice in 1996, although there had been a Division of Clinical Neuropsychology within the American Psychological Association since 1980. A few states currently have a specialty licensure option for clinical neuropsychologists, but most providers hold a general psychology license. The educational background for clinical neuropsychologists varies to a certain extent. Although all providers have completed a doctoral degree in psychology after an undergraduate degree in psychology or a related field, some providers have a research-focused PhD, whereas others earn a PsyD, which is a more clinically focused curriculum. It typically takes at least 5 years to complete either of these types of doctoral programs. Optional board certification is available through the American Board of Clinical Neuropsychology and the American Board of Professional Neuropsychology. Board certification involves a review of the applicant's professional credentials, including education, postdoctoral training, and licensure; a review of practice case samples; and written and oral examinations. The postdoctoral educational and training requirements vary by graduation date, with stricter guidelines for clinicians who graduated after 2004. For more recent graduates, the requirements include a 1-year internship followed by 2 years of supervised residency. Clinicians with certification status are designated as diplomates of the credentialing organization.

Speech-language pathologists assess and treat disorders of speech, swallowing, language, and communication (Miller et al., 2010). Speech disorders result in difficulty producing sounds correctly or fluently, such as with stuttering. Swallowing disorders cause difficulty with eating and drinking as well as managing saliva. Language disorders affect a person's ability to understand and/or use words orally or in writing to convey meaning. Disorders of communication include social-communication and cognitive-communication disorders. Individuals with social-communication disorders have difficulties communicating with others, such as greeting another person, asking for help, and following culturally appropriate ways of interacting with others through language. People with cognitive-communication disorders have problems with communication that result from difficulties with cognitive functions, such as attention, planning, problem solving, or organizing one's thoughts. All of these deficits may be relevant areas of assessment and treatment for speech-language pathologists working with individuals with ABI (American Speech-Language-Hearing Association, n.d.-b).

Speech-language pathologists are required to have a state license to practice. Licensure requirements include completion of a minimum of a master's degree (either Master of Arts or Master of Science) in communication sciences and disorders from an accredited institution and passage of a national certification examination. The American Speech-Language-Hearing Association offers a Certificate of Clinical Competence in Speech-Language Pathology, which includes the completion of a speech-language fellowship (American Speech-Language Hearing Association, n.d.-a). This certificate is currently required for licensure in some states but not all.

As can be seen from the descriptions provided earlier, the greatest area of potential overlap among these three disciplines is in the area of cognitive assessment and treatment, with neuropsychology, speech-language pathology, and occupational therapy all having expertise in this area. Team communication is essential in providing effective interdisciplinary care and achieving optimal outcomes. Communication begins with establishing which of these team members will administer which assessments to minimize the duplication of services and avoid leaving out an important area (Miller et al., 2010). Shared assessment results can then contribute to interdisciplinary goal setting and treatment planning. As with other areas of rehabilitation, the different perspectives that each of these disciplines brings to the assessment and treatment of cognitive dysfunction can result in better treatment outcomes than if just one discipline were to treat alone.

For example, imagine Farhiya, whose symptoms after TBI include difficulty with her memory. The speech-language pathologist on Farhiya's treatment team works with her to set up a memory book. She uses the book to keep track of the date, time, location, and provider name and contact information for future medical and other appointments. During or immediately after each appointment, she learns to makes notes in the book to help her remember the recommendations that were made and what she is supposed to do for follow-up. She also uses the book to keep track of the names and contact information of key family members and friends.

The occupational therapy practitioner focuses treatment on functional cognition (i.e., addressing the impact of impaired memory on Farhiya's performance of everyday tasks). For example, one of Farhiya's goals relates to remembering to purchase the food she needs to prepare daily meals each week. The occupational therapy practitioner shows her how to use a system that includes rotating weekly menu plans and preprinted master grocery shopping lists. Each grocery list includes all of the items needed for the menu plans for the upcoming week. The shopping lists are set up in the same order as the aisles of the store where she typically shops from her usual entrance to the exit. Food items are identified and color coded by category. There is a place to check off an item when it is placed in the cart at the store. Each week, Farhiya posts a new shopping list on the refrigerator door along with a highlighter pen. She highlights the food items that need to be purchased for the coming week's menus and any staples her family has run out of along with a note for how many of each item are needed. The occupational therapy practitioner works with her in the clinic to set up the system and meets her at the grocery store to provide additional instruction and feedback in using the shopping list.

As a result of concerns identified on the vision screen portion of the occupational therapy evaluation, Farhiya is referred early on to the neurorehabilitative optometrist serving as a consultant to the primary rehabilitation team to ensure that she has the best vision possible while participating in her rehabilitation. The optometrist's evaluation finds that accommodative (adjusting focus for near to far and vice versa) and oculomotor (eye movement) dysfunction are contributing to the problems Farhiya is experiencing with her memory. He focuses on vision therapy to help Farhiya regain the ability to focus and track the notes she makes in her memory book and to effectively scan the shelves when looking for items in the grocery store (N. Torgerson, personal communication, July 16, 2021).

Farhiya also attends a weekly group session with other people who have sustained a TBI that is led by the team neuropsychologist. There she learns ways to manage her anger and frustration with having to work so hard to remember things that used to be automatic. She finds the experiences and insights of the other group members helpful as she works to adjust to her new life.

Conclusion

Collaborating with other professionals in the evaluation and treatment of adults with ABI is critical to effective occupational therapy practice. The neurorehabilitation team members who address visual and cognitive and perceptual dysfunction vary somewhat by setting and facility. In all instances, understanding the professional backgrounds and roles of other team members sets the foundation for good communication and provides a framework for advocating for the role of occupational therapy and the inclusion of professionals from other key disciplines.

References

American Academy of Ophthalmology. (2020). What is an ophthalmologist? https://www.aao.org/eye-health/tips-prevention/what-is-ophthalmologist

American Academy of Optometry. (n.d.). Become a fellow. https://aaopt.org/membership/candidates-fellows/

American Board of Optometry. (2019). What is board certification? http://americanboardofoptometry.org/board-certification/

American Board of Professional Psychology. (2022). American Board of Professional Psychology, American Board of Clinical Neuropsychology board certification guidelines and procedures candidate's manual. https://abpp.org/wp-content/uploads/2022/10/ABCN-Manual.pdf

American Optometric Association. (n.d.). Studying optometry. https://www.aoa.org/education/studying-optometry?sso=y

American Psychological Association. (2008). Clinical neuropsychology. https://www.apa.org/ed/graduate/specialize/neuropsychology

American Speech-Language-Hearing Association. (n.d.-a). Speech language pathway to certification. https://www.asha.org/Certification/Speech-Language-Pathology-Pathway-To-Certification/

American Speech-Language-Hearing Association. (n.d.-b). Traumatic brain injury in adults (practice portal). www.asha.org/Practice-Portal/Clinical-Topics/Traumatic-Brain-Injury-in-Adults/

Association of Schools and Colleges of Optometry. (2019). Residency programs. https://optometriceducation.org/students-future-students/residency-programs/

Belanger, G. G., Uomoto, J. M., & Vanderploeg, R. D. (2009). The Veterans Health Administration System of Care for mild traumatic brain injury: Costs, benefits, and controversies. *Journal of Head Trauma Rehabilitation, 24*, 4-13. https://doi.org/10.1097/HTR.0b013e3181957032

Berne, S. A. (1990). Visual therapy for the traumatic brain-injured. *Journal of Optometric Vision Development, 21*, 13-16.

Berryman, A., & Rasavage, K. G. (2011). The interdisciplinary approach to vision rehabilitation following brain injury. In P. S. Suter & L. H. Harvey (Eds.), *Vision rehabilitation: Multidisciplinary care of the patient following brain injury* (pp. 31-44). CRC Press.

Berryman, A., Rasavage, K., Politzer, T., & Gerber, D. (2020). Brief report—Oculomotor treatment in traumatic brain injury rehabilitation: A randomized controlled pilot trial. *American Journal of Occupational Therapy, 74*, 7401185050. https://doi.org/10.5014/ajot.2020.026880

Bouska, M. J., & Gallaway, M. (1991). Primary visual deficits in adults with brain damage: Management in occupational therapy. *Occupational Therapy Practice, 3*(1), 1-11.

Braddom, R. L. (2005). Medicare funding for inpatient rehabilitation: How did we get to this point and what do we do now? *Archives of Physical Medicine and Rehabilitation, 86*, 1287-1292. https://doi.org/10.1016/j.apmr.2005.01.004

Centers for Medicare & Medicaid Services. (2017). Medicare benefit policy manual (Revision 234). https://www.cms.gov/Regulations-and-Guidance/Guidance/Manuals/Downloads/bp102c01.pdf

Cilo, M., Politzer, T., Ripley, D. L., & Weintraub, A. (2010). Vision examination of TBI patients in an acute rehabilitation hospital. *NeuroRehabilitation, 27*, 237-242. https://doi.org/10.3233/nre-2010-0603

Ciuffreda, K. J., Ludlam, D. P., & Kapoor, N. (2009). Clinical oculomotor training in traumatic brain injury. *Optometry & Vision Development, 40*, 16-23.

Cohen, A. H., & Rein, L. D. (1992). The effect of head trauma on the visual system: The doctor of optometry as a member of the rehabilitation team. *Journal of the American Optometric Association, 63*, 530-536.

Cohen, A. H., & Soden, R. (1981). An optometric approach to the rehabilitation of the stroke patient. *Journal of the American Optometric Association, 52*, 795-800.

College of Optometrists in Vision Development. (n.d.). Fellowship certification for optometrists. https://www.covd.org/page/Fellowship

Conrad, J. S., Mitchell, G. L., & Kulp, M. T. (2017). Vision therapy for binocular dysfunction post brain injury. *Optometry and Vision Science, 94*, 101-107. http://doi.org/10.1097/OPX.0000000000000937

D'Amour, D., Ferrada-Videla, M., San Martin Rodriguez, L., & Beaulieu, M. D. (2005). The conceptual basis for interprofessional collaboration: Core concepts and theoretical frameworks. *Journal of Interprofessional Care, 19*(Suppl.), 116-131. https://doi.org/10.1080/13561820500082529

Gianutsos, R., Perlin, R., Mazerolle, K. A., & Trem, N. (1989). Rehabilitative optometric services for persons emerging from coma. *Journal of Head Trauma Rehabilitation, 4*(2), 17-25. https://doi.org/10.1097/00001199-198906000-00005

Gianutsos, R., & Ramsey, G. (1988). Enabling rehabilitation optometrists to help survivors of acquired brain injury. *Journal of Vision Rehabilitation, 2*(1), 37-58.

Gianutsos, R., Ramsey, G., & Perlin, R. R. (1988). Rehabilitative optometric services for survivors of acquired brain injury. *Archives of Physical Medicine and Rehabilitation, 69*, 573-578.

Goodrich, G. L., Kirby, J., Cockerham, G., Ingalla, S. P., & Lew, H. L. (2007). Visual function in patients of a polytrauma rehabilitation center. *Journal of Rehabilitation Research and Development, 44*, 929-936. https://doi.org/10.1682/jrrd.2007.01.0003

Greenwood, E. (1957). Attributes of a profession. *Social Work, 2*(3), 45-55. https://doi.org/10.1093/sw/2.3.45

Hall, P. (2005). Interprofessional teamwork: Professional cultures as barriers. *Journal of Interprofessional Care, 19*(Suppl. 1), 188-196. https://doi.org/10.1080/13561820500081745

Hannay, H. J., Bieliauskas, L. A., Crosson, B. A., Hammeke, T. A., Hamshser, K., & Koffler, S. P. (1998). Proceedings of the Houston Conference on specialty education and training in clinical neuropsychology [special issue]. *Archives of Clinical Neuropsychology, 13*, 157-250.

Intagliata, S., & Hollander, R. (1987). The 3-hour therapy criterion: A challenge for rehabilitation facilities. *American Journal of Occupational Therapy, 41*, 297-304. https://doi.org/10.5014/ajot.41.5.297

Ivanhoe, C. B., Durand-Sanchez, A., & Spicer, E. T. (2013). Acute rehabilitation. In N. D. Zasler, D. I. Katz, & R. D. Zafonte (Eds.), *Brain injury medicine: Principles and practice* (2nd ed., pp. 385-405). Demos Medical.

Karol, R. L. (2014). Team models in rehabilitation: Structure, function, and culture change. *NeuroRehabilitation, 34*, 655-669. https://doi.org/10.3233/nre-141080

Malec, J. (2013). Posthospital rehabilitation. In N. D. Zasler, D. I. Katz, & R. D. Zafonte (Eds.), *Brain injury medicine: Principles and practice* (2nd ed., pp. 1238-1301). Demos Medical.

Maley, M., Ray, J. S., & Greene, J. (1991, October 3). Uniting occupational therapy and optometry. *OT Week*, 14-15.

Miller, E. L., Murray, L., Richards, L., Zorowitz, R. D., Bakas, T., Clark, P., Billinger, S. A., & the American Heart Association Council on Cardiovascular Nursing and the Stroke Council. (2010). Comprehensive overview of nursing and interdisciplinary rehabilitation care of the stroke patient. *Stroke, 41*, 2402-2448. https://doi.org/10.1161/STR.0b013e3181e7512b

Mitchell, P. M., Wynia, M. K., Golden, R., McNellis, B., Okun, S., Webb, C. E., Rohrbach, V., & Von Kohorn, I. (2012). Core principles & values of effective team-based health care. Discussion paper, Institute of Medicine. http://nam.edu/wp-content/uploads/2015/06/VSRT-Team-Based-Care-Principles-Values.pdf

Neuro-Optometric Rehabilitation Association. (n.d.). Clinical skills/fellowship program. https://noravisionrehab.org/about-nora/clinical-skills-fellowship-program

North American Neuro-Ophthalmology Society. (2018). What is a neuro-ophthalmologist? https://www.nanosweb.org/m/pages.cfm?pageid=3279

Parker, G. M. (2008). *Team players and teamwork: New strategies for developing successful collaboration* (2nd ed.). Jossey-Bass.

Payne, M. (2000). *Teamwork in multiprofessional care.* Lyceum.

Powell, J. M., & Torgerson, N. G. (2011). Evaluation and treatment of vision and motor dysfunction following acquired brain injury from occupational therapy and neuro-optometry perspectives. In P. S. Suter & L. H. Harvey (Eds.), *Vision rehabilitation: Multidisciplinary care of the patient following brain injury* (pp. 351-396). CRC Press.

Reinstein, L. (2014). The history of the 75-percent rule: Three decades past and an uncertain future. *PM&R: The Journal of Injury, Function, and Rehabilitation, 6*, 973-975. https://doi.org/10.1016/j.pmrj.2014.08.950

Ripley, D. L., Politzer, T., Berryman, A., Rasavage, K., & Weintraub, A. (2010). The Vision Clinic: An interdisciplinary method for assessment and treatment of visual problems after traumatic brain injury. *NeuroRehabilitation, 27*, 231-235. https://doi.org/10.3233/NRE-2010-0602

Roberts, P. S., Rizzo, J., Hreha, K., Wertheimer, J., Kaldenberg, J., Hironaka, D., Riggs, R., & Colenbrander, C. (2016). A conceptual model for vision rehabilitation. *Journal of Rehabilitation Research and Development, 53*, 693-704. https://doi.org/10.1682/JRRD.2015.06.0113

Rothberg, J. S. (1981). The rehabilitation team: Future directions. *Archives of Physical Medicine and Rehabilitation, 62*, 407-411.

Schaadt, A., Schmidt, L., Reinhart, S., Adams, M., Garbacenkaite, R., Leonhardt, E., Kuhn, C., & Kerkhoff, G. (2014). Perceptual relearning of binocular fusion and steroacuity after brain injury. *Neurorehabilitation and Neural Repair, 28*, 462-471. https://doi.org/10.1177/1545968313516870

Scheiman, M. (2011). *Understanding and managing vision deficits: A guide for occupational therapists* (3rd ed.). SLACK Incorporated.

Scheiman, M., & Gallaway, M. (2001). Vision therapy to treat binocular vision disorders after acquired brain injury: Factors affecting prognosis. In I. B. Suchoff, K. J. Ciuffreda, & N. Kapoor (Eds.), *Visual & vestibular consequences of acquired brain injury* (pp. 89-101). Optometric Extension Program.

Schlageter, K., Gray, B., Hall, K., Shaw, R., & Sammet, R. (1993). Incidence and treatment of visual dysfunction in traumatic brain injury. *Brain Injury, 7*, 439-448. http://doi.org/10.3109/02699059309029687

Schlageter, K., & Shaw, R. (1991, July 11). Vision therapy. *OT Week*, 13-14.

Schnell, R. D. (1992). An innovative connection between rehabilitation optometry and occupational therapy: Solving visual problems associated with brain injury. *Journal of Cognitive Rehabilitation, 10*(4), 34-36.

Simpson-Jones, M. E., & Hunt, A. W. (2019). Vision rehabilitation interventions following mild traumatic brain injury: A scoping review. *Disability and Rehabilitation, 41*, 2206-2222. https://doi.org/10.1080/09638288.2018.1460407

Suter, P. S. (2017). Rehabilitation and management of visual dysfunction following traumatic brain injury. In M. J. Ashley & D. A. Hovda (Eds.), *Traumatic brain injury: Rehabilitation, treatment, and case management* (4th ed., pp. 451-486). CRC Press.

Taylor, R. R. (2020). *The intentional relationship: Occupational therapy and use of self.* F.A. Davis.

Thiagarajan, P., & Ciuffreda, K. J. (2013). Effect of oculomotor rehabilitation on vergence responsivity in mild traumatic brain injury. *Journal of Rehabilitation Research and Development, 50*, 1223-1240. https://doi.org/10.1682/jrrd.2012.12.0235

Thiagarajan, P., & Ciuffreda, K. J. (2014a). Effect of oculomotor rehabilitation on accommodative responsivity in mild traumatic brain injury. *Journal of Rehabilitation Research and Development, 51*, 175-191. https://doi.org/10.1682/JRRD.2013.01.0027

Thiagarajan, P., & Ciuffreda, K. J. (2014b). Short-term persistence of oculomotor rehabilitative changes in mild traumatic brain injury (mTBI): A pilot study of clinical effects. *Brain Injury, 29*, 1475-1479. https://doi.org/10.3109/02699052.2015.1070905

Thiagarajan, P., & Ciuffreda, K. J. (2014c). Versional eye tracking in mild traumatic brain injury (mTBI): Effects of oculomotor training (OMT). *Brain Injury, 7*, 930-943. https://doi.org/10.3109/02699052.2014.888761

Thiagarajan, P., Ciuffreda, K. J., Capo-Aponte, J. E., Ludlam, D. P., & Kapoor, N. (2014). Oculomotor rehabilitation for reading in mild traumatic brain injury (mTBI): An integrative approach. *NeuroRehabilitation, 34*, 129-146. https://doi.org/10.3233/NRE-131025

U.S. Bureau of Labor Statistics. (2021, April 9). *Opticians: Occupational Outlook Handbook*. https://www.bls.gov/ooh/healthcare/opticians-dispensing.htm#tab-4

Chapter 3

The Visual System

Vision plays a major role in our ability to adapt to the environment. It serves as a primary receptor for information necessary for motor, cognitive, communicative, and emotive functions (Helvie, 2018). It is an important prerequisite to perception and cognition and influences both motor planning and postural control (Cuiffreda et al., 2001). It allows us to anticipate situations, which is necessary for successful adaptation to the environment (Warren, 2018). Before being able to understand the impact of a brain injury on visual functioning, it is essential for occupational therapy practitioners to understand how the visual system typically functions. Following is a brief overview of the visual system, along with a description of some of the common visual dysfunctions that can occur after damage to different parts of the visual system. For more in-depth information on the anatomical and neuroanatomical structures of the visual system, the reader is referred to the references.

The Eyeball, Pupil, Cornea, and Lens

Information enters the visual system through the eye (Figure 3-1). The first step in the ability to perceive visual information begins when structures of the eye act in concert to focus light onto the retina, the layer of tissue containing photoreceptor cells at the back of the eye (Lundy-Ekman, 2018). The amount of light that enters the eye is controlled by the size of the pupil. Pupillary size is controlled through a combination of action from the parasympathetic and sympathetic nervous systems. Parasympathetic fibers carried by cranial nerve III, the oculomotor nerve, control constriction of the pupil, whereas pupil dilation is controlled by the sympathetic nervous system (Lundy-Ekman, 2018; Scheiman, 2011a). Therefore, abnormalities in pupillary size and/or reaction times can indicate damage to the central nervous system (CNS) and can be important for doctors in diagnosing the presence and severity of a brain injury (Lussier et al., 2019; Saliman et al., 2021).

Kaminsky, T. A., & Powell, J. M.
Zoltan's Vision, Perception, and Cognition: Evaluation and Treatment of the Adult With Acquired Brain Injury, Fifth Edition (pp. 33-56).

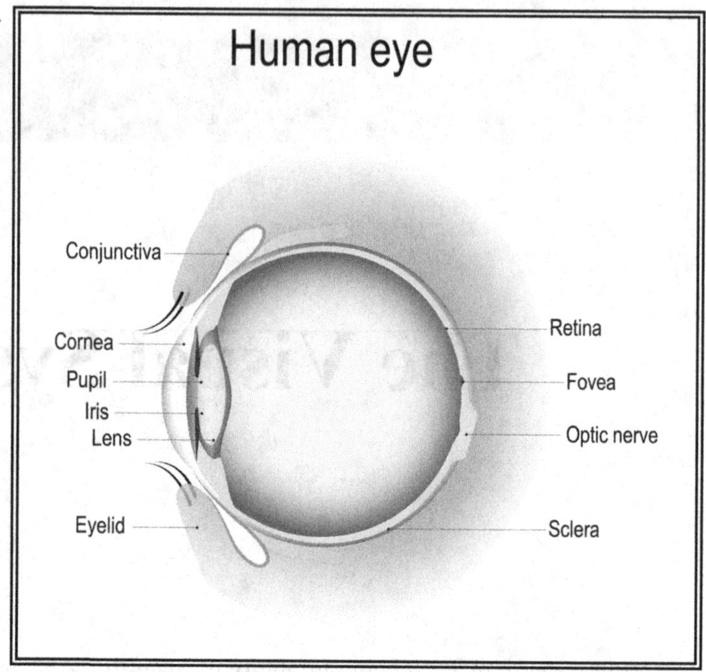

Figure 3-1. Structures of the eye. (Designua/shutterstock.com)

The cornea and lens are the primary structures involved in focusing light onto the retina. The shape of the cornea has an impact on the direction of light. For light to be focused correctly, the cornea should be smoothly and evenly curved. The lens changes its shape to assist in focusing light rays on the retina depending on the distance of the object being viewed (Scheiman, 2011a). As described in more detail later in this chapter, this process is called *accommodation*. Accommodation enables the angle of the light coming into the eye to be adjusted so that it lands directly on the surface of the retina. The lens takes on a rounder shape to allow focus on near objects and a flatter shape for focusing on objects at a distance. The lens shape changes as a result of action from zonular fibers and ciliary muscles (Scheiman, 2011a). After passing through the lens, light then travels through the vitreous gel within the eyeball (see later) and stimulates photoreceptor cells called *rods* and *cones*, which are housed in the retina (Scheiman, 2011a).

Refractive Errors

A number of eye conditions called *refractive errors* can negatively impact the ability of the eye to focus light on the retina (National Eye Institute [NEI], 2022c). Three of the most common types of refractive errors, myopia, hyperopia, and astigmatism, result from structural irregularities in the eye. A fourth, presbyopia, results from age-related changes (NEI, 2022c). We discuss each of these briefly. None of these conditions is caused by brain damage; rather, they are common pre-existing conditions that can have an impact on visual functioning, so the treating occupational therapy practitioner should be aware of them. One risk factor for developing refractive errors is heredity, with the likelihood of developing refractive errors increasing if they are present in family members (NEI, 2022c). Other risk factors are not as clearly understood, although there is growing evidence that time spent outdoors and/or playing sports may decrease the likelihood of developing myopia (nearsightedness), one of the most common refractive errors (Jones et al., 2007;

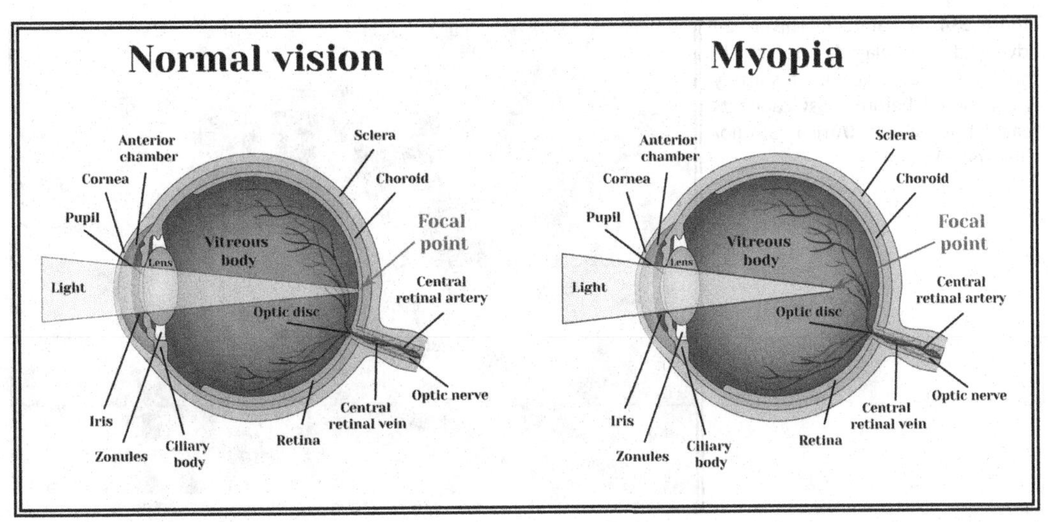

Figure 3-2. Myopia. (Mrs_Bazilio/shutterstock.com)

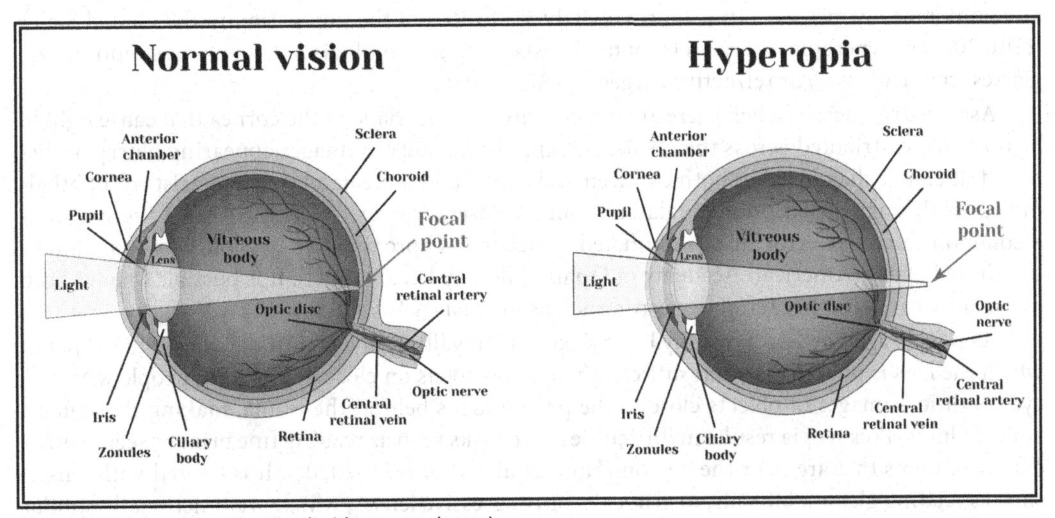

Figure 3-3. Hyperopia. (Mrs_Bazilio/shutterstock.com)

Jones-Jordan et al., 2011). At one time, engagement in close work, including increased time spent reading, was considered a risk factor for developing myopia but that has been questioned by more recent research (Jones et al., 2007; Jones-Jordan et al., 2011; Sivak, 2012).

Myopia, or nearsightedness, can occur either when the cornea is too steeply curved or when the eye is longer than normal. In this condition, the image is focused in front of the retina (Figure 3-2). The result of myopia is that images at a distance will appear blurred, whereas images that are near will be clear. Myopia is a common eye condition, impacting approximately 25% of the population in the United States. It is most commonly diagnosed in children between the ages of 8 and 12 (NEI, 2010b). It is treated by optometrists or ophthalmologists through prescription eyeglasses, contact lenses, or refractive surgery (NEI, 2020b).

For those with hyperopia, or farsightedness, the cornea is either not curved enough or the eye is shorter than normal. In this condition, the focal point lands behind the retina (Figure 3-3). The result is that objects that are closer to the person appear blurry, whereas objects that are farther away look clear. This eye condition, which can first occur either in childhood or later in life, is not

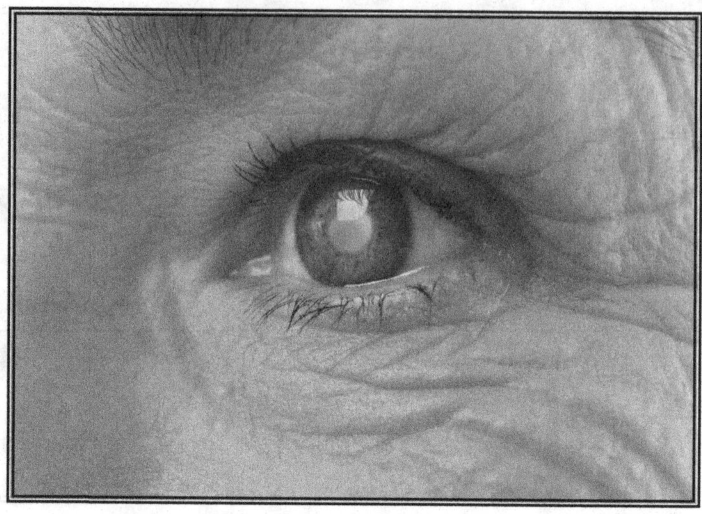

Figure 3-4. A cataract. This is an advanced age-related cataract. In the United States, cataract surgery is completed before most cataracts reach this stage. (Africa Studio/shutterstock.com)

as common as myopia, affecting approximately 5% to 10% of the population in the United States (NEI, 2010a). Hyperopia is treated by optometrists or ophthalmologists through prescription eyeglasses, contact lenses, or refractive surgery (NEI, 2020a).

Astigmatism occurs when there are irregularities in the shape of the cornea that cause light to be unevenly distributed across the retina. Astigmatism results in images appearing blurry or distorted. It can be diagnosed in both children and adults and is treated by optometrists or ophthalmologists through prescription eyeglasses, contact lenses, or surgery (NEI, 2019a). Astigmatism is a common refractive error that is estimated to occur in approximately 33% of the population in the United States (American Academy of Ophthalmology [AAO], 2011). It is possible to have both astigmatism and another refractive error, such as myopia (AAO, 2011).

As people age, the lens typically loses flexibility, resulting in a condition called *presbyopia* in which the lens is unable to round sufficiently to allow focus on close objects. For people with this eye condition, images of objects close to the person focus behind the retina, making those items appear blurry. Presbyopia results in difficulties with tasks such as reading fine print or seeing other details of items that are near the person (Hunt et al., 2018; NEI, 2020c). It is treated with lenses, such as reading glasses, bifocals, or trifocals, or progressive lenses, which are functionally similar to bifocals or trifocals but with smooth transitions in the eyeglass lenses without any demarcation lines (Hooper & Bello-Haas, 2009; NEI, 2019b). Environmental changes, such as having more light or increasing print size, can also help reduce symptoms (Warren, 2018).

Cataracts

Another eye condition that causes difficulties with the lens and impacts clarity of vision is a cataract. A cataract is a progressive opacity of the lens of the eye (Figure 3-4; Scheiman, 2011b). Cataracts are most commonly diagnosed in older adults, and the number of people with cataracts increases with age. More than half of the people over the age of 80 in the United States have or have had cataracts (AAO, 2011). In addition to older age, risk factors for the development of cataracts include smoking, excessive exposure to ultraviolet light, and family history. Symptoms of cataracts include progressive loss of vision (which can lead to blindness in severe cases) and glare sensitivity. Cataracts are treated through surgical extraction and lens replacement with an artificial lens (Scheiman, 2011b), with cataract surgery being the third most commonly performed ambulatory surgical procedure in the United States in recent years (Cullen et al., 2009).

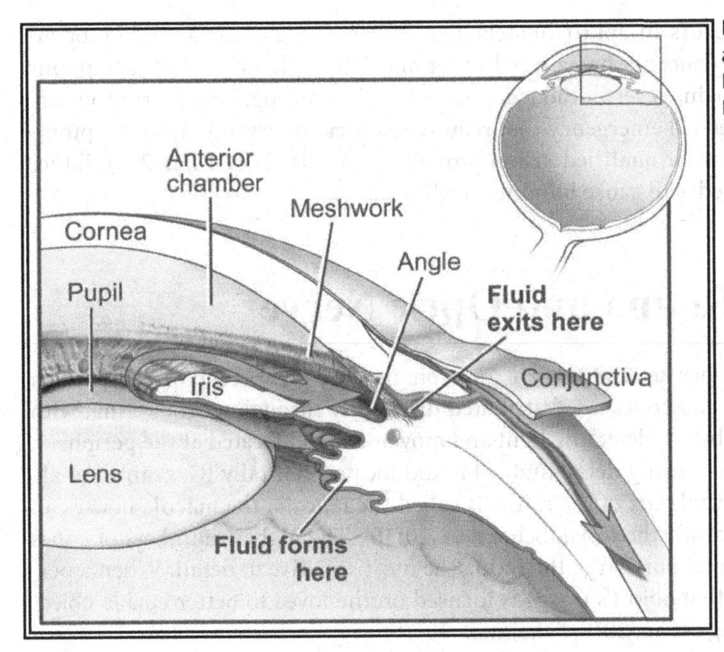

Figure 3-5. Normal fluid flow in the anterior chamber of the eye. (Courtesy: National Eye Institute, National Institutes of Health [NEI/NIH].)

Anterior Chamber and Vitreous

There are two chambers in the eye that contain fluid. The first is between the cornea and the lens and is called the *anterior chamber.* This area is filled with a clear, watery fluid called the *aqueous humor,* which is continually produced and circulated (Figure 3-5; Scheiman, 2011b). The *vitreous* is the second fluid-filled space and is located behind the lens. Light must travel through it to reach the retina. It is filled with a thick clear fluid called *vitreous humor.* Vitreous humor is mostly made up of water and also contains collagen. It helps to give the eye shape, support the lens, and hold the retina in place. Unlike the aqueous humor, the vitreous humor does not circulate (Scheiman, 2011a).

Glaucoma

Glaucoma is a group of diseases that cause an increase in intraocular pressure in the eye that can ultimately damage the optic nerve (NEI, 2022b; Scheiman, 2011b). In the United States, more than 2.7 million people over the age of 40 have been diagnosed with glaucoma (AAO, 2011). There are many types of glaucoma. Two of the most common are open-angle and angle-closure glaucoma. Open-angle glaucoma, the most common type, is caused by resistance to the outflow of aqueous fluid from the eye, although the cause is not fully understood. Its onset is gradual and initially asymptomatic until the increase in intraocular pressure causes damage to the optic nerve. This damage causes loss of vision initially in the peripheral fields, resulting in tunnel vision. Open-angle glaucoma can gradually and permanently affect the entire field of vision if untreated. Open-angle glaucoma is usually successfully treated through medicated eye drops and, in some cases, surgery. Because vision loss can be delayed or prevented with treatment, it is essential for people to be screened regularly for open-angle glaucoma. This screening, called *tonometry,* is part of a routine eye examination. A common type of tonometry consists of administering a puff of air onto the surface of the eye in order to measure intraocular pressure.

Angle-closure glaucoma occurs in approximately 10% of cases of glaucoma. Unlike open-angle glaucoma, angle-closure glaucoma has a rapid onset and is symptomatic, with symptoms including redness in the eye, pain, severe headache, nausea and vomiting, and blurred vision. Angle-closure glaucoma is a medical emergency that requires surgical intervention, so symptoms should be reported to a physician or qualified vision provider immediately (NEI, 2022b). Either type of glaucoma, if left untreated, can cause blindness (NEI, 2022b).

The Retina and Optic Nerve

The retina makes up the inner layer of the eye and contains the photoreceptor cells, which are called *rods* and *cones*. Rods and cones are distributed differently throughout the retina, with larger numbers of rods responsible for detecting light and movement and located at the periphery, and the cones responsible for discerning detail and color and located centrally (Gazzaniga et al., 2019; Scheiman, 2011a). The central part of the retina is called the *macula*; the macula houses an even smaller part of the retina called the *fovea* (Scheiman, 2011b). The highest numbers of cones are found in the fovea, making that portion of the retina the most sensitive to detail. When a person looks directly at an object, that object's image is focused on the fovea to better enable object identification to occur (Gazzaniga et al., 2019; Scheiman, 2011b).

Information from the photoreceptors leaves the eye through the optic nerve (Gazzaniga et al., 2019). The optic nerve (cranial nerve II) has a meningeal cover, and the subarachnoid space that surrounds it is continuous with the subarachnoid space surrounding the brain. When there is an increase in intracranial pressure from trauma to the brain, the optic disc can swell, a phenomenon called *papilledema*. As a result, physicians are able to use visualization of the retina as one diagnostic indicator of a brain injury (Saliman et al., 2021).

There are a number of disorders than can cause damage to the retina and/or optic nerve, including glaucoma, which was discussed previously. Although some of these conditions can be caused by trauma, most are common diseases that may be preexisting conditions for clients with acquired brain injury (ABI; Hellerstein & Scheiman, 2011). In addition, there are some health conditions, such as diabetes, that are risk factors for both stroke (i.e., cerebrovascular accident) and vision loss, so it is not unusual for the clients seen in rehabilitation to present with multiple vision-related conditions (Goodman, 2009). Because of their potentially enormous impact on visual functioning, it is essential for occupational therapy practitioners to be aware of the presence of these eye disorders and consider the impact they can have on occupational functioning (Hellerstein & Scheiman, 2011). The major disorders that affect the retina in adults, especially older adults, are age-related macular degeneration (ARMD) and diabetic retinopathy. There are other less common conditions as well, such as retinitis pigmentosa; the interested reader is referred to the references for more details.

Macular Degeneration

Low vision is defined as having visual acuity of 20/70 or worse in the better eye with optimal correction and is a health condition that can lead to limitations in functioning and quality of life (Freeman, 2011). ARMD is the most common cause of low vision (Scheiman, 2011b), affecting approximately 1.75 million people in the United States (Eye Diseases Prevalence Research Group, 2004). ARMD causes damage to the macula of the retina, thereby impacting the central visual field, which is responsible for detail and color vision. Because the periphery is left undamaged, people do not go completely blind, although functioning can be seriously negatively impacted

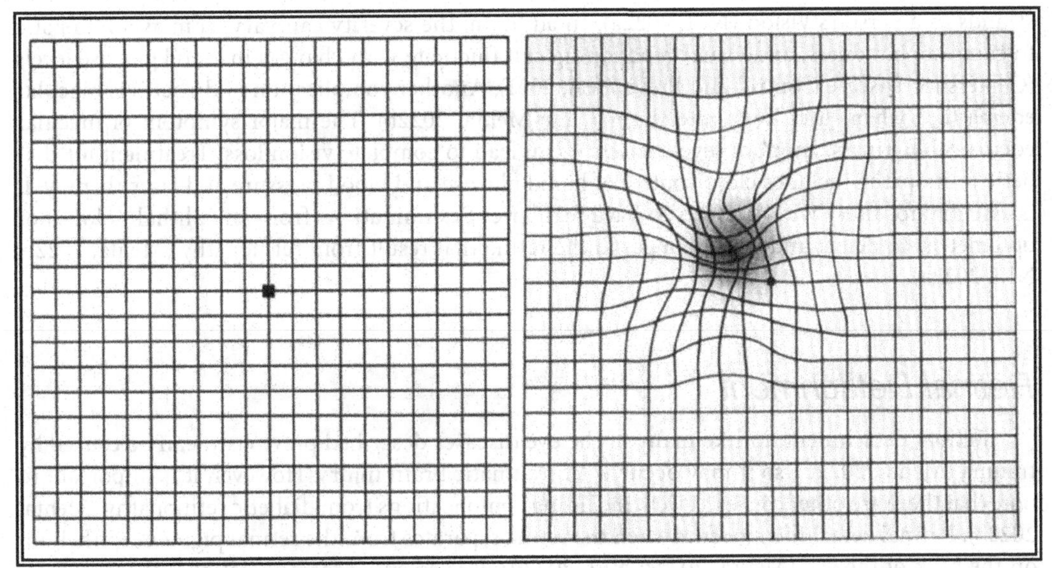

Figure 3-6. An Amsler grid. Without distortion (left). As a person with wet ARMD may see it (right). (Courtesy: National Eye Institute, National Institutes of Health [NEI/NIH].)

as a result of the disorder (Scheiman, 2011b). There are two types of ARMD: dry and wet. In the early stages of dry ARMD, yellow deposits called *drusen* form on the macula (Mehta, 2022a). At this point, especially if only one eye is affected, ARMD can be asymptomatic. It can be diagnosed during routine eye examinations, so it is essential for all people to receive screening regularly, especially as they age, so that the condition can be detected and monitored (NEI, 2021). There is no treatment for dry ARMD, although there is some evidence that dietary supplementation may slightly delay the progression of the disease (Age-Related Eye Disease Study Research Group, 2001; Evans & Lawrenson, 2017).

Wet ARMD is caused by abnormal blood vessel growth in the macula (Mehta, 2022a; NEI, 2021). It is not inevitable for people with dry ARMD to develop wet ARMD, but all who have wet ARMD had dry ARMD first (Mehta, 2022a). One of the first symptoms of wet ARMD is visual distortion (i.e., when straight lines appear wavy). As a way to detect the onset or worsening of wet ARMD early, people with dry ARMD may be given an Amsler grid (Figure 3-6). They are instructed to view the Amsler grid regularly to monitor if visual distortion appears. If a client reports visual distortion, an immediate referral to an ophthalmologist should be made because this is a medical emergency (Freeman, 2011; NEI, 2021). Wet ARMD is treated with laser surgery, photodynamic therapy, and/or medication (NEI, 2021). In addition to the medical treatments for both types of macular degeneration, low vision rehabilitation should be prescribed if occupational functioning is impacted to better enable independence in areas of occupation (NEI, 2021).

Diabetic Retinopathy

Diabetes can cause retinopathy, one of the common causes of low vision and the leading cause of blindness for working-age adults in the United States (Centers for Disease Control and Prevention, 2021). Diabetic retinopathy can cause damage in any area of the retina through weakening, dilation, and rupture of retinal blood vessels and/or growth of abnormal blood vessels (NEI, 2022a). Because the damage can occur throughout the retina, there is not a predictable pattern of visual loss, although there are common symptoms, including blurriness, floaters, and cobweblike strands in a person's vision (NEI, 2022a). In addition, the severity can vary from asymptomatic to complete blindness, and visual functioning can fluctuate with changes in blood glucose levels (Centers for Disease Control and Prevention, 2021). Another complication of diabetes is macular edema (i.e., when fluid leaks into the macula; Mehta, 2022b). The major symptom of macular edema is blurriness. In more severe cases, it can lead to complete vision loss. Treatment for diabetic retinopathy includes close control of blood glucose and blood pressure and laser therapy. It is essential for those with diabetes to have regular eye examinations from an ophthalmologist or optometrist to detect and treat changes to the retina that result from retinopathy (Mehta, 2022b; NEI, 2022a).

Retinal Detachment

Retinal detachment, unlike many of the eye diseases described previously, can be caused by trauma (Mehta, 2022c), so it may occur with traumatic brain injury. However, it is important to note that there are other causes as well, including complications from diabetic retinopathy (Mehta, 2022b). Retinal detachment occurs when the retina separates from the retinal pigment epithelium on the back of the eye (Mehta, 2022c; NEI, 2022d). It is essential for occupational therapy practitioners and others to understand that retinal detachment is a medical emergency that requires early treatment (NEI, 2022d). Retinal detachments that are untreated can lead to permanent vision loss. The symptoms of retinal detachment are a sudden occurrence of or an increase in floaters; flashes of light, especially on the periphery; and/or a block in the visual field, which is described by some as a "curtain" dropping over a part of the vision (Mehta, 2022c; NEI, 2022d). Treatment depends on the extent of the detachment and includes laser surgery or cryopexy to fuse the retina to the underlying tissue; scleral buckling in which a silicone band is placed around the outside of the eye to push the back of the eye back onto the retina; and vitrectomy, which is an extraction of the vitreous humor followed by laser surgery and a refilling of the eye (NEI, 2020).

Visual Pathway to the Occipital Lobe

Once the photoreceptors in the retina are stimulated by light, they generate a neural signal that is sent to the brain through the optic nerve (Gazzaniga et al., 2019; Lundy-Ekman, 2018). As the light rays enter the eye, the image is reversed, both vertically and horizontally. As a result, the image is positioned on the retina upside down and mirrored, so information from the superior visual field is received by the inferior part of the retinal field and vice versa. Similarly, information from the right visual field is received by the left retinal field and vice versa. This topographical organization is maintained throughout the visual pathway (from the eye to the visual cortex) and enables the brain to ultimately create a visual map of what is in the environment. This map is needed for object identification and determining location, both of the person in relation to the objects and of the objects in relation to each other (Gazzaniga et al., 2019).

Axons leave the retina via the optic nerve to the optic chiasm, which is located anterior to the pituitary gland in the brain. At the optic chiasm, the nasal fibers, which carry information about the temporal visual fields, cross to the opposite side of the brain. As a result, after the optic chiasm, all of the information about the right visual field is processed on the left side of the brain, whereas all information about the left visual field is processed on the right side of the brain (Gazzaniga et al., 2019; Lundy-Ekman, 2018).

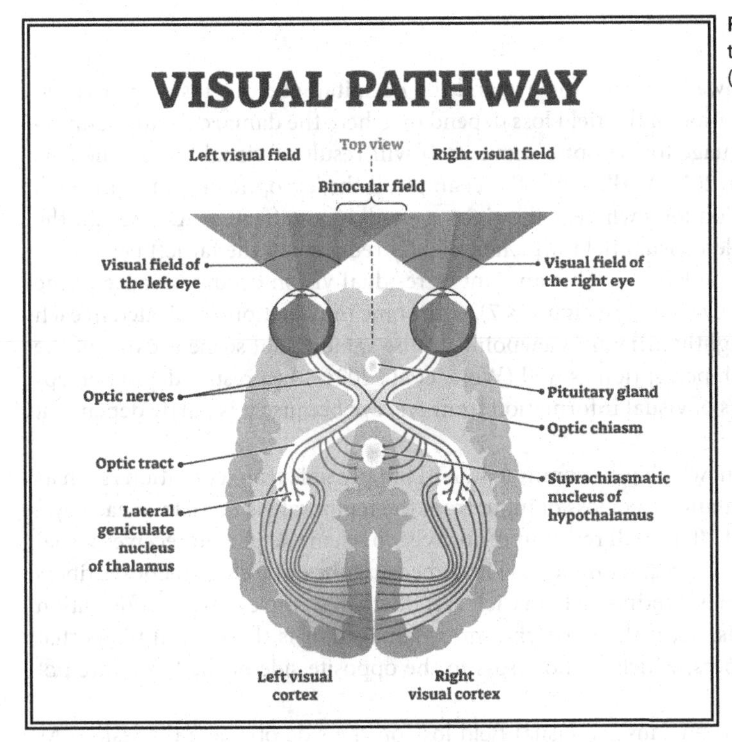

Figure 3-7. The visual pathway from the retina to the primary visual cortex. (VectorMine/shutterstock.com)

After the optic chiasm, fibers travel along the optic tract to the lateral geniculate nucleus (LGN) in the thalamus where they synapse (Gazzaniga et al., 2019; Lundy-Ekman, 2018). This is the first synapse after the fibers leave the eye. The LGN maintains the topographical organization of visual information through distribution across six layers of cells called *parvocellular* and *magnocellular layers*. There are four parvocellular layers that carry information about color and form from the cones in the macula. This information is especially important for object identification. The other two layers are magnocellular and receive information about movement and contrast. These layers are especially important for spatial relations (i.e., locating where objects are in space; Gazzaniga et al., 2019). From the LGN, fibers travel as optic radiations through the internal capsule to the primary visual cortex in the occipital lobe on the border of the calcarine fissure. This projection is also called the *geniculocortical* or *geniculocalcarine tract* (Gazzaniga et al., 2019; Lundy-Ekman, 2018). Figure 3-7 provides a depiction of the visual pathway from the retina to the visual cortex.

It is important to note that not all visual information follows this pathway. Some fibers leave the retina and travel to the pulvinar nucleus in the thalamus and the superior colliculus in the brainstem (Helvie, 2018; Lundy-Ekman, 2018). These are essential for other, subconscious activities, such as aiding with visual startle and protective reflexes. These pathways enable people to move away from an object approaching at high speed before the brain has time to fully identify what the object is. They also contribute to coordinating head, neck, and eye movements, as well as assisting in directing gaze to objects in the periphery so that object identification can occur (Gazzaniga et al., 2019). Other fibers travel to the hypothalamus where they influence circadian rhythms (Gazzaniga et al., 2019).

Visual Field Deficits

Damage to the visual pathway between the eye and the occipital lobe can result in a visual field deficit. The extent and location of the field loss depend on where the damage occurs (Lundy-Ekman, 2018; Wall, 2021). Damage to the optic nerve itself will result in visual loss in the corresponding eye (Lundy-Ekman, 2018; Wall, 2021). For example, if the left optic nerve is damaged, the left eye will experience vision loss, whereas the right eye will be unaffected. As a result, the person will see close to a complete visual field, which is slightly reduced on the far left because of loss of peripheral vision from the left eye. This amount of residual vision occurs because of the amount of overlap in what each eye sees (see Figure 3-7), with some information duplicated in each eye (Wolfe et al., 2021). The slightly different viewpoints of the same visual scene are one of the factors that contributes to depth perception as well (Wolfe et al., 2021). As a result, depth perception will be impacted by the loss of visual information from one eye because it is partly dependent on this binocularity.

Damage to the optic chiasm, which is uncommon in ABI but possible from conditions such as a tumor, causes bitemporal hemianopsia (a loss of input from the temporal visual field in each eye; Lundy-Ekman, 2018; Wall, 2021). This will result in tunnel vision when the person receives visual input from the central, but not the peripheral, fields. This is because the optic chiasm houses fibers carrying information from the nasal retinal field in each eye, fibers that convey visual information about the temporal visual fields. So, if the optic chiasm is damaged, it is these nasal fibers that are impacted. The temporal fibers, which do not cross to the opposite side of the brain, are not affected (Wall, 2021).

Damage after the optic chiasm causes a visual field loss on the side opposite the lesion. As noted previously, the extent of the field loss depends on the location and scope of the damage to the cerebrum (Lundy-Ekman, 2018; Wall, 2021). The deficit is described by identifying what part of the visual field is no longer perceived. For example, a person with a left homonymous hemianopsia no longer perceives information in the left half of the visual field from both eyes. The visual field loss affects both eyes in roughly the same way in this case (Lundy-Ekman, 2018; Wall, 2021). A person may also have a quadrantanopsia (i.e., when one quadrant of the upper or lower visual field is affected; Lundy-Ekman, 2018; Wall, 2021). A common cause of superior quadrantanopsia occurs when the Meyer's loop, a portion of the optic radiations that travel inferiorly in the temporal lobe, is damaged. This can commonly happen after traumatic brain injury because of the vulnerability of this portion of the brain being damaged as the brain moves within the skull and scrapes on the temporal bony ridges. If the Meyer's loop is damaged, inferior fibers that carry visual information are affected. As a result, the superior visual field on one side (contralesionally to the infarct) is lost (Wall, 2021). For example, if the left Meyer's loop is damaged, a person will present with a right superior quadrantanopsia (i.e., when information that appears in the upper right portion of space is not perceived).

Those who experience a field cut, such as a quadrantanopsia or hemianopsia, can display macular sparing, when the central visual field is unaffected by the field loss (Luu et al., 2010). This happens more often when the damage is in the occipital lobe because there may be an overlap in vascular supply to that portion of the brain from both the posterior and middle cerebral arteries (Luu et al., 2010). Figure 3-8 depicts a model showing common visual field cuts that may occur with damage to the visual pathway.

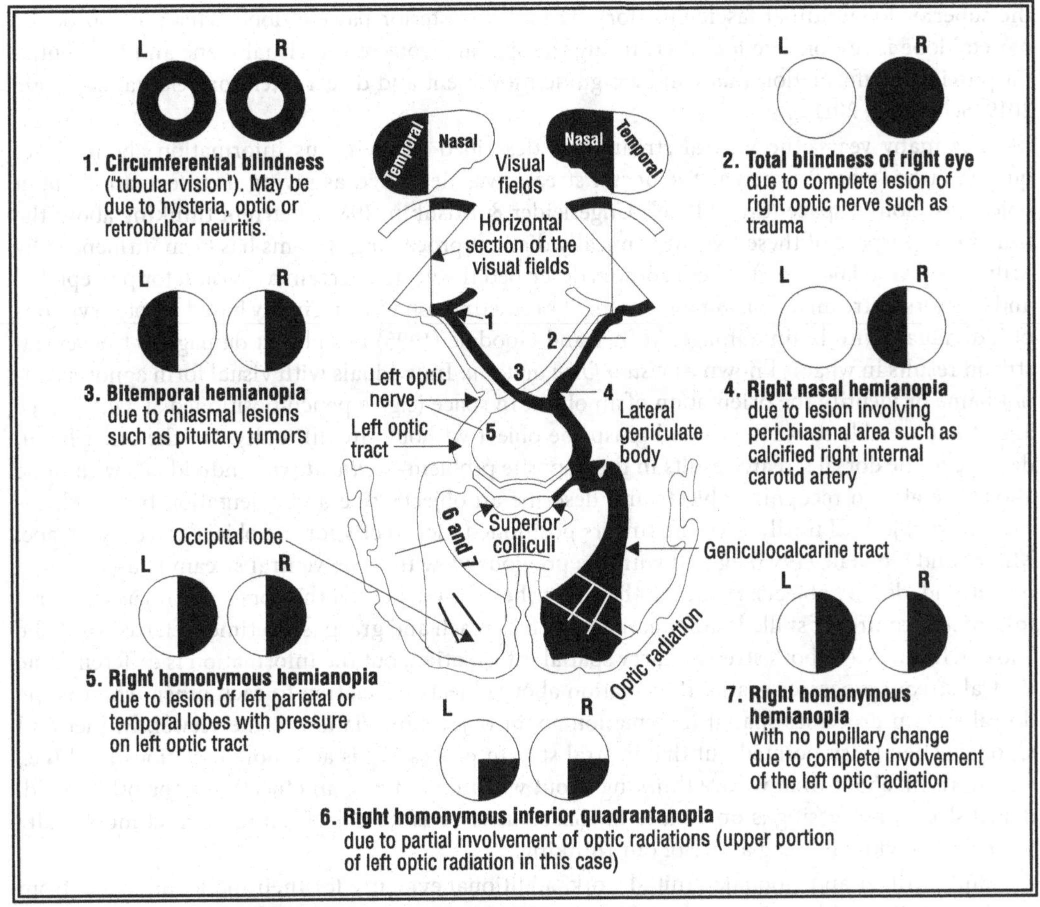

Figure 3-8. Common visual field cuts that can occur after ABI.

Higher-Level Visual Processing

Visual information does not stop when it reaches the primary visual cortex. Rather, the visual signals are routed on to other parts of the brain so that the information can be processed further. This processing allows the brain to identify the objects that have been seen in the environment and determine where they are in relation to each other and the person (Gazzaniga et al., 2019). Visual information is also used by other parts of the brain to aid in motor planning and other cognitive processing, such as decision making (Gazzaniga et al., 2019; Warren, 2018). All of this visual processing is complex, and the ways in which all parts of the brain are involved in visual processing or how visual information is used are not fully understood. It is known, however, that there are multiple different areas of the brain that are involved with vision (Gazzaniga et al., 2019).

Visual information follows one of two major pathways after leaving the primary visual cortex (Gazzaniga et al., 2019; Scheiman, 2011a). The first pathway, called the *ventral stream* after its anatomical location in the brain, contains information from the parvocellular fibers and travels along the inferior longitudinal fasciculus ventrally to the temporal lobe. This portion of the temporal lobe is responsible for object identification and also contributes greatly to visual memory (Gazzaniga et al., 2019; Scheiman, 2011a). The second pathway, called the *dorsal stream* because it is more dorsal in the brain, contains information from the magnocellular fibers and travels along the superior longitudinal fasciculus dorsally to the posterior parietal lobe. This portion of the parietal lobe is responsible for determining the spatial layout of the visual scene and is essential for providing information that can help guide movement and direct attention (Gazzaniga et al., 2019; Scheiman, 2011a).

For many years, the ventral stream was described as giving us information about object qualities (the "what"), whereas the dorsal stream was described as giving us information about object position in space (the "where"; Ungerleider & Mishkin, 1982). Current thinking about the functional purpose of these two anatomically distinct processing streams has been influenced by Milner and Goodale (1995). These authors described the ventral stream as "vision for perception" and the dorsal stream as "vision for action." This distinction was originally based on observations of individuals with brain damage. Milner and Goodale (1995) found that damage to the ventral stream results in what is known as *visual form agnosia*. Individuals with visual form agnosia cannot name or identify the orientation of an object in space (e.g., a pencil positioned at a 45-degree angle) but are able to reach out and grasp the object without any difficulty. On the other hand, damage to the dorsal stream results in the opposite problem—*optic ataxia*. Individuals with optic ataxia are able to recognize objects and describe an object's size and orientation but reach for and grasp objects clumsily with the fingers positioned incorrectly for the object's size and shape. Milner and Goodale (1995) agreed with the previous view that the ventral stream is used to recognize and identify objects. However, they described the purpose of the dorsal stream as moment-to-moment control of skilled motor actions, such as reach and grasp (sometimes referred to as the "how"). In this view, both streams carry spatial information, but the information is different. The ventral stream processes spatial information about objects in relation to each other, whereas the dorsal stream processes spatial information about objects in relation to the viewer. Milner and Goodale (1995) also pointed out that ventral stream processing is at a more conscious level (i.e., we can think about what we are thinking about when identifying an object). On the other hand, dorsal stream processing is on a more unconscious level as we use vision to interact motorically with objects without being aware of our thinking.

Since Milner and Goodale's initial work, additional evidence for their model has come from primate studies (Milner & Goodale, 2006) and comparisons of the perceptual judgments and motor actions people make when viewing optical illusions (Goodale & Westwood, 2004). Other researchers have challenged their conclusions, with some, such as Pisella et al. (2006), arguing that visual processing is much more complicated than these two-stream processing models suggest, with the possibility that there are multiple visual-motor connections working in parallel with each other. At any rate, we know that visual information continues on from the visual processing streams to other parts of the brain, including the prefrontal cortex, where visual information is essential for cognitive processing, including making plans and decision making (Scheiman, 2011a; Warren, 2018).

Oculomotor Control

Oculomotor control is necessary to allow people to move their eyes in a controlled manner so that the image that needs to be seen is focused on the fovea. This is primarily accomplished through saccadic eye movements, which are rapid eye movements that change the line of sight. The saccadic eye movement system is responsible for rapidly directing the eyes so that the visual information from a target of interest in visual space lands directly on the fovea, the area of the retina that can see the greatest amount of detail (Gouras, 1985). Saccades allow the individual to inspect some previously uninspected part of the environment (Abrams, 1992) and are used in all functional tasks, from reading (Figure 3-9) to driving (Suter, 2018). Visual stimuli that reach the

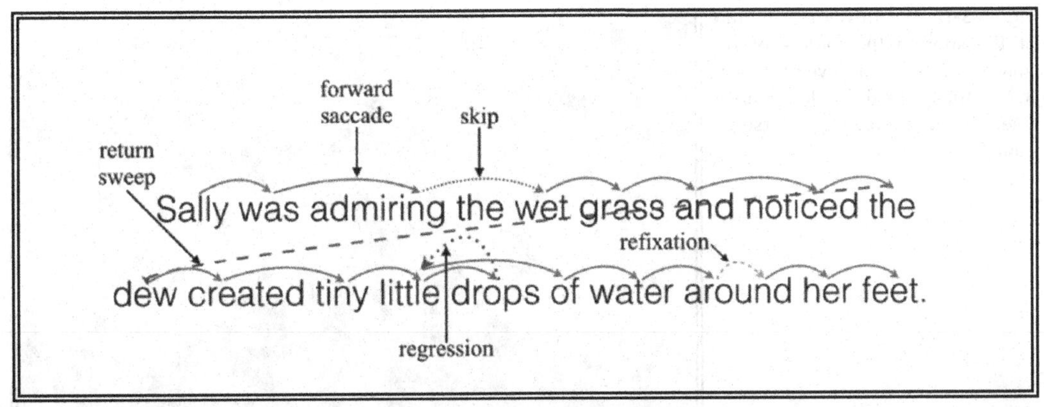

Figure 3-9. Schematic diagram of eye movements during reading. (Reproduced with permission from Rayner, K., Schotter, E. R., Masson, M. E. J., Potter, M. C., & Treiman, R. [2016]. So much to read, so little time: How do we read, and can speed reading help? *Psychological Science in the Public Interest, 17*[1], 4-34.)

periphery of the retina and attract attention will often elicit saccadic eye movements toward the stimulus (Vogel, 1992). The saccade will place the image on the fovea and keep it there as long as the eye is fixated on it. Saccades are extremely fast and, once initiated, are extremely difficult to correct (Abrams, 1992; Gouras, 1985). Numerous parts of the CNS are involved with saccadic eye movement, including cranial nerves III, IV, and VI (Lundy-Ekman, 2018; Scheiman, 2011a); the pontine gaze center (Gouras, 1985); the frontal lobe (Frohman & Zee, 1999; Heide & Kompf, 1997); the parietal lobe (Heide & Kompf, 1997); and the cerebellum (Herdman & Clendaniel, 2000; Scheiman, 2011c). Saccadic eye movement can be affected differently after ABI depending on the location of the damage. For example, damage to the cerebellum can cause overshooting of the saccade (Herdman & Clendaniel, 2000; Scheiman, 2011c). Clients with parietal lobe damage sometimes are unable to break fixation and look away from a target to generate a saccade to a new location (Fischer, 1992). On the other hand, frontal lobe damage can make it difficult for the client to suppress saccades even when instructed to look away from a suddenly appearing visual stimulus (Freeman, 2011). Bilateral frontal lesions can result in the client having difficulty with rapidly alternating their gaze between two stationary targets (Kennard, 1999).

Even when our gaze is fixed on an object, our eyes continue to move (Martinez-Conde et al., 2004). These tiny eye movements are outside our conscious awareness and control (Rolfs, 2009). Although we experience our eyes as holding steady when fixated, they are actually trembling slightly in a wavelike motion while simultaneously slowly drifting a very small distance. Then, once or twice per second, the eyes rapidly jump back with a microsaccade (Martinez-Conde et al., 2004). These fixational eye movements are needed to keep the visual image from fading from view. Just as our perception of clothing against our skin fades quickly through a process called *neural adaptation*, if a visual image is stabilized on the exact same place on the retina, it fades from view within a few seconds (Martinez-Conde et al., 2004). Continuous retinal stabilization of an image can only be achieved in the laboratory (e.g., by using a tiny slide projector or mirror on a contact lens attached to the eye; Martinez-Conde et al., 2004), but it is possible for people outside a laboratory environment to experience fading of peripheral vision. In the early 1800s, Troxler was the first to notice that stationary objects in the periphery of vision tend to fade and disappear when the eyes are fixated on an object (Martinez-Conde et al., 2004). This phenomenon, called the *Troxler effect* in recognition of his role in the discovery, can be seen in Figure 3-10. To experience this effect, fixate on the central dot while paying attention to the surrounding ring. After a few seconds, the outer ring will fade from vision until you move your eyes again. Because the receptive fields for our peripheral vision are larger than the small eye movements that occur when fixating

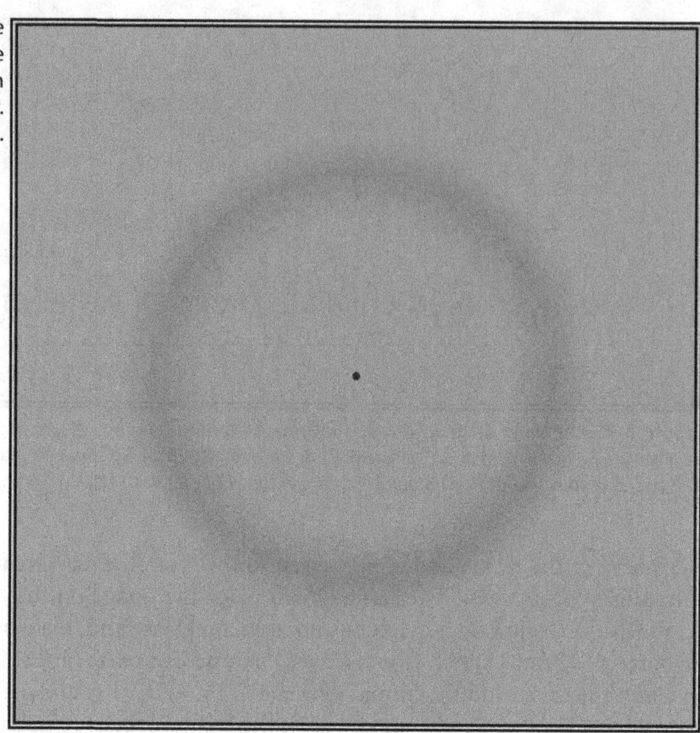

Figure 3-10. The Troxler effect. Stare at the spot in the middle of the image and keep your eye fixated on it. Eventually, the ring will disappear. (Melissa Wiederrecht/shutterstock.com)

on the central dot, there is not enough stimulation of the retina to prevent the fading of the ring, especially when the contrast between the two stimuli is relatively low.

Another type of eye movement is smooth pursuit. Smooth pursuits are those movements that keep a moving image on the retina. These smooth pursuits are not possible without a target to follow. They are limited in speed to 30 degrees/second and are complementary to the vestibulo-ocular reflex in holding images stationary on the retina when an individual is moving (Suter, 2018). This system works for stationary as well as moving objects and uses different processes for each kind of target (Gouras, 1985). Smooth pursuit movements allow people to follow a moving image or object across the visual field without compensatory head movement (Whitney & Herdman, 2000). Saccadic eye movements are used for activities such as reading, whereas smooth pursuit movements are the type of eye movements used in activities such as watching a football in the air (Cormican, 2004). Clients with temporo-occipital lesions or trauma are often unable to make accurate smooth pursuits, generally as a result of selective deficits in the detection of motion (Frohman & Zee, 1999). Clients with smooth pursuit deficits will require the help of corrective saccadic eye movements to maintain the image of the target on the retina. As a result, when these people attempt to visually follow a target moving through space, their eyes will jump (Bouska et al., 1990; Scheiman, 2011c). This jerky interruption of smooth pursuits is typically considered a cause for concern.

Vergence and Accommodation

The vergence system aligns the eyes to maintain binocular fixation and binocular vision by making the eyes move in opposite directions. Convergence occurs when the eyes move toward each other (when focusing on something close). Divergence occurs when the eyes move away from each other (when focusing on something far away; Von Noorden, 1985). The nearest point on which the eyes can converge before one eye loses focus on an object is termed the *near point of convergence.*

Accommodation is the process by which the refractive power of the eye changes through the curvature of the lens to ensure a clear retinal image when changing focus from distant to near objects and vice versa (Von Noorden, 1985). There are two types of accommodation: (a) dynamic, which occurs when a target changes its distance or when people shift attention between targets of different distances, and (b) static, which takes place after the completion of dynamic accommodation (Cuiffreda et al., 2001). The static, or steady-state, response occurs to maintain the newly acquired target in focus (Cuiffreda et al., 2001). During accommodation, vergence helps to maintain the image of an object aligned on precise corresponding points on both retinas (Wolfe et al., 2021). This, in turn, ensures that a single image is seen. Warren (2018) summarizes the process of accommodation when shifting focus from a distance object to one that is closer as follows:

> When an object approaches the eye, its point of focus on the retina is pushed further back, eventually causing the image to go out of focus. The eye adjusts for this situation through the process of accommodation. There are three basic steps to the process. As the object comes closer, (1) the eyes converge (turn inward) to ensure that the light rays entering the eye stay parallel and in focus; (2) the crystalline lens of the eye thickens to refract the light rays more strongly and shorten the focal distance; and (3) the pupil constricts to reduce scattering of the light rays. (p. 603)

The coordinated function of both eyes and visual processing in general requires ocular alignment. Normal alignment of the eyes is guaranteed by a normally functioning sensory and motor fusion system (Von Noorden, 1985). The motor system that moves each eye is made up of six muscles (the superior rectus, inferior rectus, lateral rectus, medial rectus, superior oblique, and inferior oblique) and controlled by three cranial nerves (III [oculomotor], IV [trochlear], and VI [abducens]). Therefore, when considering both eyes, there are a total of 12 muscles and 6 cranial nerves that need to work together (Helvie, 2018; Lundy-Ekman, 2018; Scheiman, 2011a). These 12 extraocular muscles are responsible for aligning the eyes, enabling them to be pointed at the same object, and moving the eyes to different positions of gaze (Lundy-Ekman, 2018; Scheiman, 2011a). This allows for ongoing perception of a single image. Injury to any of these muscles or nerves can affect ocular alignment (Lundy-Ekman, 2018; Scheiman, 2011a). In addition to lesions affecting the individual cranial nerves and muscles, brainstem lesions affecting the medial longitudinal fasciculus can cause ocular misalignment. This occurs because the medial longitudinal fasciculus is essential for allowing communication between the abducens nucleus from one eye and the oculomotor nucleus from the other eye. This communication is what enables the two eyes to move together (Lundy-Ekman, 2018). There are also cortical and cerebellar influences over eye movement (Scheiman, 2011a), including the prefrontal eye fields, which are responsible for directing a voluntary visual search (Warren, 2018). Cognition will influence how people direct their eyes as well. This is discussed further later in this chapter.

The term used for the condition in which the eyes are misaligned is called *strabismus*. Common types of strabismus are esotropia (one or both eyes turning in), exotropia (one or both eyes turning out), hypertropia (one eye turning up), and hypotropia (one eye turning down; Scheiman, 2011c). A strabismus is comitant if the magnitude of the deviation remains relatively constant regardless of where the person's gaze is directed. In a noncomitant strabismus, the magnitude of the deviation changes when the person looks up, down, or to the side, resulting in diplopia (double vision) almost all of the time (Aloisio, 2004; Scheiman, 2011c). If the strabismus is intermittent, then, for at least a portion of the time, the client can have binocular vision (i.e., use both eyes together effectively) without diplopia (Scheiman, 2011c). With intermittent strabismus, the client alternately switches use to the right or left eye or unconsciously suppresses just the right or left eye to eliminate the diplopia (Aloisio, 2004). Newly acquired strabismus as the result of ABI is usually noncomitant, in which case the degree of the eye turn changes depending on the direction in which the eyes are looking (Aloisio, 2004). When ocular deviation is relatively stable, a vision provider may be able to prescribe prisms, which can be used to move the image to compensate for misalignment (Suter, 2018).

If both eyes are not aligned, the client may close one eye, ask for a patch, or develop a head turn to reduce symptoms of diplopia by eliminating the input from one eye to compensate for the lack of action of the paralyzed muscle (Scheiman, 2011c; Suter, 2018). In some instances, the client may not be aware of the diplopia or the compensation they are making and thus may not be able to accurately report what they are experiencing. In addition to diplopia, the client with issues with eye alignment may experience vertigo, confusion, clumsiness, headache, motion sickness, and/or poor spatial judgment (Aloisio, 2004; Bouska et al., 1990).

There are other deficits, in addition to strabismus, that cause diplopia, difficulties with binocular vision, and problems with moving the eyes in a smooth, coordinated, and controlled fashion (Scheiman, 2011b). These deficits can include convergence insufficiency (i.e., when the person has difficulty moving the eyes inward to focus on a near object), which leads to nonstrabismic diplopia and ocular motility deficits (i.e., when a person has difficulty controlling eye movement). These can be caused by damage to the cerebellum and/or the cerebral cortex. These disorders are common after ABI (Scheiman, 2011b) and are discussed further in Chapter 4.

Peripheral Vision

Although much of our conscious attention is focused on our central vision (i.e., what we see when we look directly at an object), peripheral vision also plays a key role in everyday functioning. This is not surprising given that 80% of the retina is devoted to peripheral vision (Gallop, 1996). The role of peripheral vision is very different from that of central vision. Although we experience the world around us as being in focus, we cannot see detail well with our peripheral vision. Everything we see, except what we are looking at directly, is actually quite vague and unfocused. Our peripheral vision only gives us a general idea of the shape and color of larger objects. You can experience this for yourself by looking directly forward while sitting or standing still. Notice how much detail you see of whatever is directly in front of where you are looking. Keeping your eyes in the same position, notice how much detail you can see in the rest of the visual scene. Then, shift your gaze to one of the objects in the periphery of your vision and notice how much more detail you can see. Although our peripheral vision is not good at perceiving detail, it is very good at detecting movement along with a general idea of the properties of the objects in the environment. These functions are critical in noticing what is around us and detecting any changes that occur (Gallop, 1996).

One important role of peripheral vision is to organize our visual scanning (Whittaker et al., 2016). When we enter a new environment, our peripheral vision picks up larger objects of higher contrast and things that are moving. In response, saccadic eye movements occur with a series of brief glances directly at objects and other elements in the visual scene. These direct glances allow us to quickly pick up the necessary detail, shape, and color information for precise identification and understanding of the scene or area.

Peripheral vision also serves as an early warning system to inform us of threats to our safety (Gallop, 1996; Whittaker et al., 2016). This is part of a phylogenetically ancient system oriented toward survival. By picking up on high-contrast moving objects out to the side, peripheral vision lets us know if there is something we need to attend to in order to remain safe while also helping direct our movements in response (Gallop, 1996).

Another important role of peripheral vision is to guide us when moving through space, such as when walking or driving. Peripheral vision tells us how big the space is around us and what is in that space (Gallop, 1996). It tells us how fast objects are moving and in what direction. As a result, we are able to avoid collisions with stationary and moving objects and people as we walk or move in other ways (e.g., driving) through space.

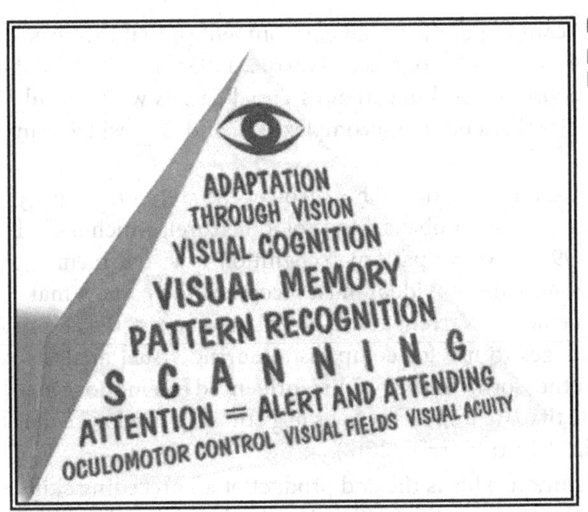

Figure 3-11. Warren's hierarchical model of visual processing. (Reproduced with permission from https://www.visabilities.com)

Peripheral vision is also much better than central vision for seeing in low-light situations (Whittaker et al., 2016). People with eye conditions that affect bilateral peripheral vision, such as glaucoma or retinitis pigmentosa, find it difficult to navigate through a space at night even though they may do fine during the day. This is a result of differences in the distribution of rod and cone cells in the retina. The fovea is primarily made up of cone cells, which do not work well in low light. In contrast, the retina outside the foveal areas is primarily made of rod cells, which do work well in low-light conditions. As a result, under low-light conditions, we actually see better with our peripheral vision (Whittaker et al., 2016).

Warren's Hierarchal Model of Visual Processing

One model of visual processing that is used widely by occupational therapy practitioners was created by Warren (1993b) and describes visual processing as a hierarchy (Figure 3-11). According to this model, visual processing occurs within a hierarchy of skills rather than a series of independent skills. Skills at the bottom of the hierarchy form the foundation for each level above it. Higher-level skills "evolve from the foundation skills and depend on complete integration of the lower-level skills for their development" (Warren, 1993a, p. 43).

At the most basic level of the hierarchy is the registration of visual input through oculomotor control, visual fields, and acuity. These three primary skills are essential for visual attention and the higher-level skills in the hierarchy. For instance, oculomotor control, through enabling quick and accurate eye movements, provides perceptual stability and also allows the retina to be positioned appropriately, such that it can gather visual information, ultimately enabling accurate object recognition and spatial positioning (Warren, 2018). Visual fields and acuity are also essential for getting accurate visual information into the system by enabling the person to get a complete and fully focused picture of the environment. These basic visual skills control the quality and quantity of visual input. Without intact skills at this level of the hierarchy, the brain does not have accurate visual information to process (Warren, 2018).

The next two levels, scanning and attention, are closely associated with each other. Scanning (i.e., searching the visual environment) is one observable application of the visual skills lower in the hierarchy. Attention is the ability of the person to focus on the visual information presented. Higher visual processing is dependent on both of these skills. For example, recognizing patterns in the visual world is dependent on organized scanning of the visual environment so that the visual system has the information it needs for an object to be recognized (Warren, 1993a, 1993b). Visual attention is the ability to concentrate on the visual world to gather essential details while simultaneously ignoring irrelevant information. Visual attention is a complex skill and is considered in depth in Chapter 6.

The next level up in the hierarchy is pattern recognition. This involves the ability to identify shape, contour, and general and specific features of an object (e.g., color, texture), which are all required for object recognition (Warren, 1993a). Above pattern recognition is visual memory, which is higher than pattern recognition because an individual must recognize the pattern making up the image before it can be stored in memory (Warren, 2018). Visual memory is "the ability to create, retain, and recall memories of images to use for comparison during visual analysis" (Warren, 2018, p. 598). Visual memory, like other forms of memory, is influenced by emotions and meaningfulness. It is easier to picture objects that are important to us (e.g., the face of a loved one) than those that are not (e.g., the face of a bus driver; Warren, 2018).

At the top of the hierarchy is visual cognition. This is the end product of all preceding skills and is the highest level of visual skills integration within the CNS. It "can be defined as the ability to manipulate visual input and integrate vision with other sensory information to gain knowledge, solve problems, formulate plans, and make decisions" (Warren, 2018, p. 598). Visual cognition fosters complex visual analysis and, for many people, serves as the foundation for all occupations (Warren, 2018). Disorders of visual cognition can include agnosia (the inability of the brain to identify stimuli visually), alexia (the inability to recognize words), decreased visual closure (difficulties with identifying an object when only a portion is visible), disorders of spatial analysis, decreased figure ground (the ability to distinguish an item from the background), and decreased position in space (Warren, 1995).

It is important to appreciate that the visual system is more dynamic in nature than Warren's model may imply. As a result, a disruption of any level of the hierarchy can affect the total structure of the hierarchy. According to Warren (1993a),

> Each skill level depends on the integration of those before it and cannot function effectively without the assistance of its predecessors. Thus, visual cognition cannot maintain its integrity without the support provided by visual memory, scanning, attention and so on. (p. 44)

In other words, the integrity of the skills on the lower levels of the hierarchy will impact higher-order visual perception (Cate & Richards, 2000). However, the functioning of the upper levels of the hierarchy can influence how the skills on the lower levels are used as well. For example, a person with limitations in visual cognition may not recognize the need to gather additional details about a visual scene and will not use oculomotor skills, even fully functional ones, to move the eyes in the direction of objects of importance.

The critical role that cognition plays in vision can be seen in the influence of cognition on saccadic eye movements. In the early 1960s, Yarbus (1967), a Russian psychologist, was the first to record the eye movements people made when viewing static images, such as paintings and photographs. As seen in Figure 3-12, when viewers were asked to look at a painting of a young girl (left) for 3 minutes and a photograph of a woman (right) for 1 minute, their saccadic eye movement patterns were remarkably similar. The eye movements were not oriented more toward brighter or darker elements, elements with more details, or contours or borders. Rather, the eye movements occurred in a cyclical pattern with the viewers going back, again and again, to the eyes, mouth, and, to a lesser extent, the nose where relevant information about the person (e.g., their mood) could be found.

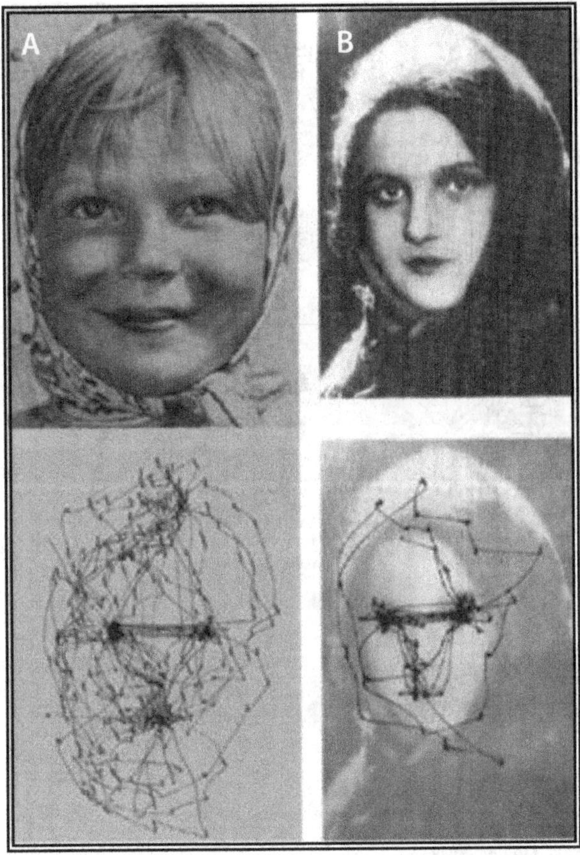

Figure 3-12. Eye fixations when viewing photographs of faces without any instructions. (A) Viewed for 3 minutes. (B) Viewed for 1 minute. (Reproduced with permission from Yarbus, A. L. [1967]. Eye movements during perception of complex objects. In *Eye movements and vision* [pp. 179-180]. Springer Nature.)

Yarbus (1967) continued his research by examining the influence of instructions on viewers' eye movements when viewing a static scene. Using a painting by Ilya Repin called *Unexpected Visitors,* which shows a visitor coming into a room where people had been sitting at a table, he recorded eye movements of viewers for 3 minutes under 7 different conditions. As seen in Figure 3-13, the first condition was free examination (i.e., no specific instructions). In the next six conditions, the viewer was given specific instructions before viewing the scene. Clear differences in eye movement patterns can be seen in each condition, ranging from movements focused on the objects in the room when viewers were asked to estimate the family's material circumstances to movements focused on the faces of each of the people in the painting when asked to estimate their ages. Yarbus (1967) concluded "that the pattern in the examination of pictures is dependent not only on what is shown on that picture, but also on the problem facing the observer and the information that he hopes to gain" (p. 194).

Eye movement research was restricted to these types of static viewing tasks for 20 more years. Then, in the 1980s, head-mounted eye tracking systems were developed. These new tools allowed researchers to examine how eye movements were used in unstructured dynamic situations in which a person performed an everyday functional task while moving through space. One of the first tasks to be examined was making tea (which likely reflected the location of researchers in the United Kingdom; Land et al., 1999) followed by a study of making a peanut butter and jelly sandwich (for a United States version of simple food preparation; Hayhoe & Ballard, 2005; Hayhoe et al., 2003). Eye movements have also been examined in driving (e.g., steering on winding roads, driving in urban environments, learning to drive, car racing), ball sports (e.g., table tennis, cricket,

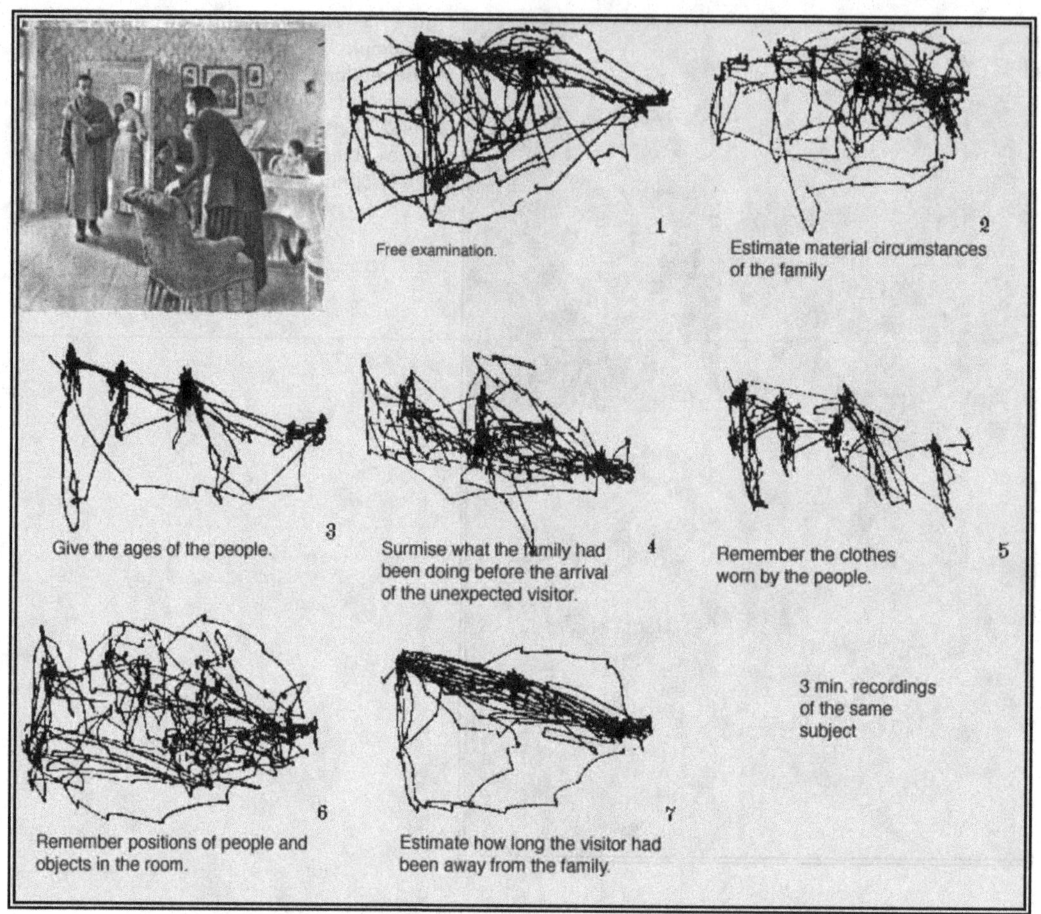

Figure 3-13. A demonstration of the changes in visual scanning pattern with a variety of instructions. A research participant was directed to examine a reproduction of *Unexpected Visitors* by Ilya Repin. The same person examined the painting for 3 minutes after receiving different sets of instructions as follows: (1) no directions given (free examination), (2) determine the financial status of the family, (3) determine the ages of the people, (4) guess what the family had been doing before the visitor arrived, (5) remember the clothes worn by the people, (6) remember the position of the people and objects, and (7) guess how long the visitor had been away. (Reproduced with permission from Yarbus, A. L. [1967]. Eye movements during perception of complex objects. In *Eye movements and vision* [pp. 179-180]. Springer Nature.)

baseball), operating heavy equipment (e.g., a lift truck), and crossing complex intersections (see Land, 2006 for review). Similar to the conclusions of Yarbus from his experiments with static tasks, researchers found that scanning in dynamic tasks was directed at objects in the environment that were relevant to the task being performed rather than those that were visually conspicuous (e.g., brightly colored; Land et al., 1999).

Land and colleagues (1999) further noted that saccadic eye movements in everyday tasks are used for four primary functions: locating, directing, guiding, and checking. Eye movements for locating objects used in a task are often done by surveying the task environment before starting the task but may also occur during a task. Eye movements for directing the hand to a task object are nearly always preceded by a single fixation on the object of interest. The eyes typically move away from the object just before the hand reaches it and rarely move to fixate on the hand itself. When guiding two or more task objects relative to each other (e.g., the teakettle and cup or the knife, bread, and peanut butter), the eyes move between the objects as they approach each other until the action is completed. Checking to determine if a condition is met is often done in relation to stopping an action (e.g., turning off the water when the teakettle is full). In these situations, there are longer fixations or multiple, repeated fixations on the object that is being checked (e.g., the teakettle). When the condition is met, the person may act on the other object of interest (e.g., turn off the water) while still looking at the checked object (e.g., the teakettle). As seen in these studies, saccadic eye movements used for scanning and searching in natural tasks are proactive, goal directed, and outside our conscious control.

Additional Influences on Visual Functioning

This visual skills hierarchy is a useful tool for considering various visual and perceptual skills. However, it is important to understand that there are other influences on visual functioning, including input from other sensory systems, cognition, environment, and prior experience (Scheiman, 2011d). These factors help people to focus on relevant information, ignore irrelevant information, interpret visual information, and make decisions about how to respond (Scheiman, 2011d). These influences can both help and hinder visual processing. For example, a woman may see the outline of a large object on a chair in a darkened room. Remembering that her son was sitting in the chair studying 1 hour earlier, the woman may think that she sees her son curled up on the chair asleep. Her cognition and prior experience coupled with the poor lighting in the environment lead her to "see" her son in the chair. Upon turning on the light, she may discover that the large object is actually a pile of laundry. In this case, the factors that surround her visual processing system led her to misinterpret the visual scene.

As a result of the influence that these factors can have on visual functioning, it is important to always consider the internal and external circumstances that surround the person with potential visual deficits and consider how those circumstances may impact visual functioning.

> Visual processing involves the ability to extract and select information from the environment.... Once information is extracted or selected from the environment, meaning has to be attached to the visual stimuli. This process involves a complex interaction between visual processing and cognitive factors that are influenced by past experiences, motivation, and development. (Scheiman, 2011d, pp. 79-80)

Conclusion

The visual system is complex and involves numerous structures and portions of the brain. As a result, it is extremely common for visual disorders to be present after a person sustains an ABI. In the next chapter, the assessment and treatment of some of these visual disorders are discussed.

References

Abrams, R. A. (1992). Planning and producing saccadic eye movements. In K. Rayner (Ed.), *Eye movements and visual cognition: Scene perception and reading* (pp. 66-88). Springer Verlag.

Age-Related Eye Disease Study Research Group. (2001). A randomized, placebo-controlled, clinical trial of high-dose supplementation with vitamins C and E, beta carotene, and zinc for age-related macular degeneration and vision loss. *Archives of Ophthalmology, 119*, 1417-1436. https://doi.org/10.1001/archopht.119.10.1417

Aloisio, L. (2004). Visual dysfunction. In G. Gillen & A. Burkhardt (Eds.), *Stroke rehabilitation: A function-based approach* (2nd ed., pp. 338-357). Mosby, Inc.

American Academy of Ophthalmology. (2011). Eye health statistics at a glance. www.aao.org/newsroom/upload/Eye-Health-Statistics-April-2011.pdf

Bouska, M. J., Kauffman, N. A., & Marcus, S. E. (1990). Disorders of the visual perceptual system. In D. A. Umphred (Ed.), *Neurological rehabilitation* (2nd ed., pp. 522-585). CV Mosby.

Cate, Y., & Richards, L. (2000). Relationship between performance on tests of basic visual functions and visual-perceptual processing in persons after brain injury. *American Journal of Occupational Therapy, 54*, 326-334. https://doi.org/10.5014/ajot.54.3.326

Centers for Disease Control and Prevention. (2021). Diabetes and vision loss. https://www.cdc.gov/diabetes/managing/diabetes-vision-loss.html

Cormican, D. (2004). Seeing the whole picture. *OT Practice, 9*(7), 14-17.

Cuiffreda, K. J., Suchoff, I. B., Kapoor, N., Jackowski, M. M., & Wainapel, S. F. (2001). Normal vision function. In E. G. Gonzales, S. Myers, J. Edelstein, J. Lieberman, & J. Downey (Eds.), *Downey and Darling's physiological basis of rehabilitation medicine* (3rd ed., pp. 241-261). Butterworth Heimann.

Cullen, K. A., Hall M. J., & Golosinskiy, A. (2009). Ambulatory surgery in the United States, 2006. *National Health Statistics Reports, 11*, 1-28.

Evans, J. R., & Lawrenson, J. G. (2017). Antioxidant vitamin and mineral supplements for slowing the progression of age-related macular degeneration. *Cochrane Database of Systematic Reviews*. https://doi.org//10.1002/14651858.CD000254.pub4

Eye Diseases Prevalence Research Group. (2004). Prevalence of age-related macular degeneration in the United States. *Archives of Ophthalmology, 122*, 564-572. https://doi.org/10.1001/archopht.122.4.564

Fischer, B. (1992). Saccadic reaction time: Implications for reading, dyslexia, and visual cognition. In K. Rayner (Ed.), *Eye movements and visual cognition: Scene perception and reading* (pp. 31-45). Springer Verlag.

Freeman, P. B. (2011). Low vision: Overview and review of low vision evaluation and treatment. In M. Scheiman (Ed.), *Understanding and managing vision deficits: A guide for occupational therapists* (pp. 277-299). SLACK Incorporated.

Frohman, E., & Zee, D. (1999). Supranuclear eye movement abnormalities. In D. L. Easty & J. M. Sparrow (Eds.). *Oxford textbook of ophthalmology* (Vol. 2, pp. 866-871). Oxford University Press.

Gallop, S. (1996). Peripheral visual awareness: The central issue. *Journal of Behavioral Optometry, 7*, 151-155.

Gazzaniga, M. S., Ivry, R. B., & Mangun, G. R. (2019). *Cognitive neuroscience: The biology of the mind* (5th ed.). W. W. Norton & Company.

Goodale, M. A., & Westwood, D. A. (2004). An evolving view of duplex vision: Separate but interacting cortical pathways for perception and action. *Current Opinion in Neurobiology, 14*, 201-211. https://doi.org/10.1016/j.conb.2004.03.002

Goodman, C. C. (2009). The endocrine and metabolic systems. In C. C. Goodman & K. S. Fuller (Eds.), *Pathology: Implications for the physical therapist* (3rd ed., pp. 453-518). Saunders Elsevier.

Gouras, P. (1985). Oculomotor system. In E. R. Kandel & J. H. Schwartz (Eds.), *Principles of neural science* (2nd ed., pp. 571-583). Elsevier Science.

Hayhoe, M., & Ballard, D. (2005). Eye movements in natural behavior. *Trends in Cognitive Sciences, 9*, 188-194. https://doi.org/10.1016/j.tics.2005.02.009

Hayhoe, M. M., Shrivastava, A., Mruczek, R., & Pelz, J. B. (2003). Visual memory and motor planning in a natural task. *Journal of Vision, 3*, 49-63. https://doi.org/10.1167/3.1.6

Heide, W., & Kompf, D. (1997). Specific parietal lobe contribution to spatial constancy across saccades. In P. Tier & H. O. Karnath (Eds.), *Parietal lobe contributions to orientation in 3D space* (pp. 149-172). Springer Verlag.

Hellerstein, L. F., & Scheiman, M. (2011). Visual problems associated with acquired brain injury. In M. Scheiman (Ed.), *Understanding and managing vision deficits: A guide for occupational therapists* (pp. 189-200). SLACK Incorporated.

Helvie, R. E. (2018). Disruptions in physical substrates of vision following traumatic brain injury. In M. J. Ashley & D. A. Hovda (Eds.), *Traumatic brain injury: Rehabilitation, treatment, and case management* (4th ed., pp. 135-156). CRC Press.

Herdman, S. J., & Clendaniel, R. A. (2000). Assessment and treatment of complete vestibular loss. In S. J. Herdman (Ed.), *Vestibular rehabilitation* (pp. 424-450). F.A. Davis.

Hooper, C. R., & Bello-Haas, V. D. (2009). Sensory function. In B. R. Bonder & V. D. Bello-Haas (Eds.), *Functional performance in older adults* (3rd ed., pp. 101-129). F.A. Davis.

Hunt, L. A., Stead, A., & Nijjar, B. (2018). Sensory function and function related to the skin. In B. R. Bonder & V. D. Bello-Haas (Eds.), *Functional performance in older adults* (4th ed., pp. 129-143). F.A. Davis.

Jones, L. A., Sinnott, L. T., Mutti, D. O., Mitchell, G. L., Moeschberger, M. L., & Zadnik, K. (2007). Parental history of myopia, sports and outdoor activities, and future myopia. *Investigative Ophthalmology and Vision Science, 48*, 3524-3532. https://doi.org/10.1167/iovs.06-1118

Jones-Jordan, L. A., Mitchell, G. L., Cotter, S. A., Kleinstein, R. N., Manny, R. E., Mutti, D. O., Twelker, J. D., Simms, J. R., & Zadnik, K. (2011). Visual activity before and after the onset of juvenile myopia. *Investigative Ophthalmology and Vision Science, 52*, 1841-1850. https://doi.org/10.1167/iovs.09-4997

Kennard, C. (1999). Disorders of visual perception. In D. L. Easty & J. M. Sparrow (Eds.), *Oxford textbook of ophthalmology* (Vol. 2, pp. 857-859). Oxford University Press.

Land, M. F. (2006). Eye movements and the control of actions in everyday life. *Progress in Retinal and Eye Research, 25*, 296-324. https://doi.org/10.1016/j.preteyeres.2006.01.002

Land, M., Mennie, N., & Rusted, J. (1999). The roles of vision and eye movements in the control of activities of daily living. *Perception, 28*, 1311-1328. https://doi.org/10.1068/p2935

Lundy-Ekman. L. (2018). *Neuroscience: Fundamentals for rehabilitation* (5th ed.). Elsevier.

Lussier, B. L., Olson, D. M., & Aiyagar, V. (2019). Automated pupillometry in neurocritical care: Research and practice. *Current Neurology and Neuroscience Reports, 19*(10), 1-11. https://doi.org/10.1007/s11910-019-0994-z

Luu, S., Lee. A. W., Daly, A., & Chen, C. S. (2010). Visual field defects after stroke: A practical guide for GPs. *Australian Family Physician, 39*, 499-503.

Martinez-Conde, S., Macknik, S. L., & Hubel, D. H. (2004). The role of fixational eye movements in visual perception. *Nature Reviews Neuroscience, 5*, 229-40. https://doi.org/10.1038/nrn1348

Mehta, S. (2022a). Age-related macular degeneration (AMD or ARMD). *Merck manual professional version*. Merck & Co., Inc. http://www.merckmanuals.com/professional/eye_disorders/retinal_disorders/age-related_macular_degeneration_amd_or_armd.html?qt=&sc=&alt=

Mehta, S. (2022b). Diabetic retinopathy. *Merck manual professional version*. Merck & Co., Inc. https://www.merckmanuals.com/professional/eye-disorders/retinal-disorders/diabetic-retinopathy

Mehta, S. (2022c). Retinal detachment. *Merck manual professional version*. Merck & Co., Inc. http://www.merckmanuals.com/professional/eye_disorders/retinal_disorders/retinal_detachment.html

Milner, A. D., & Goodale, M. A. (1995). *The visual brain in action*. Oxford University Press.

Milner, A. D., & Goodale, M. A. (2006). *The visual brain in action* (2nd ed.). Oxford University Press.

National Eye Institute. (2010a). Farsightedness. https://www.nei.nih.gov/sites/default/files/health-pdfs/Farsightedness.pdf

National Eye Institute. (2010b). Nearsightedness. https://www.nei.nih.gov/sites/default/files/nehep-pdfs/Nearsightedness.pdf

National Eye Institute. (2019a). Astigmatism. https://www.nei.nih.gov/learn-about-eye-health/eye-conditions-and-diseases/astigmatism

National Eye Institute. (2019b). Eyeglasses for refractive error. https://www.nei.nih.gov/learn-about-eye-health/eye-conditions-and-diseases/refractive-errors/eyeglasses-refractive-errors

National Eye Institute. (2020a). Farsightedness (hyperopia). https://www.nei.nih.gov/learn-about-eye-health/eye-conditions-and-diseases/farsightedness-hyperopia

National Eye Institute. (2020b). Nearsightedness (myopia). https://www.nei.nih.gov/learn-about-eye-health/eye-conditions-and-diseases/nearsightedness-myopia

National Eye Institute. (2020c). Presbyopia. https://www.nei.nih.gov/learn-about-eye-health/eye-conditions-and-diseases/presbyopia

National Eye Institute. (2020d). Surgery for retinal detachment. https://www.nei.nih.gov/learn-about-eye-health/eye-conditions-and-diseases/retinal-detachment/surgery-retinal-detachment

National Eye Institute. (2021). Age-related macular degeneration. https://www.nei.nih.gov/learn-about-eye-health/eye-conditions-and-diseases/age-related-macular-degeneration

National Eye Institute. (2022a). Diabetic retinopathy. https://www.nei.nih.gov/learn-about-eye-health/eye-conditions-and-diseases/diabetic-retinopathy \

National Eye Institute. (2022b). Glaucoma. https://www.nei.nih.gov/learn-about-eye-health/eye-conditions-and-diseases/glaucoma

National Eye Institute. (2022c). Refractive errors. https://www.nei.nih.gov/learn-about-eye-health/eye-conditions-and-diseases/refractive-errorshttps://www.nei.nih.gov/learn-about-eye-health/eye-conditions-and-diseases/refractive-errors

National Eye Institute. (2022d). Retinal detachment. https://www.nei.nih.gov/learn-about-eye-health/eye-conditions-and-diseases/retinal-detachment

Pisella, L., Binkofski, F., Lasek, K., Toni, I., & Rossetti, Y. (2006). No double-dissociation between optic ataxia and visual agnosia: Multiple sub-streams for multiple visuo-manual integrations. *Neuropyschologica, 44*, 2734-2748. https://doi.org/10.1016/j.neuropsychologia.2006.03.027

Rolfs, M. (2009). Microsaccades: Small steps on a long way. *Vision Research, 49*, 2415-2441. https://doi.org/10.1016/j.visres.2009.08.010

Saliman, N. H., Belli, A., & Blanch, R. J. (2021). Afferent visual manifestations of traumatic brain injury. *Journal of Neurotrauma, 38*, 2778-2789. https://doi.org/10.1089/neu.2021.0182

Scheiman, M. (2011a). Review of basic anatomy, physiology, and development of the visual system. In M. Scheiman (Ed.), *Understanding and managing vision deficits: A guide for occupational therapists* (3rd ed., pp. 9-16). SLACK Incorporated.

Scheiman, M. (2011b). Three component model of vision, part one: Visual integrity. In M. Scheiman (Ed.), *Understanding and managing vision deficits: A guide for occupational therapists* (3rd ed., pp. 17-56). SLACK Incorporated.

Scheiman, M. (2011c). Three component model of vision, part two: Visual efficiency skills. In M. Scheiman (Ed.), *Understanding and managing vision deficits: A guide for occupational therapists* (3rd ed., pp. 57-78). SLACK Incorporated.

Scheiman, M. (2011d). Three component model of vision, part three: Visual information processing skills. In M. Scheiman (Ed.), *Understanding and managing vision deficits: A guide for occupational therapists* (3rd ed., pp. 79-94). SLACK Incorporated.

Sivak, J. (2012). The cause(s) of myopia and the efforts that have been made to prevent it. *Clinical and Experimental Optometry, 95*, 572-582. https://doi/org/10.1111/j.1444-0938.2012.00781.x

Suter, P. S. (2018). Rehabilitation and management of visual dysfunction following traumatic brain injury. In M. J. Ashley & D. A. Hovda (Eds.), *Traumatic brain injury: Rehabilitation, treatment, and case management* (4th ed., pp. 451-486). CRC Press.

Ungerleider, L. G., & Mishkin, M. (1982). Two cortical visual systems. In D. J. Ingle, M. A. Goodale, & R. J. W. Mansfield (Eds.), *Analysis of visual behavior* (pp. 549-586). MIT Press.

Vogel, M. S. (1992). An overview of head trauma for the primary care practitioner: Part II—ocular damage associated with head trauma. *Journal of the American Optometric Association, 63*, 532-546.

Von Noorden, G. K. (1985). *Binocular vision and ocular motility* (3rd ed.). Mosby.

Wall, M. (2021). Perimetry and visual field defects. In J. J. S. Barton & A. Leff (Eds.), *Handbook of clinical neurology: Neurology of vision and visual disorders* (pp. 51-77). Elsevier.

Warren, M. (1993a). A hierarchical model for evaluation and treatment of visual perceptual dysfunction in adult acquired brain injury, part 1. *American Journal of Occupational Therapy, 47*, 42-54. https://doi.org/10.5014/ajot.47.1.42

Warren, M. (1993b). A hierarchical model for evaluation and treatment of visual perceptual dysfunction in adult acquired brain injury, part 2. *American Journal of Occupational Therapy, 47*, 55-65. https://doi.org/10.5014/ajot.47.1.55

Warren, M. (1995). Providing low vision rehabilitations services with occupational therapy and ophthalmology: A program description. *American Journal of Occupational Therapy, 49*, 877-883. https://doi.org/10.5014/ajot.49.9.877

Warren, M. (2018). Evaluation and treatment of visual deficits after brain injury. In H. M. Pendleton & W. Schultz-Krohn (Eds.), *Pedretti's occupational therapy: Practice skills for physical dysfunction* (8th ed., pp. 594-630). Mosby Elsevier.

Whitney, S. L., & Herdman, S. J. (2000). Physical therapy assessment of vestibular hypofunction. In S. J. Herdman (Ed.), *Vestibular rehabilitation* (pp. 333-372). F.A. Davis.

Whittaker, S. G., Scheiman, M., & Sokol-McKay, D. A. (2016). *Low vision rehabilitation: A practical guide for occupational therapists* (2nd ed.). SLACK Incorporated.

Wolfe, J. M., Kluender, K. R., Levi, D. M., Bartoshuk, L., M., Herz, R. S., Klatzky, R. L., & Merfeld, D. M. (2021). *Sensation & perception* (6th ed.). Oxford University Press.

Yarbus, A. L. (1967). *Eye movements and vision*. Plenum Press.

Chapter 4

Assessment and Treatment of Visual Dysfunction

The occurrence of visual dysfunction after acquired brain injury (ABI), including traumatic brain injury (TBI) and cerebrovascular accident (CVA), is high (Bryan et al., 2018; Cormican, 2004). Incidence reports vary depending on the study, but between 50% and 68% of TBI survivors (Bulson et al., 2012; Goodrich et al., 2013; Magone et al., 2014; Schlageter et al., 1993) and between 30% and 85% of CVA survivors (Khan et al., 2008) have been reported to have lasting visual changes after their injury. Visual deficits can have a significant effect on all areas of occupation, including activities of daily living (ADLs), instrumental activities of daily living (IADLs), work, leisure, and social participation (Hellerstein & Freed, 1994). Without efficient and accurate visual functioning, the rehabilitation process can also be adversely affected (Falk & Askionoff, 1992). Therefore, visual system disorders and their rehabilitation should be viewed as an integral part of the rehabilitation program.

Visual Changes After Traumatic Brain Injury

Many of the areas of the brain related to the primary and associated visual systems, including the cortex and brainstem, are very vulnerable to injury (Jacobs & Van Stavern, 2013; for details about the visual system, refer to Chapter 3). Some visual deficits are so common after TBI that they have been grouped together in a classification called *post-traumatic vision syndrome* (PTVS; Padula & Argyris, 1996; Padula & Shapiro, 1993). Common symptoms of PTVS include blurred vision, diplopia (double vision), perceived movement of print or stationary objects, eye pain, headaches, difficulty reading, and poor concentration (Greenwald et al., 2012; Padula & Argyris, 1996; Padula & Shapiro, 1993). People with PTVS may also experience changes in balance and/or posture and spatial disorientation. Visual abnormalities associated with PTVS include convergence insufficiency (i.e., difficulty bringing the eyes toward each other to focus on close work), accommodative dysfunction (i.e., difficulty changing the focal distance of the eye from near to

Kaminsky, T. A., & Powell, J. M.
Zoltan's Vision, Perception, and Cognition: Evaluation and Treatment of the Adult With Acquired Brain Injury, Fifth Edition (pp. 57-104).

far and vice versa), decreased near visual acuity, exophoria or exotropia (i.e., malalignment of the eyes with one or both eyes tending to or consistently turning out), oculomotor dysfunction (i.e., difficulty with visual fixation, saccadic eye movements, and pursuits), and low blink rate (Padula & Argyris, 1996; Padula & Shapiro, 1993). Other visual symptoms after a brain injury include eyestrain and tearing. There may be binocular dysfunction that affects the ability to use the eyes together effectively, nystagmus, and/or pupillary abnormalities (Adams, 2009; Jacobs & Van Stavern, 2013; Padula et al., 1994).

Damage to the brain can cause other types of visual dysfunction. For example, the visual pathway (described in Chapter 3) can be impacted, which can result in visual field loss. The vestibulo-ocular reflex can also be damaged, causing gaze-stabilizing deficits when moving (Greenwald et al., 2012). In addition to damage to the brain, those with TBI can have an injury to the eye itself and/or the surrounding bony structures (Greenwald et al., 2012). Therefore, the occupational therapy practitioner should have at least a basic understanding of the components of the eye (see Chapter 3).

Visual Changes After Cerebrovascular Accident

Individuals with CVA also frequently experience visual system deficits because of cortical and/or brainstem damage (Cormican, 2004; Khan et al., 2008). Because efficient visual processing depends on contributions from each cortical hemisphere and vision is represented in approximately 30 visual cortical areas, it is common for clients with CVA to have some degree of visual system impairment (Warren, 1993a). In addition, although there is not a high occurrence of specific injury to the ocular structures of the eye with CVA, many clients who have sustained a CVA are older adults and may have preexisting conditions that have caused damage to the eye itself, such as age-related macular degeneration, glaucoma, and cataracts (Scheiman, 2011; Warren, 2018).

Visual deficits as a result of a CVA, such as TBI, can include deficits in near and distant acuity, accommodation, convergence, quality of saccade, visual pursuit, fixation, functional searching, color perception, stereopsis (i.e., the sense of space and depth perception that results from the disparity in the retinal information from the two eyes with binocular vision; Sanet & Press, 2011), visual fields, and conjugate gaze (i.e., movement of the eyes in the same direction; Khan et al., 2008; O'Dell et al., 1998).

Screening of Visual Skills

Vision and visual processing skills will ideally be evaluated by several team members, although the specific professionals who are a standard part of the team will vary. As described in more detail in Chapter 2, professionals who evaluate the visual system in depth include ophthalmologists, optometrists, neuro-ophthalmologists, and rehabilitative (also called *behavioral* or *neuro-*) optometrists (Warren, 2018). As a member of the vision team, the occupational therapy practitioner screens for visual or visual processing dysfunction. It is important to note that the primary role of the evaluating occupational therapy practitioner is not to diagnose visual disorders but rather to identify how visual impairment is impacting occupational performance and communicate those findings with other members of the rehabilitation team (Bryan et al., 2018; Warren, 2018). The visual screening can also help to identify visual strengths that can aid in functional independence. Warren (2018) outlined the three purposes of the occupational therapy visual screening as follows: (a) identifying the occupational limitations, (b) linking the occupational limitations to the presence of a visual impairment, and (c) determining an appropriate treatment intervention based on the results of the assessment. However, it is essential to appreciate that the visual screening that can be conducted by the occupational therapy practitioner is rudimentary compared with the thorough evaluation completed by vision providers. As a result, it is important for the occupational therapy practitioner to understand that a primary purpose of the screening is to provide documentation regarding the need for a referral to an eye care provider, who can then determine the cause of the visual impairment and make an accurate diagnosis to serve as the basis for intervention (Warren, 2018). Moving forward to intervention without an accurate diagnosis can result not only in wasted time and resources but also in harm to the client. For example, an occupational therapy practitioner may decide that a client's peripheral field loss is due to a stroke and move forward with compensatory interventions when the field loss is actually caused by glaucoma. Without the accurate diagnosis and medically necessary treatment, this client is at risk for irreversible vision loss. As Scheiman (2011) stated, "such a screening is not a substitute for a comprehensive examination by an optometrist, [but] it can be helpful in establishing the need for such an examination" (p. 96).

Although people with ABI need a thorough evaluation from an eye care provider for true diagnosis, the clinical screening of the component skills within the hierarchy of visual processing (described in Chapter 3) and how they affect functional adaptation is well within the occupational therapy practitioner's role (Warren, 2018). Although there is some variation in the scope and methods of the various vision screening procedures that have been proposed for use by occupational therapy practitioners, there is general agreement that the assessment of oculomotor control, far and near acuity, and peripheral visual fields should be included (Powell & Torgerson, 2011; Radomski et al., 2014; Scheiman, 2011; Warren, 2018). It is important to begin with these foundational visual functions before screening for deficits in higher-order visual (and cognitive) processing. Research has shown that deficits in one of these visual components can predict difficulties with higher-order visual processing, and it is important to understand which aspects of visual functioning are impacted when creating treatment plans (Cate & Richards, 2000). It is also essential that before and during screening the occupational therapy practitioner observe the client during functional activity.

In presenting the information for how to conduct a screen of visual functioning, we have followed the recommendations of Radomski and colleagues (2014) for the types of tests and the administration order for the most part. Their screening protocol was developed for use with service members with TBI using a modified nominal group technique with a panel of nine experts, including two optometrists and seven occupational therapy practitioners with extensive experience working with people with visual impairment. We have included a wider variety of methods for some aspects of the screen, changed the order of the oculomotor screening, and added an assessment of eye range of motion.

Occupational Performance

Visual impairment can often be observed during the performance of functional activities. Although there are times when it is easy to identify that there is an issue with visual skills, it can often be difficult to determine the specific underlying issue or combination of issues. It is also possible for visual impairment to be confused with cognitive (Scheiman, 2011) or psychological (Adams, 2009) impairments, and it is essential that the treating clinician screen for a variety of conditions. A visual deficit (indeed, any deficit involving sensation and/or perception) can present as a cognitive impairment because the person is getting only a portion of the information available and, therefore, is making decisions based on incomplete data (Scheiman, 2011). For example, if people have impaired visual acuity, they will be unable to see details and may not be able to easily identify objects, especially if the objects are unfamiliar and are presented in an unfamiliar environment. In this case, clients may appear to be confused when, in fact, the issue is a sensory one. Without an adequate evaluation, it is easy to assume that clients have cognitive impairment and devise treatment that may not be appropriate (Warren, 2018).

It is vitally important to consider areas of occupation that may be affected by changes in visual performance. Many activities can be impacted by visual impairment, including but not limited to those related to information access (e.g., reading books, signs, or computer screens), mobility (within the home environment, in addition to in the community), social participation (for tasks such as face recognition and recognizing nonverbal cues), and tasks that require decision making or problem solving (Warren, 2018). It is also important to consider the environment in which clients are completing activities. Different visual skills and levels of visual processing are needed for engagement in dynamic environments (e.g., crowded department stores during the holiday season) than in more static environments (e.g., a person's home). As a result, clients should be observed in different environments if possible (Warren, 2018).

Some examples of what may be observed during the occupational therapy assessment include the following:

- Visual acuity deficits can present as a person missing details in the environment. For example, during a medication management assessment, a person with near visual acuity deficits may be unable to accurately read the print on medication bottles. Deficits with distance acuity may be observed with tasks such as reading signs in a grocery store or hospital corridors. Acuity (near or distance) deficits can also have an impact on social participation (e.g., people may have difficulty with facial recognition or reading body language).
- During assessment, those with oculomotor control deficits may complain of double vision (i.e., diplopia). The person may also complain of headache or eye fatigue or strain. Other behaviors that the clinician should look for in the course of assessment that may indicate an oculomotor deficit are clients adopting an atypical head tilt or turn, displaying increased agitation during activities, or closing an eye during activity. People may also have difficulty judging distance in space when reaching out for objects or navigating the environment.
- Visual field loss may impact function differently depending on which portion of the visual field is affected. Central field loss, which can occur in macular degeneration, may be suspected during assessment if clients have difficulty with object identification (including with reading) and color perception. For example, a clinician completing a dressing assessment with a client with macular degeneration may observe that the client has difficulty distinguishing between navy blue and black slacks. Peripheral field loss, which can happen with a visual field cut such as homonymous hemianopsia, can lead to missing information from one area of space. This can be seen during assessment when a person collides with obstacles on one side, is unable or slow to locate food on certain parts of a food tray, misses seeing signs that are positioned in the impaired field, and so forth. Loss of peripheral vision can also have a negative impact on balance.

If the occupational therapy practitioner suspects that the client may be experiencing visual dysfunction based on an occupational performance assessment, a vision screen should be conducted. Given the frequency of visual dysfunction after ABI and the prevalence of eye conditions in older adults, an increasing number of occupational therapy practitioners routinely include a vision screen in their standard assessment protocols for those populations.

Interview and Visual History

The occupational therapy practitioner should begin a vision screen by asking the client and/or the family or caregiver if the client had any premorbid visual conditions, such as strabismus, amblyopia (clients may use the lay term *lazy eye*), glaucoma, macular degeneration, myopia, hyperopia, astigmatism, presbyopia, ocular trauma, or retinopathy associated with diabetes and/or hypertension. (See Chapter 3 for a discussion of these visual conditions.) The practitioner should ask about the date of the client's last eye examination; the use of prescription and over-the-counter eyeglasses and/or contact lenses (including monovision, which is the use of one contact lens for near vision and one for far); and any surgical correction of vision, including surgically induced monovision. After gathering this background information, the occupational therapy practitioner should ask the client and/or the family or caregiver about their perceptions of any visual problems the client may be having post–brain injury, how these problems compare with visual function before the brain injury, and how they are impacting the person's functioning and/or quality of life (Radomski et al., 2014). A sample of an interview is presented in Figure 4-1. A standardized screening tool with established test–retest reliability with adults, such as the College of Optometrists in Vision Development Quality of Life Outcomes Assessment (Maples, 2000; Figure 4-2), can also be used to learn about the client's perspective about the impact visual dysfunction is having on everyday life (Radomski et al., 2014). It is important to note that people do not typically have good "metavision" (i.e., the ability to think about their vision). As a result, clients may not always be able to report the specific nature or the functional impact of visual impairment accurately, especially in the acute phase of ABI rehabilitation.

Visual Acuity

As described in Chapter 3, visual acuity affects the quality of the visual input that reaches the central nervous system and contributes to the central nervous system's ability to identify details in the environment as needed for processing information and making decisions (Warren, 1993b, 2018). Decreased acuity will result in blurred near and/or far vision, which, in turn, can result in visual fatigue and eyestrain and decrements in occupational performance (Aloisio, 2004). Individuals with visual acuity loss have also been found to be at risk for falls and injury, such as hip fracture (Ivars et al., 2003). A discrepancy in visual acuity between the two eyes results in the greatest risk even when one eye is not impaired (Felson et al., 1989).

Impaired visual acuity can be the result of premorbid disorders, such as structural abnormalities of the eye that cause myopia, hyperopia, astigmatism, and presbyopia, or premorbid eye conditions, such as macular degeneration. It can also result from injury to the eye or the brain (Scheiman, 2011). For example, in TBI, scarring on the cornea, which may be caused by direct trauma to the eye, can result in a deficit in the ability of the eye to focus light on the retina (Warren, 2018). Trauma to the eye can also result in bleeding into the vitreous humor, which impedes light passing through to the retina and may, in some cases, cause the development of a trauma-related cataract in the lens of the eye (Warren, 2018). Visual acuity can also be impacted if the brain injury limits the ability of the zonular fibers and ciliary muscles to change the shape of the lens when changing focus, resulting in accommodative dysfunction, or when the eyes do not come together to focus up close, as with convergence insufficiency. In addition, acuity can be affected with brainstem damage; if cranial nerve III is injured, deficits in accommodation may be present (Warren, 2018).

Visual acuity is typically divided into near and distance acuity, although it is also important to consider the person's ability to focus on objects at an intermediate distance, such as computer screens. Near visual acuity is the ability to see detail close to the person, at approximately arm's length or less. Distance acuity is the ability to see detail at a distance. Near vision deficits will affect reading, writing, and any other functional activities requiring close work. Distance acuity deficits will affect the client functionally in areas such as depth perception, spatial judgments, identification of information at a distance (e.g., on street signs), and facial recognition (Scheiman, 2011).

Visual Symptoms Checklist

Prescription glasses: Yes________ No ________

If yes: Were glasses worn prior to injury?________________
Since the injury only? ________________
Last vision examination? ________________
New prescription? ____________ Date: ____________

Answer yes or no to the following questions:	**Yes**	**No**
1. Do you have blurred or double vision?	_____	_____
2. Do you tilt you head to see more clearly?	_____	_____
3. Do you squint or close an eye to see?	_____	_____
4. Do you get a headache while reading, watching television, or riding in or driving a car? Other?__________	_____	_____
5. Do your eyes feel "tired"?	_____	_____
6. Do you lose your place while reading?	_____	_____
7. Do you hold objects or reading material close to see?	_____	_____
8. Do you avoid reading or not read as often as you did before the injury?	_____	_____
9. Do you miss words, letters, or numbers while reading?	_____	_____
10. Do you have difficulty distinguishing colors?	_____	_____
11. Do you avoid dark areas or avoid driving after dark?	_____	_____
12. Do you sometimes confuse which direction is right or left?	_____	_____
13. Do you reverse letters, numbers, or words?	_____	_____
14. Do you have difficulty recognizing road or street signs before it is too late to turn?	_____	_____
15. While you are standing still, do objects seem to jump or move?	_____	_____
16. While you are walking, do objects seem to jump or move?	_____	_____
17. Do you bump into objects on one side or the other?	_____	_____

Figure 4-1. Visual symptoms checklist. This guide could be used in an interview with a client about their perceptions of their visual functioning. (Reproduced with permission from Morton, R. L. [2004]. Visual dysfunction following traumatic brain injury. In M. J. Ashley [Ed.], *Traumatic brain injury rehabilitative treatment and case management*. CRC Press.)

Distance visual acuity is most often described by the testing distance at which the individual recognizes the test stimulus compared with the distance at which the test stimulus being viewed could be identified by an individual with normal visual acuity (Scheiman, 2011). One of the most common distance acuity tests is the Snellen chart, which was designed to be used at a distance 20 feet from the client (Figure 4-3). Results from this chart are reported in a ratio with 20 as the numerator, indicating the 20-feet testing distance. Good visual acuity for the purposes of assessments based on Snellen notation is considered 20/20. However, many people without impaired visual acuity have better than 20/20 vision (e.g., 20/15). For this reason, 20/20 visual acuity is referred to as standard vision rather than typical or normal acuity. The denominator gives

Quality of Life Questionnaire

Name:______________________________ **Date:**__________

Name of person filling out form:______________________________

Mark the column that best describes how often each symptom occurs.

	Never	Seldom	Occasional	Frequently	Always	Score
Headaches with near work	0	1	2	3	4	
Words run together when reading	0	1	2	3	4	
Burning, itchy, watery eyes	0	1	2	3	4	
Skips/repeats lines when reading	0	1	2	3	4	
Head tilt/close one eye when reading	0	1	2	3	4	
Difficulty copying from chalkboard/ overhead	0	1	2	3	4	
Avoids near work/reading	0	1	2	3	4	
Omits small words when reading	0	1	2	3	4	
Writes uphill or downhill	0	1	2	3	4	
Misaligns digits/columns of numbers	0	1	2	3	4	
Reading comprehension down	0	1	2	3	4	
Holds reading material too close	0	1	2	3	4	
Trouble keeping attention on reading	0	1	2	3	4	
Difficulty completing assignments on time	0	1	2	3	4	
Always says "I can't" before trying	0	1	2	3	4	
Clumsy, knocks things over	0	1	2	3	4	
Does not use his/her time well	0	1	2	3	4	
Loses belongings/things	0	1	2	3	4	
Forgetful/poor memory	0	1	2	3	4	
					Total Score	

20 – 24 points = suspect 25 points or more = refer for care

Figure 4-2. College of Optometrists in Vision Development Quality of Life Outcomes Assessment. (Reproduced with permission from the College of Optometrists in Vision Development.)

information about the smallest stimulus size on the chart that the client can see at 20 feet in relation to the performance of a person with 20/20 vision (International Council of Ophthalmology, 1984). For example, 20/100 distance visual acuity indicates that the smallest stimuli that the individual being tested can identify at 20 feet could be seen by a person with 20/20 visual acuity at 100 feet. Results from other assessments can be converted into a Snellen fraction called a *Snellen fraction equivalent*, which makes the comparison of visual acuity easier (International Council of Ophthalmology, 1984). Many screening tools, including vision cards for the assessment of near visual acuity, include Snellen fractions.

As previously stated, it is not the role of the occupational therapy practitioner to discern the underlying cause of a detected visual acuity deficit during visual screening. Instead, it is the occupational therapy practitioner's role to determine the impact of the visual impairment on

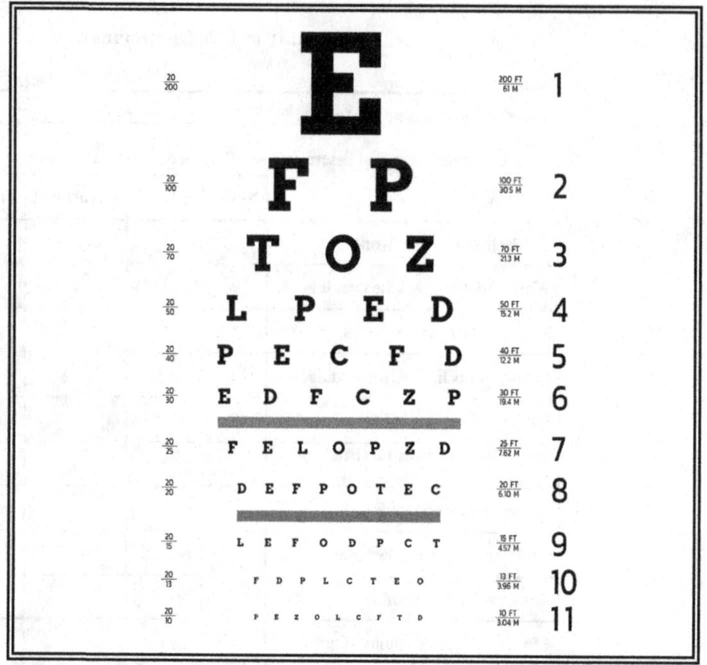

Figure 4-3. The Snellen acuity chart. (shopplaywood/shutterstock.com)

occupation (Warren, 2018). Clients who typically wear eyeglasses or contacts should do so during the screen to allow for the assessment of functional vision. If a deficit is suspected, the occupational therapy practitioner should refer the client to the appropriate eye specialist (Scheiman, 2011; Warren, 2018). When the occupational therapy practitioner refers the client to the eye specialist, it is extremely helpful to describe, orally or in writing, how the deficit is affecting the client's performance during functional activities, what screening tests were performed, and the observations made during screening (Kaldenberg, 2014).

General Guidelines for Screening Acuity

1. The distance for screening acuity will be determined by the specific screening tool, so instructions should be read carefully before administering the screen (Gianutsos et al., 1988).
2. Clients should wear eyeglasses or contacts during the screening if they typically do so. It is also important to position clients so that they are maximally able to attend and concentrate.
3. Screening should be performed in a well-lit room with full and even illumination of the acuity chart. Eliminate any sources of glare (Warren, 1998). Adequate illumination is important because when illumination decreases so does acuity (Warren, 2018). However, it is important to note that clients who are able to pass a screening test under these conditions may not be able to see adequately in natural environments where the lighting is less optimal (or where there is less contrast between the stimuli and the background).
4. Screen each eye individually (monocular vision) and then both eyes together (binocular vision; Warren, 1998; Weisser-Pike, 2014). It is important to measure both monocular and binocular vision because the acuity in the better-seeing eye cannot always predict binocular visual acuity, even in healthy older adults (Schneck et al., 2010). In addition, it is important to know if the acuity in each eye is different because discrepancies can lead to difficulties with depth perception and can also indicate that an eye condition, such as a cataract, is present.

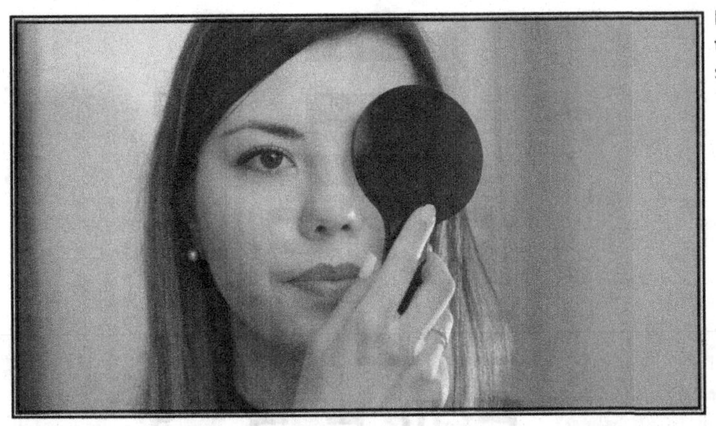

Figure 4-4. An occluder for vision testing. (KONSTANTIN_SHISHKIN/shutterstock.com)

5. An occluder to cover the eye not being tested is the best option (Figure 4-4). If an occluder is not available, other options to cover one eye include using a sturdy paper cup or note card large enough to completely cover the eye. Note that it is best not to ask clients to close one eye or hold it shut.
6. A standard Snellen chart with letters is typically used for English speakers without speech/language impairments or barriers. A Tumbling E chart (Figure 4-5), Landolt C chart, Lighthouse Picture Symbols test, or Lea Symbols test (Figure 4-6) is especially useful for the client with aphasia or for clients for whom English is not a first language because neither of these screening tools is language dependent (Scheiman, 2011). One study that compared the Lea Symbols test with the Bailey-Lovie logMAR letter chart found that the two charts produced similar results in children and adults without a brain injury, although acuity was reported as slightly better with the Lea Symbols test (Vision in Preschoolers Study Group, 2003).
7. If a client is unable to follow the instructions using typical administration procedures, modify the screening by presenting one visual stimulus at a time and identify the stimulus by pointing. Make careful note of any deviations made to the standard administration procedures.
8. The instructions provided by Hellerstein and Freed (1994; see Visual Acuity Screening section) specify starting with the largest stimulus on the chart and moving down line by line until the client reaches a line where they are unable to correctly identify more than half of the items on that line. To save time, the occupational therapy practitioner can start testing with the 20/40 line because 20/40 is considered functional vision and typically serves as the basis for referral for more in-depth testing (Scheiman, 2011; Wagener et al., 2015). According to Hellerstein and Freed (1994), unless the occupational therapy practitioner wants to determine the exact visual acuity, it is not necessary to test with the larger stimuli.
9. Radomski and colleagues (2014) recommend testing distance acuity before near acuity. Others have suggested that the assessment of visual acuity with a client with ABI who has cognitive and perceptual problems should be performed at near distance before far because it may be easier to teach the test procedure and maintain the client's attention at near (Scheiman, 2011). Note that slowness of response from the client with language, cognitive, and/or perceptual problems does not necessarily mean the client lacks the visual acuity to identify the stimulus. If the client has difficulty with identifying the stimulus on each line but does so accurately, then continue the test until the client reaches a line for which they can no longer identify half of the items on that line (e.g., three of five correct; Warren, 2018).

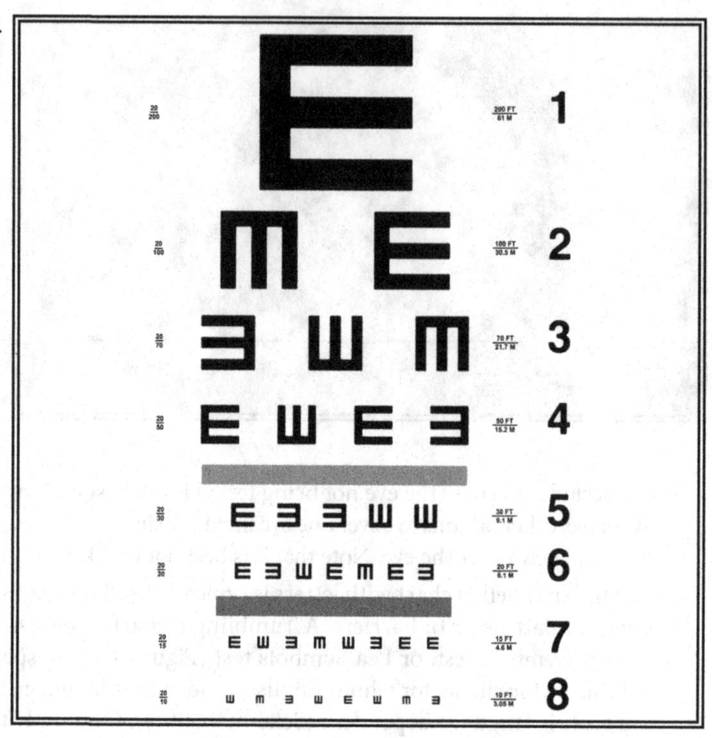

Figure 4-5. The Tumbling E test. (grebeshkovmaxim/shutterstock.com)

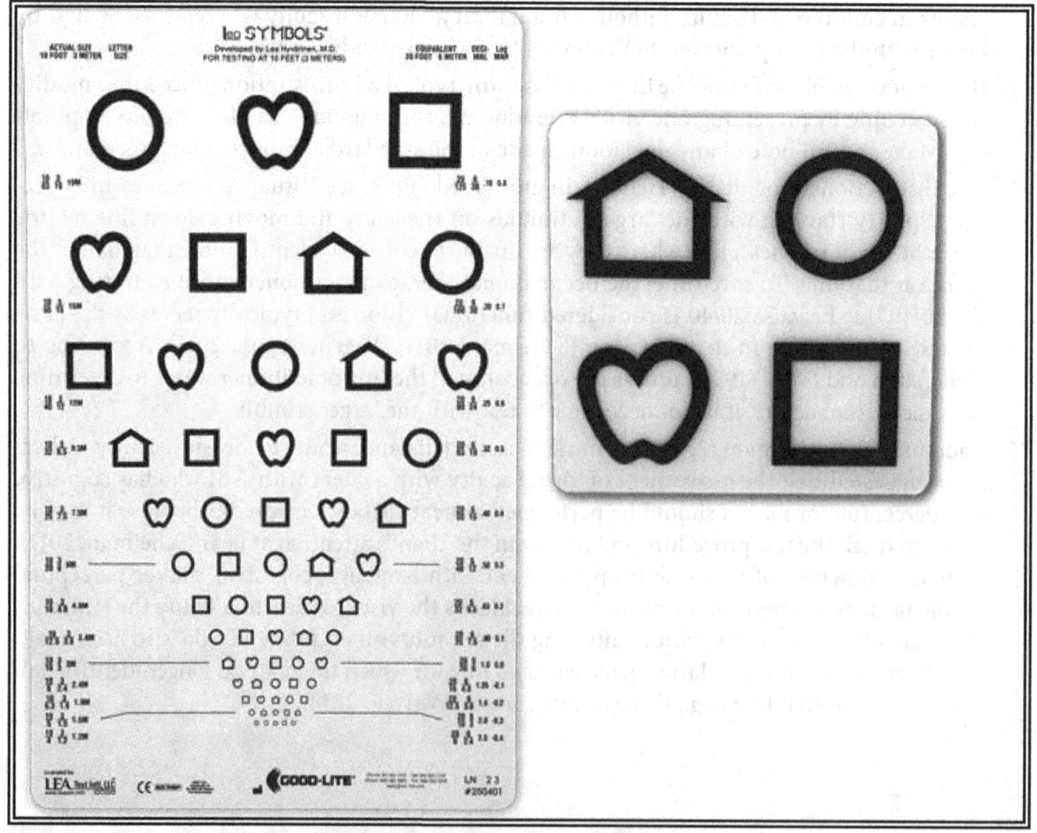

Figure 4-6. The Lea Symbols test. (Reproduced with permission from Lea Test Intl, LLC.)

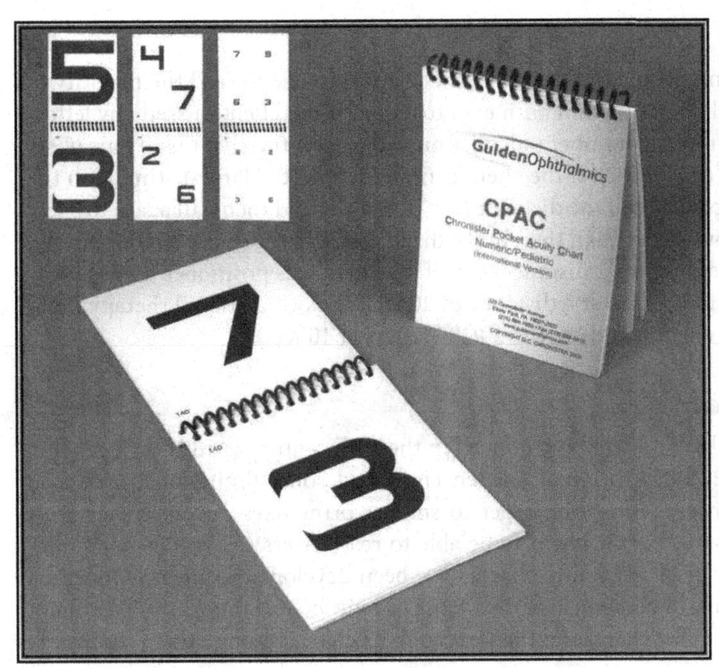

Figure 4-7. The Chronister Pocket Acuity Chart can be used to screen visual acuity. (Reproduced with permission from GuldenOphthalmics. Chronister Pocket Acuity Book. https://guldenophthalmics.com/product/pediatric-chronister-pocket-acuity-chart/)

Visual Acuity Screening

Distance Visual Acuity (Hellerstein & Freed, 1994)

Description

The purpose of screening distance visual acuity is to determine the level of detail that can be seen at a distance (e.g., as used to identify people or objects). Distance visual acuity can be affected by a variety of conditions, including damage to the cornea, lens, or retina; uncorrected refractive error; and amblyopia. The specific underlying condition should be thoroughly assessed by an eye care provider.

As indicated previously, there are a variety of distance acuity charts that are available. One should be chosen that is appropriate for the client's speech/language abilities (see #6 in General Guidelines for Screening Acuity). Radomski and colleagues (2014) recommend use of a Chronister Pocket Acuity Chart because the smaller size makes it easier to transport (Figure 4-7). An occluder or other means of covering one eye is also needed (see #5 in General Guidelines for Screening Acuity).

Procedure

The client may be seated or standing at the appropriate distance from the chart as specified in the test instructions (usually 20 feet). Note that clients with any degree of standing imbalance should be tested in sitting.

1. Cover the left eye to test the right eye first.
2. Starting with the line with the largest stimulus at the top of the card, instruct the client to read each line in turn until they miss more than half of the stimuli on one line (e.g., three of five or three of four). Observe the client for behaviors that may indicate visual dysfunction, such as head tilt or squinting.
3. Cover the right eye to test the left eye following the same procedure.
4. Test both eyes together following the same procedure.

Scoring

Record the Snellen notation for the last line where the client was able to read the majority of the stimuli with the right eye, the left eye, and both eyes together. If the client missed any letters on that line, record the ratio minus the number of letters missed (e.g., if the client read four of six letters on the 20/20 line, record as 20/20-2). If the client cannot identify the largest stimuli on the chart, move the client closer (typically half the distance to 10 feet away and then half again to 5 feet if needed). If the client must move closer than the standardized distance to see the largest stimuli, report what line the client read and at what distance (e.g., if the client was positioned 10 feet away from a chart that was designed to be used at a distance of 20 feet, the occupational therapy practitioner would document that a client could see the 20/100 letters at 10 feet).

Psychometric Properties

The Snellen visual acuity chart was first introduced in the 19th century (Arditi & Cagenello, 1993; Azzam & Ronquillo, 2022). The original Snellen chart had some limitations, including a lack of standardization for progression from larger to smaller print sizes, inconsistency with letter spacing on lines, and reliance on the client to be able to read letters (Azzam & Ronquillo, 2022). Since that time, a variety of visual acuity charts have been developed to address concerns about the original Snellen chart. These include the Bailey-Lovie chart, the Early Treatment Diabetic Retinopathy Study (ETDRS) chart, and the Lea Symbols chart, among others (Azzam & Ronquillo, 2022).

Studies examining test–retest reliability of various charts have found it to vary, depending on the chart that is used and the population that is tested. The ETDRS chart has been studied by multiple researchers who have found test–retest reliability of $r = 0.94$ (Camparini et al., 2001) and $r = 0.895$ (Arditi & Cagenello, 1993). One study by Chaikitmongkol and colleagues (2018) examined the test–retest reliability of three different charts with populations of people with different eye conditions (no diagnosed eye impairment, age-related macular degeneration, age-related cataract, or diabetic retinopathy with macular edema). These researchers found test–retest reliability ratings of $r = 0.7$ to 0.93 for the ETDRS chart with letters, $r = 0.61$ to 0.87 for the ETDRS chart with numbers, and $r = 0.73$ to 0.91 for the Landolt C, which is a chart that uses symbols instead of letters (Chaikitmongkol et al., 2018). Some researchers point out that reliability may be lower for practitioners in clinical practice than it is in research studies, depending on the practitioner's training and experience (Arditi & Cagenello, 1993).

Chaikitmongkol and colleagues (2018) examined inter-chart reliability among the ETDRS chart with letters, the ETDRS chart with numbers, and the Landolt C. These researchers found that agreement among the charts ranged from ICC = 0.72 to 0.99 (Chaikitmongkol et al., 2018).

Referral

Clients with visual acuity of 20/40 or worse in one or both eyes (Weisser-Pike, 2014) or whose binocular vision is worse than their monocular vision (Powell & Torgerson, 2011) should be referred to an eye care provider. In addition, the occupational therapy practitioner should report any behaviors that may indicate visual dysfunction, such as adopting a head tilt or squinting.

Alternative Method

In some settings, the occupational therapy practitioner may not have access to the acuity charts described previously. In these situations, a gross estimate of visual acuity can be made using materials available in many environments (Powell & Torgerson, 2011). For example, distance acuity can be estimated by having the client identify individual letters in the smallest print on a wall sign or poster that the examiner can read at 20 feet. This method assumes that the examiner has either corrected or uncorrected 20/20 distance vision.

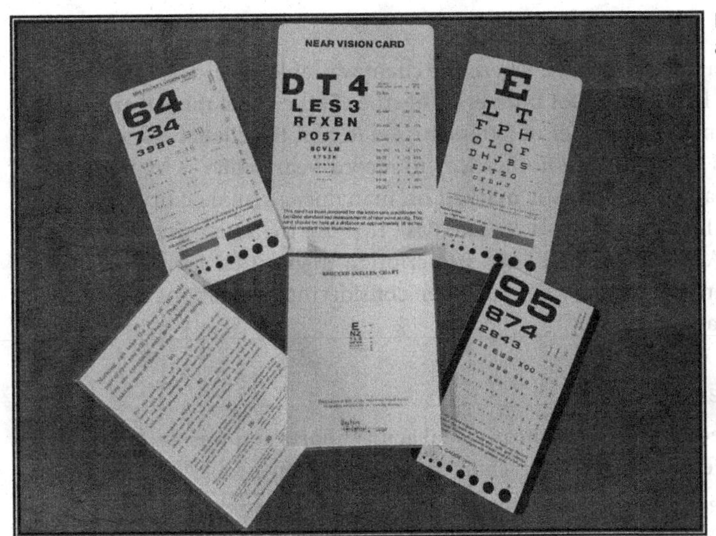

Figure 4-8. Examples of near visual acuity charts.

Near Visual Acuity (Hellerstein & Freed, 1994)

Description

The purpose of screening near visual acuity is to determine the level of detail that can be seen up close (e.g., the smallest size of print that can be read). Near visual acuity can be affected by a variety of conditions, including damage to the lens, cornea, or retina; uncorrected refractive error; accommodation dysfunction; and convergence insufficiency. The specific underlying condition should be thoroughly assessed by an eye care provider.

A near visual acuity card is needed as appropriate for the client's speech/language abilities (see #6 in General Guidelines for Screening Acuity). Radomski and colleagues (2014) recommend use of a Chronister Pocket Acuity Chart reading card. An occluder or other means of covering one eye is needed (see #5 in General Guidelines for Screening Acuity). String or cord for positioning the card at the correct distance is also needed. Figure 4-8 provides examples of near visual acuity charts.

Procedure

The client should be sitting. Hold the card at the appropriate distance as indicated by test instructions (usually 14 to 16 in.). One way to ensure that the distance from the eye to the card is correct is to place two knots in a soft string or cord the appropriate distance apart. Place one knot next to the eye, hold the string taut, and position the card in line with the second knot. For clients who wear bifocals or trifocals, the screening card should be in line with the portion of the glasses used for reading (i.e., the lower portion of the lens). You should be in a position to read the card the client is looking at or have a duplicate card available to check for accuracy.

1. Cover the left eye to test the right eye first.
2. Starting with the line with the largest stimulus at the top of the card, instruct the client to read each line in turn until more than half of the stimuli on one line are missed (e.g., three out of five or three out of four). Observe the client for behaviors that may indicate visual dysfunction, such as head tilt or squinting.
3. Cover the right eye to test the left eye following the same procedure.
4. Test both eyes together following the same procedure.

Scoring

Record the Snellen notation for the last line where the client was able to read the majority of the stimuli for the right eye, the left eye, and for both eyes together. If the client missed any letters on that line, record the ratio minus the number of letters missed (e.g., if the client read four of six letters on the 20/20 line, record as 20/20-2). Another way to record near acuity is by noting the letter size that the client can read clearly. This is marked on many near visual acuity cards and is designated by the letter "M." Letters that are delineated as "1M" are the same size as standard newspaper text and common ADL-related text (e.g., prescription medication labels). Knowing the size of print that can be clearly seen is very helpful when considering adaptations that may be needed for reading material (Warren, 1998).

Psychometric Properties

Test–retest reliability has been studied with near visual acuity charts and was found to range from $r = 0.628$ to 0.989 (Stifter et al., 2004). Inter-chart reliability, when people had their near acuity tested with different tools, was found to range from $r = 0.635$ to 0.947 (Stifter et al., 2004).

Referral

Clients with visual acuity of 20/40 or worse in one or both eyes (Weisser-Pike, 2014) or whose binocular vision is worse than their monocular vision (Powell & Torgerson, 2011) should be referred to an eye care provider. In addition, the occupational therapy practitioner should report any behaviors that may indicate visual dysfunction, such as adopting a head tilt or squinting.

Alternative Method

If a near vision card is not available, a gross estimate of near visual acuity can be made by having the client identify individual letters in a newspaper or magazine article (Powell & Torgerson, 2011).

Ocular Alignment and Binocular Vision

Radomski and colleagues (2014) recommend that occupational therapy practitioners screen clients with TBI for ocular alignment and binocular vision using the Eye Assessment Test. The use of this assessment tool requires additional training. The interested reader should refer to Wagener and colleagues (2015) for more details.

Oculomotor Control Screening

The quality, speed, and accuracy of eye movements should all be screened (Scheiman, 2011), especially if behaviors that may indicate oculomotor dysfunction are present (e.g., complaints of diplopia, headache, or eye strain; the client adopting a head tilt or closing one eye; or observations of disconjugate gaze [when the eyes are not pointing in the same direction]). As stated earlier, it is also common for people with ABI to experience accommodative dysfunction or convergence insufficiency. It is easy to miss oculomotor control deficits, especially mild ones; thus, it is important that oculomotor control be thoroughly assessed by a vision specialist (Scheiman, 2011). The following is a general screening strategy that can aid the clinician in determining when a referral is needed, although it is essential to realize that it will not pick up all oculomotor control deficits, including the most subtle.

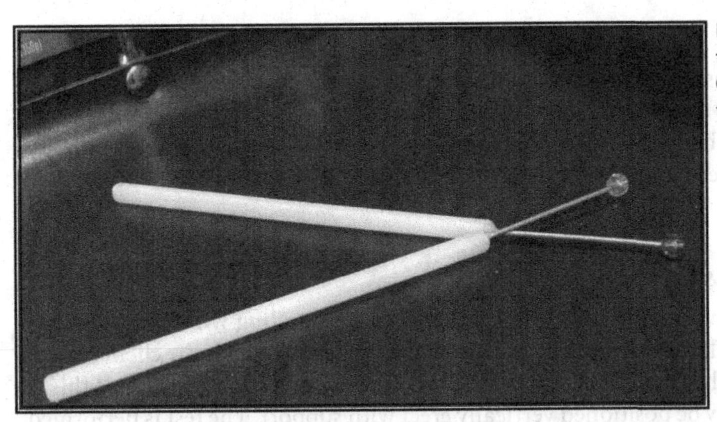

Figure 4-9. Targets to be used with the Northeastern State University College of Optometry oculomotor test.

Saccades Screenings

Visual Pursuits and Saccades Screening: Northeastern State University College of Optometry Oculomotor Test (Maples, 1995)

Description

The Northeastern State University College of Optometry (NSUCO) Oculomotor Test is a direct observation method of screening two key oculomotor skills: (a) the ability to visually track a moving object through the space (visual or smooth pursuits) and (b) the ability to accurately move the eyes quickly between two objects (saccades). The test is appropriate for clients who are at least 5 years of age. Norms for minimal acceptable performance have been established for people up to age 14 (Maples, 1995; Maples et al., 1992).

One target for screening visual pursuits and two targets for screening saccades are needed. The targets that can be purchased with the test manual are small 5-mm reflective balls that are mounted on dowels (Figure 4-9). The author of the test states that other targets can be used. Pushpins with balls of two different colors inserted into the eraser end of a standard pencil work well to give a specific target for the client to focus on. Avoid using red and green targets as those will be difficult for the client with red/green color blindness to distinguish.

Procedure for Visual Pursuits

The client should be standing with feet shoulder-width apart directly in front of the examiner. The test can also be completed with the client seated. In either position, it is best for the client's head to be erect and not supported in any way. If this is not possible, the client's head may be positioned vertically erect with support.

1. Hold one target 40 cm (16 in.) from the client's face at eye level. This distance can be measured from the side of the eye using the same string or cord used in the near acuity testing.
2. Give the following instructions: "Watch the target as it goes around. Don't take your eyes off the target." Do not give any instructions to the client to move or not to move their head.
3. Move the target clockwise for two rotations and counterclockwise for two rotations. Each rotation should be approximately 20 cm (8 in.) in diameter, with the midpoint of the circle aligned with the client's nose.
4. Observe the accuracy of the pursuit eye movements and any head or body movement. Determine if the client can maintain their attention to complete all four rotations. The attentional aspect is referred to as "ability" in the scoring criteria.

Scoring for Pursuits

In general, during this assessment, you should watch for accuracy of eye movement, making notes of any occasions of losing track of the target and/or eyes not moving in a conjugate fashion. Movements of the head and/or body should also be noted and recorded. Assign scores for ability (i.e., attention), accuracy, and head and/or body movements during the observation of pursuits as per the scoring criteria in Table 4-1.

Procedure for Saccades

As with the procedure for visual pursuits, the client should be standing with feet shoulder-width apart directly in front of the examiner. The test can also be completed with the client seated. In either position, it is best for the client's head to be erect and not supported in any way. If this is not possible the client's head may be positioned vertically erect with support. The test is performed binocularly as described below.

1. Hold targets 40 cm (16 in.) from the client's face at eye level. This distance can be measured from the side of the eye using the same string or cord used in the near acuity testing.
2. Position each target 10 cm (4 in.) from the client's midline, with one target on the client's right and one on the client's left. The targets should be 20 cm (8 in. apart; Figure 4-10). This distance can be measured using half of the distance between the knots 16 in. apart on the measuring string or cord.
3. Give the following instructions using the colors of the two targets: "Here are two balls, one yellow and one green. When I say yellow, look at the yellow ball. When I say green, look at the green ball. Do not look until I tell you to." Do not give any instructions to the client to move or not to move their head. Powell and Torgerson (2011) recommended giving the instructions using an uneven rhythm to reduce the possibility of the client anticipating when the next instruction will be given.
4. Have the client fixate on each target 5 times for a total of 10 fixations.
5. Observe the accuracy of saccades and any head or body movement. Determine if the client can maintain their attention to complete all 10 fixations. The attentional aspect is referred to as "ability" in the scoring criteria.

Scoring for Saccades

In general, during this assessment, you should watch for accuracy of eye movement, making notes of any occasions of overshooting, undershooting, or losing track of the target. Movements of the head and/or body should also be noted and recorded. Assign scores for ability (attention), accuracy, and head and/or body movements with saccadic eye movements based on the scoring criteria in Table 4-1.

Psychometric Properties for Visual Pursuits and Saccades

Inter-rater reliability testing has been conducted on the NSUCO Oculomotor Test with children. The researchers found 73.5% agreement when completing visual pursuit testing and 75% agreement between assessors when conducting testing of saccades (Maples & Ficklin, 1988). Test–retest reliability was also conducted with children. There was no significant difference between the children's scores on the first and second administration of the NSUCO Oculomotor Test with the exception of head movements with saccades. In this case, children scored significantly better with head movement on the second administration of the saccades test ($p = .005$; Maples, 1995).

Table 4-1

Scoring for Northeastern State University College of Optometry Oculomotor Test

Ability: Can the patient keep their attention under control to complete five round trips for saccades and two clockwise and then two counterclockwise rotations for pursuits?

A. Saccades

1. Completes fewer than two round trips
2. Completes two round trips
3. Completes three round trips
4. Completes four round trips
5. Completes five round trips

B. Pursuits

1. Cannot complete one-half rotation in either the clockwise or counterclockwise direction.
2. Completes one-half rotation in either direction
3. Completes one rotation in either direction but not two rotations
4. Completes one rotation in one direction but fewer than two rotations in the other direction
5. Completes two rotations in each direction

Accuracy: Can the patient accurately and consistently fixate so that no noticeable correction is needed in the case of saccades or track the target so that no noticeable refixation is needed when doing pursuits?

A. Saccades

1. Large over- or undershooting is noted one or more times
2. Moderate over- or undershooting is noted one or more times
3. Constant slight over- or undershooting notes (greater than 50% of the time)
4. Intermittent slight over- or undershooting notes (less than 50% of the time)
5. No over- or undershooting noted

B. Pursuits

1. No attempt to follow the target or requires greater than 10 refixations
2. Refixations 5 to 10 times
3. Refixations three or four times
4. Refixations two times or fewer
5. No refixations

(continued)

Table 4-1 (continued)

Scoring for Northeastern State University College of Optometry Oculomotor Test

Head and Body Movement: Can the patient accomplish the saccade or pursuit test without moving their head or body? Both saccade and pursuit scoring use the same criteria for this aspect of the testing.

1. Large movement of the head (body) at any time
2. Moderate movement of the head (body) at any time
3. Slight movement of the head (body) (greater than 50% of the time)
4. Slight movement of the head (body) (less than 50% of the time)
5. No movement of the head (body)

Reproduced with permission from Maples, W. C. (1995). *NSUCO Oculomotor Test manual.* Optometric Extension Program Foundation.

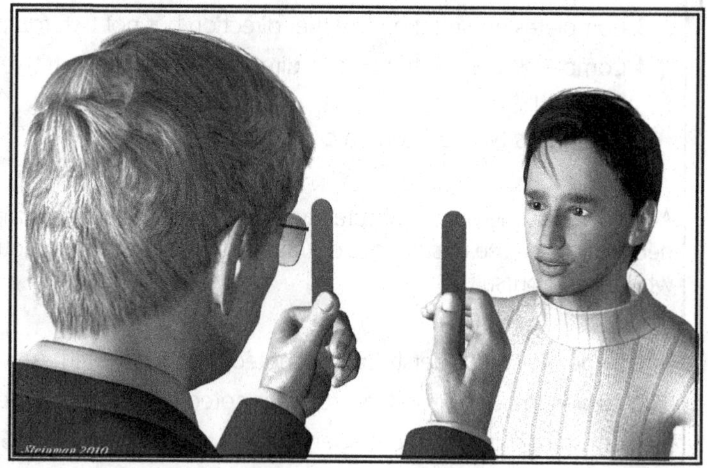

Figure 4-10. Screening of saccades. (Reproduced with permission from Scheiman, S. (2011). *Understanding and managing vision deficits: A guide for occupational therapists* [3rd ed.]. SLACK Incorporated.)

Maples and Ficklin (1989, 1990) conducted two studies examining the reliability of the NSUCO Oculomotor Test. They hypothesized that children who demonstrated oculomotor control deficits, as determined by the NSUCO Oculomotor Test, would demonstrate poorer performance in school. Both studies found that poorer scores on the assessment correlated with having a diagnosed learning disability (Maples & Ficklin, 1989) or having below-average reading scores (Maples & Ficklin, 1990).

Referral for Visual Pursuits and Saccades

There are no well-established cut-off scores for the direct observation of visual pursuits and saccades. Scheiman (2011) recommended that clinicians working with adults use the minimal acceptable NSUCO Oculomotor Test scores for children in the normative sample to determine when referral to an eye care provider is indicated. As performance in the normative sample improved with age, the scores of the oldest age group are best suited for this determination. This age group was relatively small, consisting of 45 children (28 female and 17 male) who were at least

14 years old (Maples, 1995; Maples et al., 1992). Using a 31% failure criterion for test performance in the 14 years and older group (Maples, 1995), the minimal acceptable scores for adults on visual pursuits would be 5 on ability (completes two rotations in each direction), accuracy (no refixations of gaze), and body movement (no body movement) and 4 on head movement (no more than slight movement of the head less than 50% of the time). The minimal acceptable scores on saccades would be 5 on ability (completes five round trips) and body movement (no body movement) and 4 on accuracy (no more than intermittent slight over- or undershooting less than 50% of the time) and head movement (no more than slight movement of the head less than 50% of the time).

As noted by the test author, the NSUCO Oculomotor Test is a simple screen that is not sufficient for a definitive diagnosis of oculomotor dysfunction (Maples, 1995). While oculomotor dysfunction is likely if the person scores below the minimal acceptable level, a passing score does not rule out problems with visual pursuits or saccades. Therefore, the clinician should interpret test results in the context of all other relevant information.

The occupational therapy vision screen for adults with ABI developed by Powell and Torgerson (2011) also includes direct observation of visual pursuits and saccades with recommendations for referral to an eye care provider. This screen sets higher expectations for visual pursuits and saccades than the NSUCO Oculomotor Test. When performing the visual pursuits subtest, adult clients are expected to have smooth eye movements when following the target up, down, side to side, diagonally in both directions, clockwise, and counter-clockwise. Both eyes are expected to maintain gaze on the target with no loss of target, no jerkiness of motion, no under- or overshooting of the target, and no movement of the head. For the saccades portion of the screen, clients are expected to have quick, accurate eye movements for five full sets, no under- or overshooting of the target, and no movement of the head.

As normal limits for this method of assessing eye movements have not been established, occupational therapy practitioners should document their findings in terms of what they observed rather than using terminology such as "within normal limits" or WNL. If no deficits in oculomotor control were noted, "no observed difficulty with visual pursuits or saccadic eye movements" or similar language would be considered appropriate.

If the performance expectations are not met for both saccades and visual pursuits, referral to an eye care provider is recommended (Powell & Torgerson, 2011). Impaired performance of either saccades or visual pursuits is characterized as a minor finding. In this situation, referral is recommended if there is at least one other minor finding (e.g., binocular acuity worse than monocular acuity) or at least one major finding (e.g., any positive self-reported or clinician observation of vision-related symptoms or difficulties with functional activities that could be due to impaired vision, distance or near visual acuity equal to or less than 20/40, or visual field deficit).

However, these referral criteria were deliberately set to be more conservative in nature. Given the lack of objective data on the performance on adults on direct observations of visual pursuits and saccades, it seems prudent that occupational therapy practitioners consider referral to an eye care provider for any concern related to saccades or visual pursuits identified using this type of screen to ensure that clients with oculomotor dysfunction following ABI receive adequate care.

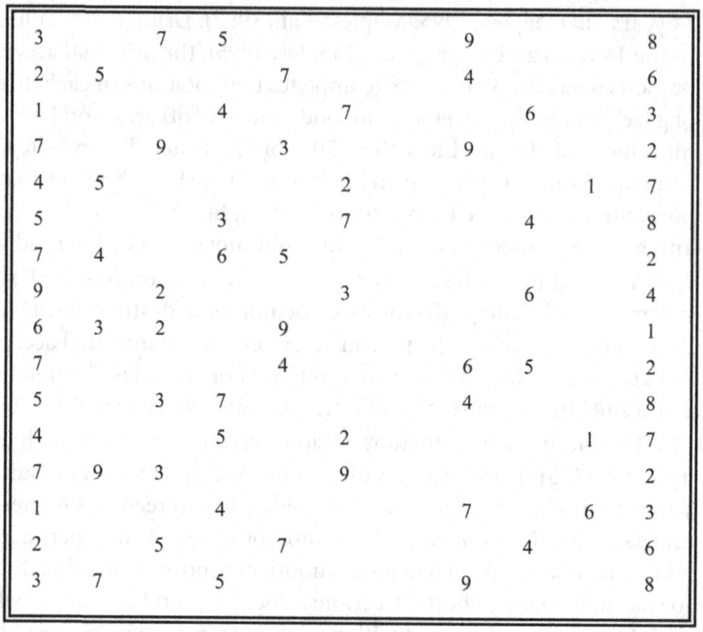

Figure 4-11. Subtest C from the DEM. (Reproduced with permission from Richman, J., & Garzia, P. [1987]. *Developmental Eye Movement Test. Test booklet*. Bernell Corporation.)

3 7 5 9 8
2 5 7 4 6
1 4 7 6 3
7 9 3 9 2
4 5 2 1 7
5 3 7 4 8
7 4 6 5 2
9 2 3 6 4
6 3 2 9 1
7 4 6 5 2
5 3 7 4 8
4 5 2 1 7
7 9 3 9 2
1 4 7 6 3
2 5 7 4 6
3 7 5 9 8

Developmental Eye Movement Test (Richman, 2009)

Description

The Developmental Eye Movement Test, or DEM (pronounced D-E-M), is the tool recommended by Radomski and colleagues (2014) to screen a client's saccadic eye movements. An adult version of the test, the Adult Developmental Eye Movement Test (A-DEM), has been described in the literature (Sampedro et al., 2003). However, there are several key differences between the DEM and the A-DEM that have raised concerns about the validity of the adult version (Powell et al., 2006). Of particular concern is the use of different numbers for the A-DEM vertical and horizontal arrays. The A-DEM also uses double-digit numbers rather than the single-digit numbers used in the DEM. As a result of these two changes in the test materials, it is not possible to account as well for the speed of number naming in the A-DEM ratio score, diminishing the logic of the measurement approach. In addition, the A-DEM was normed on Spanish-speaking adults with the potential for language-based differences in the normative scores. Based on these concerns and the lack of a commercial version of the A-DEM, Radomski et al. (2014) recommended use of the original DEM for screening with adults, rather than the A-DEM, despite a lack of adult norms.

Procedure

The DEM consists of three subtests. For subtests A and B, clients are timed while reading numbers down two vertical columns as quickly as possible. This subtest gives a baseline for how fast the client can read numbers aloud. For subtest C (Figure 4-11), they are timed while reading the same numbers as in the two vertical subtests as quickly as possible but with the numbers arranged horizontally across rows. This subtest adds a saccadic eye movement component to the number-naming task. Normative data were generated from a sample of children ages 6 to 13 years.

Scoring

A vertical score is generated by adding completion times for subtests A and B. A horizontal score is calculated with a formula that considers both the time to complete the task and errors made. The vertical score is then divided by the horizontal score to give a ratio that reflects the efficiency of horizontal saccadic eye movements as used in reading. The scores achieved are compared to the normative data from children.

Psychometric Properties

This test has undergone some validity and reliability testing with children. Those studies have found that the DEM shows good intra-rater (r=0.86-0.89), inter-rater (r=0.81-0.91), and test–retest (r=0.52-0.85) reliability (Richman, 2009). The DEM has also been shown to have good discriminative ability through studies that concluded that children who were reading at age-appropriate levels received better DEM scores than children who were academically performing lower than expected (Richman, 2009).

Referral

Some authors have suggested that even though normative data are only available up to age 13, the DEM can be used with adults with ABI because limited additional improvement is expected in performance on this test with increased age (Scheiman, 2011). Based on this recommendation, clinicians should refer clients for further evaluation based on the norms for the 13-year-old age group. A study done by Powell et al. (2005), however, indicated that these normative data may underestimate the performance of adults on the DEM. As a result, clinicians should consider referring clients for further evaluation if their score on this screen is close to the cut-off, especially if the client is demonstrating difficulties in functional activities, such as reading, that might be due to saccadic eye movement dysfunction.

Saccades and Visual Pursuits: Direct Observation Method

Direction of Gaze/Range of Motion (Chusid, 1979)

Description

All six muscles that move each eye are tested by having the client look in different directions. These muscles include the four rectus muscles (superior, inferior, lateral, and medial) and the two oblique muscles (superior and inferior).

Procedure

The client is seated opposite the examiner with the client's head positioned vertically.

1. Instruct the client to look first to one side and then to the other to test the medial and lateral rectus muscles.
2. Next, instruct the client to look up and down while looking to the side. In this position, the adducted eye (i.e., the eye directed toward the nose) is elevated by the superior rectus muscle and depressed by the inferior rectus muscle. The abducted eye (i.e., the eye directed away from the nose) is elevated by the inferior oblique muscle.
3. Repeat the procedure with the opposite side to test the opposite muscles.

Scoring

Observations should be made about the client's ability to look in different directions and whether or not the eyes are moving together. To improve validity, rule out aphasia and poor visual attentiveness as causes of poor performance.

- *Intact*—The client is able to direct their gaze in all directions as instructed.
- *Impaired*—The client is unable to direct their gaze in one or more directions. (Specify which movements are impaired. The occupational therapy practitioner can also make note of whether or not the eyes are moving together.)
- *Unable to perform*—The client is unable to direct their gaze in any direction as instructed.

Psychometric Properties

No information about psychometric testing for this assessment could be found in the literature.

Referral

Clients should be referred for examination by an eye care provider if any restrictions in eye movement or behavioral changes that indicate eye range of motion dysfunction are observed.

Visual Fields

An individual's visual field is the external world that can be seen while looking straight ahead without moving the head (Cate & Richards, 2000; O'Dell et al., 1998). Intact visual fields are dependent on two major portions of the visual system. First, the receptors that are housed in the retina (the rods and cones) need to be intact. Second, the visual pathway from the optic nerve to the occipital area needs to be fully functional (Ciuffreda et al., 2001).

As described in Chapter 3, the fovea, or the area of greatest acuity, is surrounded by the macular area. The portion of the visual field that is seen by this area of the retina is referred to as the *central visual field* (Gianutsos & Suchoff, 2002; Warren, 1998). The central field area is thought to extend about 5 degrees around the point of fixation (i.e., the place at which the person is focusing their gaze; Gianutsos & Suchoff, 2002). The area of space beyond the central field is defined as the *peripheral visual field* (Gianutsos & Suchoff, 2002). The peripheral field is highly responsive to motion but is unable to perceive detail (Gianutsos & Suchoff, 2002).

Central and peripheral vision are both required for a full field of vision. Loss of vision in either type of field (central or peripheral) can lead to impairments in function. An impairment of the central visual field, especially the foveal area, may cause the client to have difficulty identifying visual details, contrast, and color (Warren, 2018). Functional activities that may be impacted include tasks that require reading, writing, and fine motor coordination, such as grooming, meal preparation, financial management, medication management, and shopping (Warren, 2018). Impaired peripheral field vision can affect balance, safety for ambulation (because of problems with obstacle avoidance), awareness of the environment (including locating objects), and safe driving (Bryan et al., 2018; Warren, 2018).

The location of the visual field loss is also important to consider. For example, an inferior (lower) field loss has been linked to decreased balance, decreased mobility, difficulty seeing steps or curbs, short strides, walking near walls and using them for balance, and difficulty identifying visual landmarks (Aloisio, 2004). A superior (upper) visual field cut has been associated with issues such as difficulty with reading signs (Aloisio, 2004). A visual field loss on the same side as the client's dominant hand may result in difficulty guiding the hand in fine motor activities

(Warren, 2018). This can manifest functionally, for example, in a reduction of writing legibility or clumsiness (Warren, 2018). Additional common behavioral changes associated with visual field deficits are a narrowing of the scope of searching (the area in which a person will look for objects) and slow visual searching toward the impacted side (Warren, 1998).

Functional deficits associated with visual field loss are numerous and diverse. Warren (1994) identified four factors that influence whether field loss will affect overall function:

1. Whether the field cut is the same in each eye. This is referred to as a *homonymous* (or *congruous) field cut.*
2. The contour of the boundary between the sound and impaired field. If the boundary is abrupt, the client typically has more difficulty compensating. This is best assessed through perimetry testing (discussed later) and cannot be determined by screening by the occupational therapy practitioner.
3. The presence of macular involvement, which will result in central field cut. People have reduced levels of functioning with central field loss.
4. The client's conscious awareness of the field cut. Greater levels of awareness lead to improved outcomes.

Visual Field Screening

An individual's visual field is measured in degrees, with the center of the fixation point acting as 0 degrees (Morton, 2004). The normal field of vision for each eye is approximately 50 to 60 degrees upward, 60 degrees inward, 70 to 75 degrees downward, and 90 to 100 degrees outward (when the eyes are facing forward; Figures 4-12 and 4-13). The type of deficit the client sustains after ABI depends on the location and size of the lesion. The types of common visual field deficits after a brain injury and the associated lesion sites are illustrated in Figure 4-14. Deficits may include hemianopsias (when half of the visual field is not seen), quadrantanopsias (when a quarter of the visual field is not seen), and/or scotomas (smaller areas of decreased sensitivity; Morton, 2004). With smaller field cuts, the brain may fill in the missing information, thereby decreasing a client's conscious awareness of the deficit. Visual fields deficits may be observed in clients with or without associated visual inattention (i.e., neglect; see Chapter 6). Clients with visual field cut generally exhibit smaller saccadic eye movements, decreased speed of visual searching (particularly with saccades toward the impaired field), and a narrower scope of visual searching (Warren, 2018).

Visual fields may be evaluated by confrontation screening, which is a gross measure (Figure 4-15), or perimetry testing, which is a more refined and accurate method, but requires specialized equipment and training and is also more time consuming (Anderson et al., 2009). The major advantage of confrontation screening is that it requires no elaborate devices; therefore, it can be completed by a variety of practitioners, including occupational therapy practitioners, in any setting (Morton, 2004). Perimetry testing can require two different types of devices depending on the type of perimetry evaluation being performed. For kinetic perimetry evaluation, the stimulus presented to the client is a spot of light of a specific size and intensity that is moved toward the center of fixation until the client indicates that it is seen (Morton, 2004). Static perimetry testing uses a static device that measures the client's visual fields by increasing the brightness of a spot at a fixed location until the client indicates that it is seen (Morton, 2004). Whether perimetry testing is static or dynamic, it involves three parameters. As outlined by Warren (1998), these are (a) fixation on a central target by the client while the testing is completed, (b) presentation of a target of a specific size in a designated area of the visual field, and (c) acknowledgment of the target by the client. Perimetry testing is typically conducted by eye care practitioners, not occupational therapy practitioners.

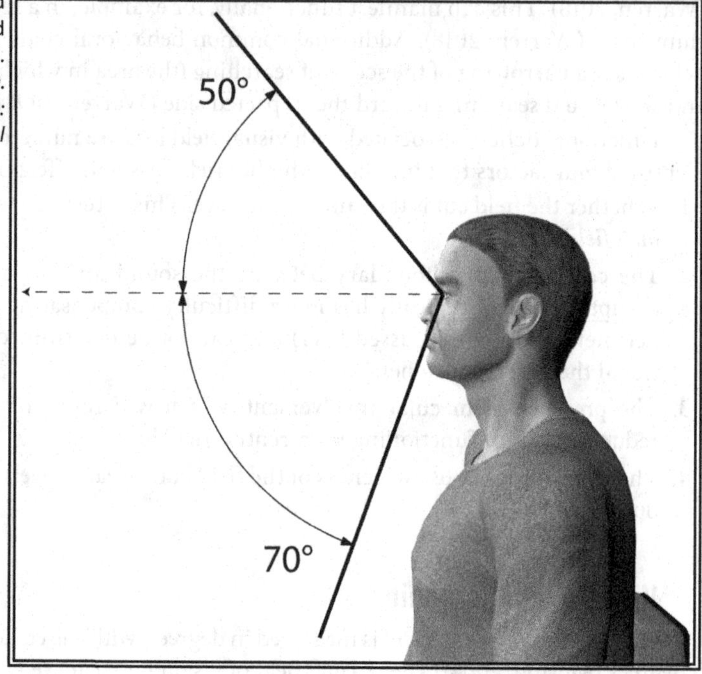

Figure 4-12. The superior and inferior visual fields. (Reproduced with permission from Whittaker, S. G., Scheiman, M., & Sokol-McKay, D. A. [2007]. *Low vision rehabilitation: A practical guide for occupational therapists*. SLACK Incorporated.)

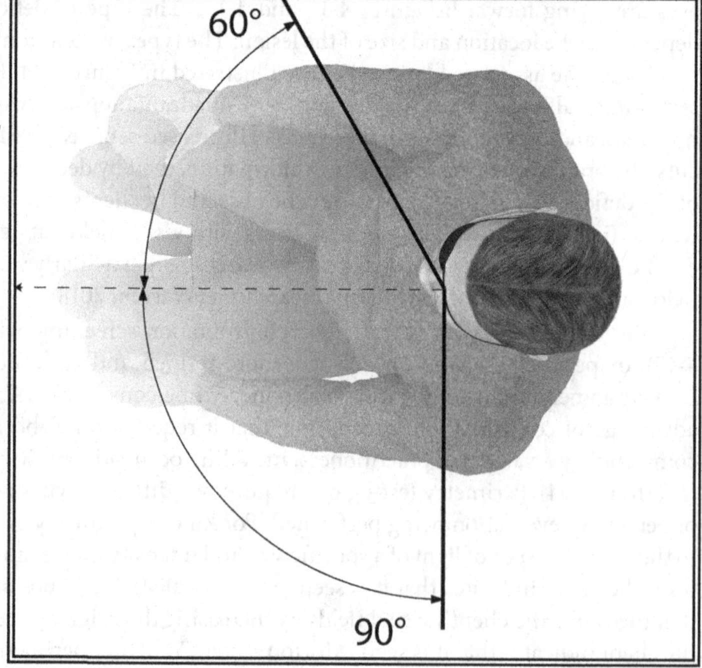

Figure 4-13. The medial and lateral visual fields. (Reproduced with permission from Whittaker, S. G., Scheiman, M., & Sokol-McKay, D. A. [2007]. *Low vision rehabilitation: A practical guide for occupational therapists*. SLACK Incorporated.)

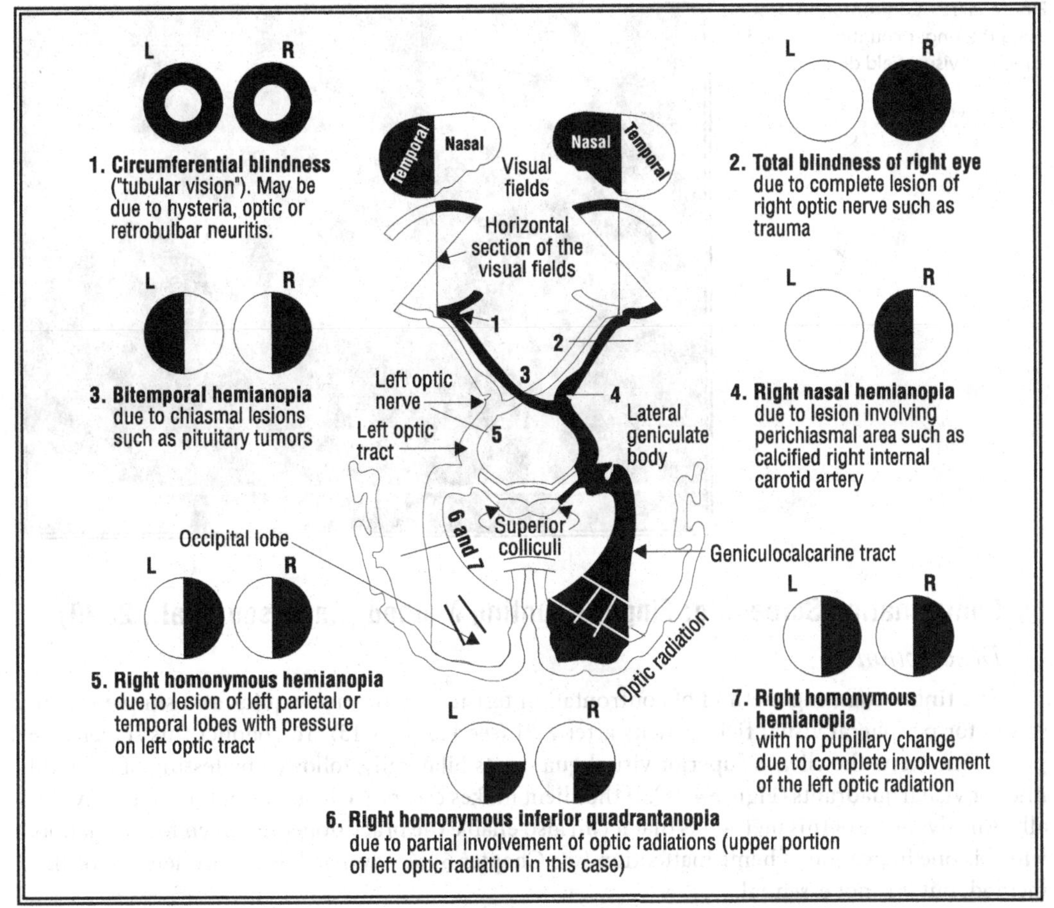

Figure 4-14. Visual field deficits and the associated lesion sites.

As previously mentioned, confrontation screening is considered to be a gross measurement of the client's peripheral visual fields. The occupational therapy practitioner should keep this in mind when using confrontation screening and use the results as a screening that can rule in a visual field problem but not completely rule one out (Anderson et al., 2009; Scheiman, 2011). Clients with positive findings on confrontation testing will likely have visual field loss, whereas those with negative findings may or may not have visual field loss. Findings that do not indicate field cut should be reported as "visual fields are grossly intact on confrontation screening" to indicate that an unidentified visual field cut may be present. In addition to screening through confrontation testing, the occupational therapy practitioner should evaluate and report any indications of potential field loss picked up through clinical observations of the client during functional activities. Examples include the client changing head position when asked to look at something placed in a certain visual plane, consistently bumping into objects on one side, misplacing objects in one field, or consistent errors in reading (e.g., leaving the first letter off of words; Warren, 2018). If there appears to be a visual field deficit on screening or clinical observations, a referral is necessary for a more precise measurement of the client's visual field.

There are a variety of methods for conducting a confrontation screen, several of which are described later in this chapter. The recommendation of Radomski et al. (2014) was to use the finger counting method. Information about other methods is included as well because they are screenings that are currently used widely in practice. Alternative methods may also be useful if a client has difficulty counting or adding numbers.

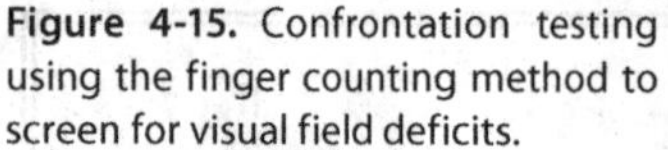

Figure 4-15. Confrontation testing using the finger counting method to screen for visual field deficits.

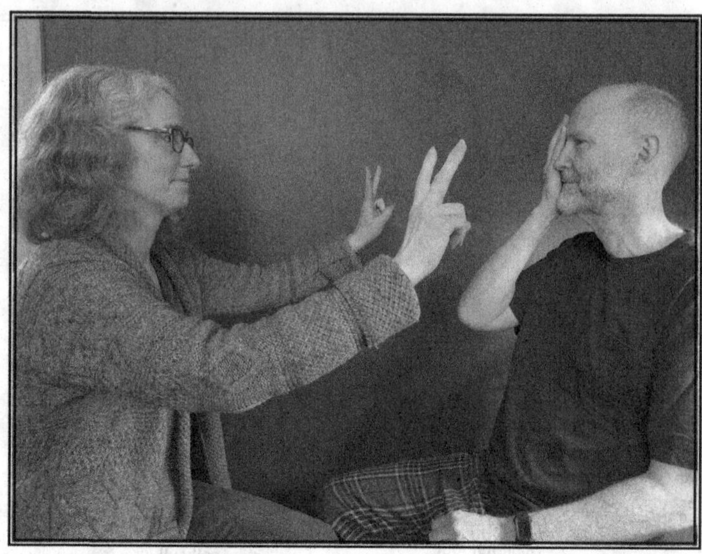

Confrontation Screening: Finger Counting Method (Anderson et al., 2009)

Description

The finger counting method of confrontation testing is a relatively quick and simple way to screen for peripheral visual field deficits after ABI (see Figure 4-15). To conduct this screen, the practitioner tests the client's superior visual quadrants bilaterally, followed by testing of bilateral inferior visual quadrants (Figure 4-16). If the client makes errors, each quadrant is tested individually. An advantage of this method is that it can also enable the practitioner to screen for extinction, which is one indication of hemi-inattention (see Chapter 6). An eyepatch is recommended for this method, but it is not essential.

Procedure

The client is seated opposite the examiner with the client's head positioned vertically.

1. Place the eye patch over the client's left eye. Alternatively, clients can use their hands or an occluder to cover their eye, although this method may result in the client inadvertently uncovering the eye. Have the client fixate on your nose or on your left eye (the eye directly in front of the uncovered right eye). Fixation should be maintained throughout the screening.
2. Starting with the superior fields, hold up one or two fingers on each hand so that the total number of fingers presented is two, three, or four. Your hands should each be 20 to 60 degrees from the point of fixation, both superiorly and laterally. Your right hand will be positioned in the client's left visual field. Your left hand will be positioned in the client's right visual field.
3. Instruct the client to indicate the total number of fingers that you are holding up by adding the number of fingers in the right visual field with the number of fingers in the left visual field.
4. Repeat these procedures while placing your hands in the inferior visual fields.
5. Remove the patch from the left eye (or have the client uncover the eye) and repeat steps 1 through 4 with the right eye occluded.
6. If the client does not report the total number of fingers accurately, screen each quadrant alone to determine the specific area that the client is not perceiving.

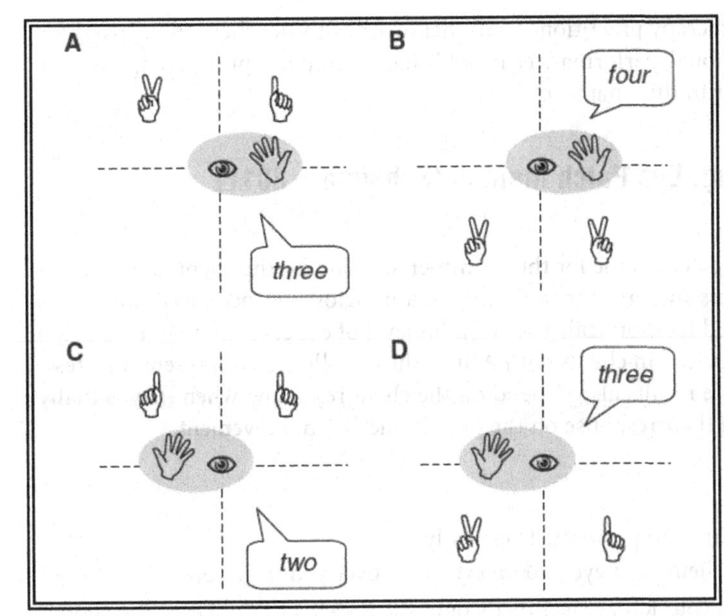

Figure 4-16. The finger counting confrontation screen. (Reproduced with permission from Anderson, A. J., Shuey, N. H., & Wall, M. [2009]. Rapid confrontation screening for peripheral visual field defects and extinction. *Clinical and Experimental Optometry, 92,* 45-48. https://doi.org/10.1111/j.1444-0938.2008.00280.x)

Scoring

The client's accuracy with this assessment should be recorded, including which quadrants were not perceived. For example, imagine that a client was inaccurate with adding fingers presented bilaterally. When each quadrant was tested on its own, the client missed the stimuli when they were presented left of midline in both superior and inferior fields. The occupational therapy practitioner would then report that the client appeared to have a field cut left of midline. As noted previously, it is important to know that this test can also indicate the presence of extinction, which is a sign of hemi-inattention (see scoring information in Chapter 6).

Psychometric Properties for All Visual Field Screening Methods

No information could be found in the literature regarding the reliability of confrontation testing. Multiple studies report on the sensitivity of these screening tools as compared to automated perimetry testing. Researchers have found that perimetry testing is much better able to pick up visual field deficits as compared to confrontation testing (Bass et al., 2007; Kerr et al., 2010; Townend et al., 2007). This is especially true when a client has a mild visual field deficit (Bass et al., 2007; Kerr et al., 2010). Perimetry testing is not always readily available, however, and confrontation tests are quick and easy to administer and require little equipment (Kerr et al., 2010). They may also be more accurate when multiple methods are combined (Kerr et al., 2010). As a result, researchers do not recommend that practitioners cease their use. Rather, confrontation testing should be used a screening tool that is best able to identify more severe visual field loss (Bass et al., 2007; Kerr et al., 2010).

Referral for All Visual Field Screening Methods

If an occupational therapy practitioner finds a deficit with visual field screening or if a field cut is suspected due to issues observed during functional activities (e.g., consistently missing information from one part of the visual space), referral to an eye care provider should be made. The eye care provider can complete more accurate visual field testing with automated perimetry and, when appropriate, provide treatment such as specialized prisms to improve the client's visual functioning. The occupational therapy practitioner will then work with the client to utilize these treatments to improve occupational performance, in addition to implementing compensatory strategy training (discussed later in this chapter).

Confrontation Screening: Eye Patch Method (Scheiman, 2011)

Description

For this screening, two eye patches (one for the examiner and one for the client) and a target (e.g., a white sphere 3 mm or less in diameter mounted on a nonglossy wand) are needed. It is important to remember that good fixation ability and a high level of concentration and attention are necessary, which may be impaired in clients with ABI. If these skills are not present, this testing will not be accurate. Accurate results also depend on the client reporting when they actually see the target rather than basing their response on the practitioner's arm movement.

Procedure

The client is seated with their head positioned vertically.

1. Place an eye patch over the client's left eye and an eye patch over your right eye.
2. Sit opposite the client so that your left eye is directly opposite the client's right eye. You should be about 20 in. from the client. It is preferable that the background for the client be dark and uniform.
3. Explain that you will be moving the target into their field of vision, and the client should report as soon as they see it. The client will need to maintain fixation on your left eye.
4. Begin at the 12 o'clock position. Slowly move the target down in an arclike motion until the client first reports seeing it. Compare the client's response to yours. If the client cannot see the target as soon as you can, it is an indication of a possible problem.
5. Move clockwise to the 2, 4, 6, 8, and 10 o'clock positions, and repeat step 4.
6. Record approximately where the client reports seeing the target in each orientation tested. Degrees are best to use, with 0 degrees being in line with the fixation point.
7. Place the eye patch over the client's right eye and an eye patch over your left eye.
8. Sit opposite the client so that your right eye is directly opposite the client's left eye, and repeat steps 3 through 6.

Scoring

Occupational therapy practitioners should report approximate degrees of field loss. To make that determination, 0 degrees is considered to be directly in front of the client, at the point of fixation. In a young adult without field loss, there is an expected 50 degrees of superior visual field, 70 degrees of inferior visual field, 60 degrees nasal visual field, and at least 90 degrees of temporal visual field for each eye (see Figures 4-12 and 4-13). The point at which the client reports seeing the stimulus is noted and approximate degrees of field loss are then reported.

Psychometric Properties

See information under the psychometric properties for the finger counting method of confrontation testing.

Referral

The client should be able to see the target at approximately the same point at which you can see it. If there appears to be a significant discrepancy, a visual field deficit may be present, and a referral is indicated for a more precise measurement of the client's visual field as described under the referral information for the finger counting method.

Confrontation Screening: Two-Examiner Method (Scheiman, 2011; Warren, 1998)

Description

In response to concerns that single-examiner methods of confrontation screening are insensitive, some authors recommend using two examiners. With this method, one examiner presents the targets from behind the client while the other examiner monitors the client's fixation. This method is more likely to result in the client responding solely to the perception of the target versus the examiner's arm movements during testing. Note, however, that in many clinical settings two examiners are often not available so this may not always be feasible. An eye patch and a target (e.g., a white sphere 3 mm or less in diameter mounted on a nonglossy wand) are needed.

Procedure

The client is seated with their head positioned vertically.

1. Place the eye patch over the client's left eye.
2. The first examiner sits in front of the client and directs the client to fixate on a target located directly in front of the client (e.g., the first examiner's nose). The first examiner is responsible for monitoring whether or not the client maintains fixation on the target and noting where the client first sees the target.
3. The second examiner is situated behind the client and moves the target forward. Begin at the 12 o'clock position and slowly move the target down until the client first reports seeing it. Repeat this step, moving clockwise to the 2, 4, 6, 8, and 10 o'clock positions.
4. Record approximately where the client reports seeing the target in each orientation tested (in degrees).
5. Place the eye patch over the client's right eye and repeat steps 2 through 4.

Scoring

Scoring for the two-examiner confrontation screen is identical to the scoring for the eye patch method as described previously.

Psychometric Properties

See information under the psychometric properties for the finger counting method of confrontation testing.

Referral

Referral for the two-examiner confrontation screen is the same as for the eye patch method as described previously.

Assessment of Vision in Clients Who Are Minimally Responsive

An accurate assessment of the visual status of clients who are in a minimally responsive state is a critical component of rehabilitation efforts (Whyte & DiPasquale, 1995). Vision is often used in tests of basic cognitive function, with visual orientation being one of the criteria for judging whether or not a client is emerging from a coma or vegetative state. However, the visual testing procedures described previously rely on the client making a specific oral (e.g., standard Snellen chart) or gestural (e.g., a Tumbling E chart) response and cannot be used with individuals who are unable to respond in these ways. Whyte and DiPasquale (1995) described a method for assessing vision (and visual attention) for clients in a minimally responsive state that is similar to the forced-choice preferential looking technique developed by Teller and colleagues (1986) to assess vision in infants.

This visual assessment protocol compares the number of eye movements a client makes toward brightly colored photographs provided by the client's family, a blank card, and no stimulus. The assessment assumes that a person is more likely to look at a brightly colored familiar photograph than a blank card and is more likely to look at a blank card than no stimulus. To perform the assessment, the examiner stands approximately 6 feet in front of the client with a photograph in one hand and the blank card in the other (both out of the client's sight). The examiner then raises one or both hands 30 to 40 degrees from midline at the level of the patient's ears. The photograph and/or card are shown in a random order to the right and/or left sides using either a single stimulus or both stimuli simultaneously. The examiner observes the client's eyes and records the first lateralized eye movement after the presentation of the stimuli as the response. If no eye movements occur within 5 seconds, the trial is recorded as "no response" (Whyte & Pasquale, 1995).

Whyte and Pasquale (1995) reported the results of using this protocol with six clients who were in a minimally responsive state. Based on observations of eye movements to the various presentations of the photograph and card, they concluded that one client had functional vision in both visual fields, one had functional fields and a monocular visual deficit, two had a homonymous hemianopsia with one of those also having a monocular visual deficit, and two had some degree of hemi-inattention (a condition described in Chapter 6).

Treatment

As described previously, the treatment of visual dysfunction after ABI should be based on an assessment by a qualified vision provider. Intervention priorities include the treatment of any medical conditions of the eye, such as glaucoma; provision of the best eyeglasses or contact lens prescription to improve visual acuity; implementation of compensatory strategies, including optical devices, such as prisms; and, in some instances, remedial vision therapy under the guidance of a qualified specialist. As described in more detail in Chapter 2, the vision provider is responsible for medical treatment of the eye, prescribing corrective and specialized lenses, and directing vision therapy. Surgical interventions may also be indicated for some clients (e.g., for correction of a strabismus [eye turn]). The role of the occupational therapy practitioner varies to some degree by setting. For many clients, the occupational therapy practitioner provides interventions aimed at improving occupational performance through the identification and implementation of compensatory strategies. However, the occupational therapy practitioner may or may not be directly involved with providing vision therapy for clients depending on the setting. In the following section, we focus on the compensatory treatment strategies typically provided by occupational therapy practitioners followed in greater detail by a description of the role of the occupational therapy practitioner in other types of interventions.

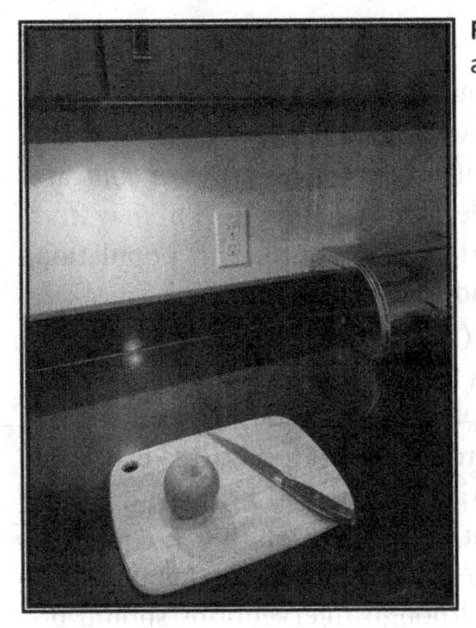

Figure 4-17. Under-cabinet lighting designed to increase the task lighting available, although it needs to be balanced with glare reduction.

Compensatory Treatment Strategies

When treating people with visual impairment of any kind, there are often some modifications that can be made to the environment that will lessen the demand that is placed on the visual system and decrease the likelihood of visual overload (Kaldenberg, 2014; Warren, 2018). This, in turn, makes it easier for people to locate and identify objects in their environments. There are six general principles that can be followed when considering environmental adaptation for people with visual impairment: provide sufficient lighting, improve contrast, limit glare, reduce patterns or visual clutter, enlarge critical features, and instruct in the use of other senses (Kaldenberg, 2014; Warren, 2018).

Provide Sufficient Lighting

Working in an environment with adequate illumination can aid the client in seeing and identifying objects. There are two types of lighting that should be considered. The first is ambient lighting, which is the general lighting present in a room. A consistent level of light throughout the space is ideal to avoid forcing the visual system to adjust rapidly to areas of light and areas of dark. Increasing the number of lamps or lighting fixtures that are available can improve ambient lighting. Lamps that point upward to reflect light off of the ceiling will provide better overall lighting and decrease the chances of pools of light and pools of dark, which can happen with table lamps. Another simple strategy that can be used to maintain sufficient levels of lighting in a person's environment is to keep light bulbs free of dust to allow the most light to shine through as possible.

The second type of lighting is task lighting, which focuses a light source onto the work surface, such as a desk or kitchen counter. Using under-cabinet lighting can be helpful for increasing task lighting in the kitchen (Figure 4-17). A gooseneck lamp, which can be adjusted to direct the light, can also be helpful so that people can direct the light onto the working surface in a way that is most comfortable for them.

For some people, such as those with macular degeneration, more lighting is usually preferred, although some other populations, such as those with TBI, are more likely to have photophobia (light sensitivity), resulting in a need for more moderate levels of lighting (Greenwald et al., 2012; Warren, 2018). As a result, close consultation with the client is essential when considering lighting. There is also no agreement on the type of lighting (e.g., florescent, halogen, incandescent) to use, and client preference should be the deciding factor, although clinicians should be aware that some people with TBI are especially sensitive to fluorescent lighting (Kapoor, 2012).

Improve Contrast

Increasing the contrast between an object and its background can make it easier to locate items and objects. The easiest contrast for most people to see is white on black or black on white, although it is important for the clinician to understand that preferences for the types of contrast vary based on the diagnosis and personal preference. For example, some people with TBI may find that black on white is too much contrast and causes visual overload. As a result, this population may prefer contrast such as dark gray on a light gray background (Niemeier, 2010).

Contrast should be considered in all areas of occupation (Figures 4-18 through 4-20). For example, when brushing teeth, it is easier to put toothpaste on a toothbrush with white bristles if using a green gel rather than a white toothpaste. For meal preparation, consider using different colored chopping boards in the kitchen; use a white cutting board for darker foods (e.g., broccoli) and a dark cutting board for lighter foods (e.g., onions). Contrast should also be considered in functional mobility, with particular attention paid to areas that are not as well lit (e.g., outdoor pathways) and stairs. Using strategies such as marking stair edges can improve functional mobility for many people with visual impairment (Warren, 2018), although interventions should be individualized because not everyone will respond in the same way (Figure 4-21).

Limit Glare

Glare occurs when light reflects off of a surface and is a major issue for many people with visual impairments. Glare in an environment forces the visual system to work harder to see and identify objects. Glare inside buildings, as well as outside, should be considered (Warren, 2018). Whenever possible, avoid shiny surfaces, such as glossy paper or highly polished floors. Adjustable blinds can reduce glare because people are able to change the angle of light coming into a room, thus eliminating this source of glare. Another option for the home is the use of translucent curtains, which filter the light coming through windows. The use of hats with brims or visors may also be helpful for someone who is impacted by glare coming from overhead, as can be the case for many people with TBI who have photophobia (Greenwald et al., 2012). Sun shields (colored glasses that are designed to filter light) may also be considered (Greenwald et al., 2012). They are available in a wide range of colors and shades and are readily available online or in stores specializing in equipment for people with visual impairment. For some clients, it can be helpful to consult a vision provider who specializes in prescribing colored lenses to identify the most effective color from a wide range of options. Also, using the monitor glare adjustment and/or attaching a computer glare screen can reduce glare on computers and improve performance with computing. Finally, yellow acetate sheets placed over written materials can help to reduce glare and maximize contrast.

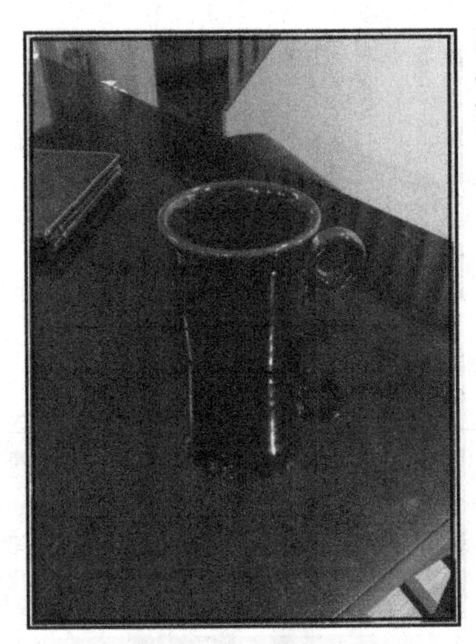

Figure 4-18. An example of poor contrast in the kitchen with a dark-colored coffee mug on a dark counter. Glare is also present on the glossy surface of the counter.

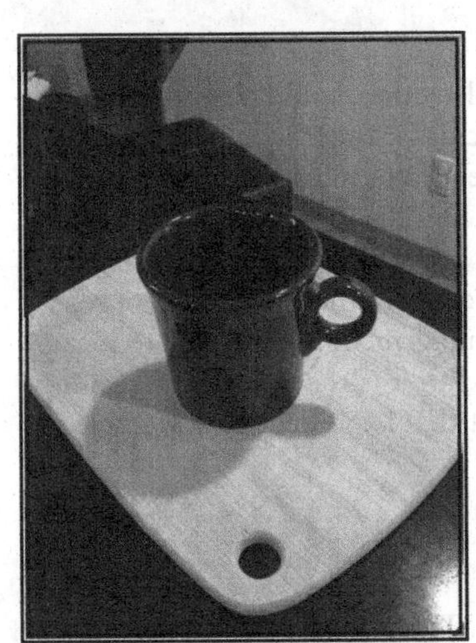

Figure 4-19. Placing the coffee mug on a light-colored cutting board improves contrast. It also helps to reduce the glare on the counter surface.

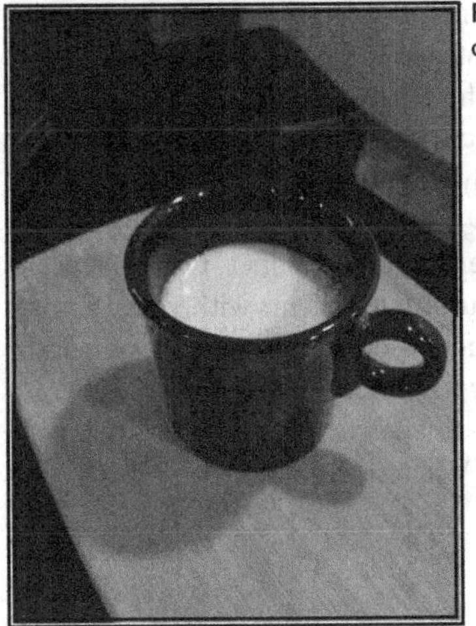

Figure 4-20. Using a dark-colored coffee mug for milk allows better use of contrast to distinguish the level of the milk in the mug.

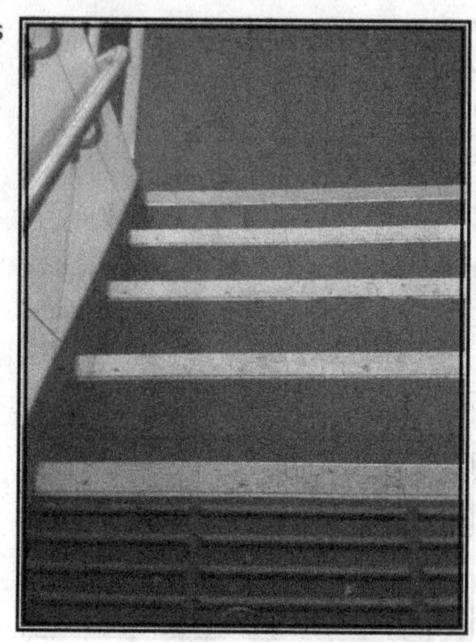

Figure 4-21. Marking the edges of stairs with a contrasting color improves the visibility of stair edges.

Reduce Patterns or Visual Clutter

Patterns, such as can be present on rugs, bedspreads, and tablecloths, should be minimized in the visual environment whenever possible because it can be difficult for those with visual impairments to locate objects when they are resting on patterned surfaces. Patterns can also cause people to believe that items are present when they are not. Surfaces to be considered include floors, tables, couches, and beds. Similarly, a highly cluttered environment will prove difficult for a person with visual loss to navigate. Simplifying the visual environment, especially in the early stages of rehabilitation, will improve the chances that a person with visual impairment will be able to locate items and decipher the visual scene. Related to reducing visual clutter is the strategy of keeping environments well organized, which reduces the time and effort that is needed to locate objects (Warren, 2018; Figures 4-22 through 4-25).

Enlarge Critical Features

When magnification is used, an object is made to look larger. There are several strategies that can be used to achieve magnification. Relative distance magnification is accomplished by bringing an item closer; it will look bigger when it is nearer. Relative size magnification refers to increasing the actual size of the object. The use of large print falls into this category. When deciding how much to enlarge print, use the smallest line on the acuity chart that the client reads easily as a starting point (Warren, 2018). For example, if a client is able to easily read 2M print on the near vision test card, standard-sized print for reading material should be roughly doubled. There are a number of devices available in large print that can be useful to clients with visual impairment, including large print calendars, clocks, watches, playing cards, checkbook registers, and telephones. Other devices, such as magnified mirrors, are also available and may prove to be useful for clients with visual acuity loss. Angular magnification refers to the use of optical devices, such as prescription glasses (including bifocals, trifocals, and reading glasses), magnifying glasses, or telescopes. There are a number of different types of devices available. The client should be referred to an eye care provider, such as a rehabilitation optometrist if the use of these devices is indicated (Warren, 2018).

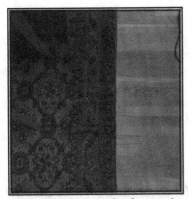

Figure 4-22. An example of a complex pattern hiding an object.

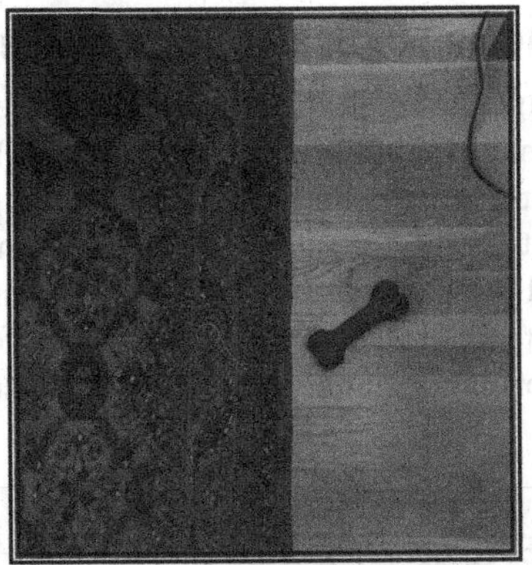

Figure 4-23. Simplifying the pattern improves the visibility of items resting on top of the surface.

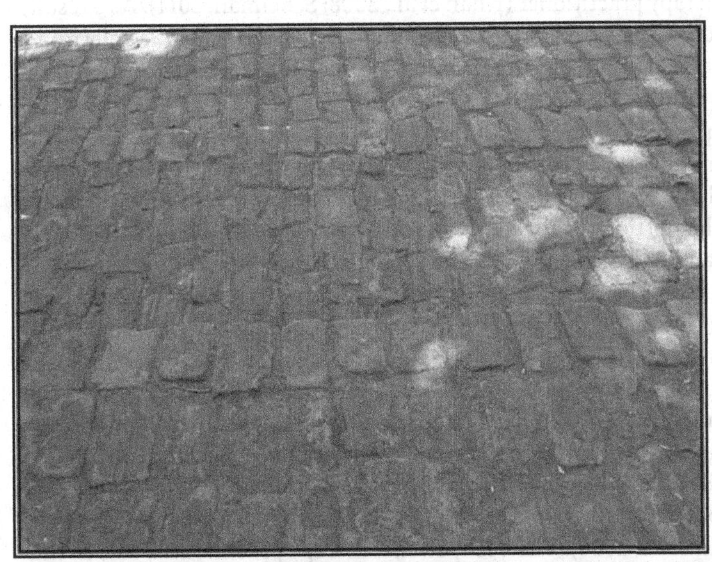

Figure 4-24. An example of how patterns and limited contrast can limit the ability to identify obstacles. This is the view from one direction.

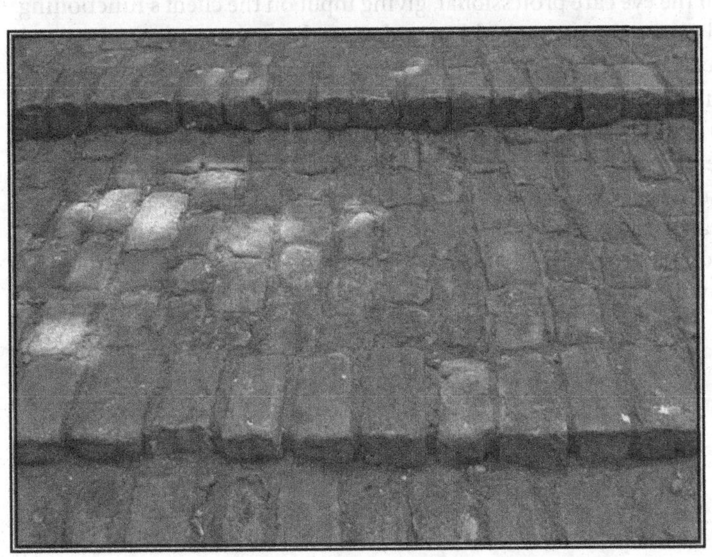

Figure 4-25. This is the same location as in Figure 4-24 viewed from the opposite direction.

Instruct in the Use of Other Senses

To compensate for visual loss, use the remaining sensory systems (i.e., hearing, tactile discrimination, kinesthesia, and proprioception) to assist in increased function (Kaldenberg, 2014). The auditory system can be used by utilizing items such as talking clocks. Clients can also be instructed to listen for signals in the environment, such as from alarms. Tactile discrimination can be used to locate objects or to identify them, feeling for distinguishing characteristic (e.g., feeling for the teeth of a comb when orienting it for use). Kinesthesia and proprioception can be used to gain information about the environment, such as the type of walking surface being navigated.

Treatment of Impaired Visual Acuity and Accommodation

As noted earlier, there are specific treatments that can assist people with impairments in visual acuity besides compensation, although these require intervention by other members of the team besides the occupational therapy practitioner (Khan et al., 2008; Scheiman, 2011). As a result, if the occupational therapy practitioner's screening of acuity indicates impairment, a referral to a vision provider for continued evaluation, lens prescription, or additional treatment should be made (Scheiman, 2011; Warren, 2018).

It is important for the occupational therapy practitioners to be aware of any lenses the client has been prescribed and use them during treatment. It is also important to understand the impact bifocal and trifocal lenses can have on function, especially if they are progressive (i.e., there is not an obvious line separating the portions of the lens). If clients are wearing bifocals or trifocals during functional mobility, it can be difficult for them to maneuver over and around obstacles, especially steps or curbs. This happens because clients may be attempting to focus on objects near their feet with the portion of the lens that is designed for focusing on reading material. It may also be difficult to change focus from one part of the lens to another quickly (e.g., when looking up to see someone coming from the opposite direction on stairs and looking back down again to the stairs). The situation is more complicated if the client wears progressive lenses, which may cause a distortion and may also have a negative impact on peripheral vision, an important contributor to balance. A client may be best served by having different sets of glasses instead, one for distance and one for near tasks, with a potential third pair needed for intermediate distances (e.g., when completing computer work; Khan et al., 2008). The occupational therapy practitioner's role in this situation is to communicate with the eye care professional, giving input on the client's functioning with different lens options, and to use the prescribed lenses during therapy in order to improve occupational performance (Scheiman, 2011; Warren, 2018).

If the client is seen by a rehabilitation optometrist and an impairment in accommodation (the ability to change focal distance) is discovered, a visual rehabilitation program may be prescribed. There is evidence that some clients with accommodative dysfunction caused by ABI can develop skills to improve their visual acuity through exercise (Thiagarajan & Ciuffreda, 2014). If a visual rehabilitation program is indicated and prescribed, the occupational therapy practitioner may assist with the implementation of the program. Further instructions should be received from the rehabilitation optometrist, who will also be responsible for supervising the program.

Treatment of Visual Field Deficits

There are several types of intervention that can be used when treating those with visual field deficits, some of which require the involvement of eye care practitioners. Intervention includes instruction in the use of organized search patterns or other compensatory techniques, the use of optical devices, and restorative training (Ajina & Kennard, 2012; Berryman et al., 2010; Grunda et al., 2013; Hellerstein et al., 2011; Kaldenberg, 2014; Khan et al., 2008; Luu et al., 2010; Pollock et al., 2011b).

Instruction in the Use of Organized Search Patterns

Occupational therapy practitioners can work directly with the client with visual field loss on establishing an effective search strategy. In this case, the client is taught to intentionally search in the impaired visual field to locate items and obstacles (Ajina & Kennard, 2012; Berryman et al., 2010; Grunda et al., 2013; Hellerstein et al., 2011; Kaldenberg, 2014; Luu et al., 2010; Pollock et al., 2011b; Warren, 2018).

Clients will need to be taught to use a highly organized search pattern in order for this to be effective, and, because this requires conscious effort, the client will need to have awareness of the presence and impact of the visual field deficit (Berryman et al., 2010; Hellerstein et al., 2011; Luu et al., 2010). The occupational therapy practitioner can assist the client in developing this awareness through prompting or cueing during functional activities. The use of the dynamic interactional approach in these situations (Toglia, 2018) can aid in this process (see Chapter 8). Using this approach, clients would be asked to predict and then reflect on their performance of activities. Cueing can also be adjusted to improve client performance, with notes made about the types of cues or adaptations that are needed (Scheiman, 2011). The types of cues that may be needed include verbal, auditory (e.g., bell ringing, finger snapping), and tactile cueing to encourage the client to look to the affected field of vision. For further details about improving the awareness of deficits after a brain injury, see Chapters 9 and 10.

Warren (2018) outlines the following components of an effective search strategy. It should be noted that more research is needed to determine the efficacy of these approaches for people with ABI.

1. Initiation of a wide head turn toward the impaired field
2. An increase in the number of head and eye movements toward the impaired field
3. Execution of an organized and efficient search pattern that begins on the impaired side
4. Attention to and detection of visual detail on the impaired side
5. Ability to quickly shift attention and search between the central visual field and the peripheral visual field on the impaired side

There are a variety of methods that the clinician can use when teaching clients with visual field deficits to use an organized searching pattern, but all would start by having clients begin the search strategy in the impaired field and then carry it out in an organized way (Warren, 2018).

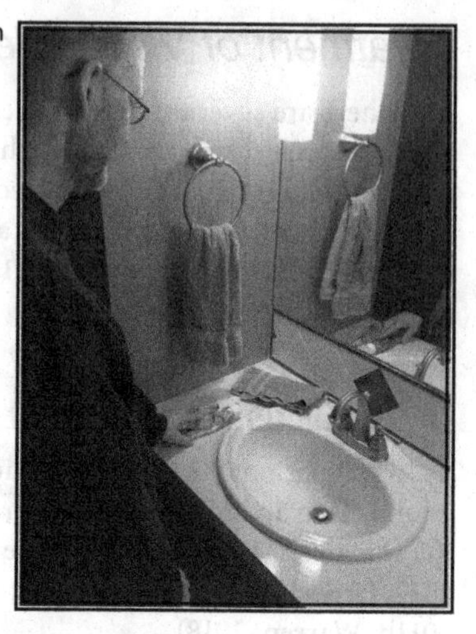

Figure 4-26. A client with left hemianopsia using an organized search strategy to locate grooming items placed in the impaired visual field.

Hellerstein and colleagues (2011) recommended starting by teaching clients to search when looking for a specific and expected object. A simple and uncluttered environment is recommended when first teaching this strategy. For example, the clinician could begin teaching a client to search in an organized way by first asking the client to search for a toothbrush placed on the side of the sink that falls in the impaired field. As the client improves, the task would be made more complex, and the client is taught to use the organized search pattern when looking for objects in a larger space. Ultimately, the clinician would work toward having the client regularly and spontaneously search all visual spaces, including dynamic and changing environments, during all tasks (Hellerstein et al., 2011).

In order to work to this end goal, it is essential for all members of the team to encourage the client to practice search strategies with tasks in a variety of contexts or environments, which will better enable the client to learn to generalize the use of an organized search pattern (Berryman et al., 2010; Kaldenberg, 2014). Using the multicontext approach to treatment is one way to guide the systematic approach to generalization (Toglia, 1991; see Chapter 9). For example, the occupational therapy practitioner could start by training the client in using an organized search strategy to locate a tube of toothpaste in a medicine cabinet where there are 10 items. Then, the occupational therapy practitioner would have the client use the same search strategy to find a bar of soap in a cupboard where there are 10 items (near transfer). The next step would be to have the client locate a carton of milk in a refrigerator where there are 10 items, again using the same search strategy (intermediate transfer). The client would then need to locate a pair of shoes in a room with 10 items on the floor (far transfer). Then, the client would practice searching for items on grocery store shelves (very far transfer).

The specific treatment activities that clinicians can use vary and include ADLs (e.g., having the client search for needed grooming or clothing items), in addition to using tasks such as tabletop activities. These activities should all be designed to encourage visual searching. Ideally, the activities will also be set up in such a way that the client needs to manipulate objects that are located in the impaired field (Kaldenberg, 2014). Some examples of activities that the clinician can use are games such as concentration or checkers, word searches, and computer games in which searching is needed (Warren, 2018). The client's general environment can also be modified to encourage searching. For example, objects needed for the completion of a task can be placed on the side of the field cut, encouraging the client to look to that side (Figure 4-26). In addition to everyday tasks, a treatment tool that can be used when training a client to search is the Dynavision, which can encourage searching over a larger array than many traditional tabletop activities (Warren, 2018; Figure 4-27).

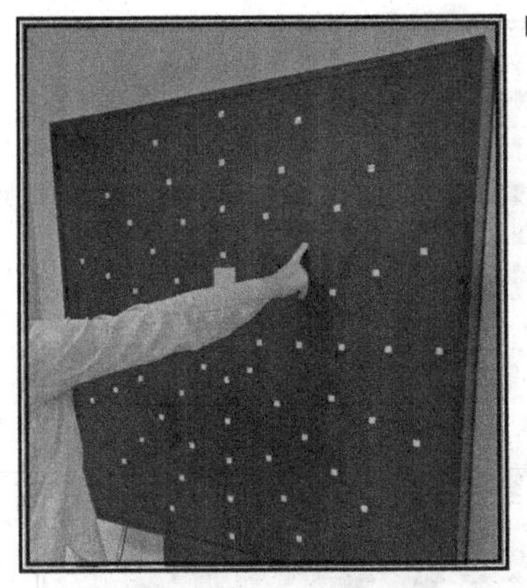

Figure 4-27. Using the Dynavision to encourage an organized search pattern.

As the client improves, the clinician should work on increased speed and accuracy of eye movements. The clinician should also use walking during searching tasks or other forms of movement to integrate vision, movement, and perception (Aloisio, 2004). For example, when walking with clients from their rooms (or from lobby areas) to the therapy gym, ask them to search for and point out all items that are red, such as fire extinguishers or emergency call boxes. Clients can also be asked to complete "narrated walks" (i.e., they describe the items that they see as they navigate a variety of environments; Warren, 2018).

The research that has been done with treatments for visual field deficits indicates that teaching visual searching is the most efficacious thus far (Grunda et al., 2013; Pollock et al., 2011b), although this is not universally agreed on. For example, a Cochrane review of randomized controlled trials conducted with those with visual field deficits concluded that there was limited evidence that the use of organized searching improved performance. Outcomes that were addressed included tasks such as reading and ADLs; the authors indicated that more research needs to be done with this technique to determine its impact on these and other areas of occupation (Pollock et al., 2011b).

Other Compensatory Strategies

In addition to teaching clients to search the environment using an organized search pattern, there are additional strategies that occupational therapy practitioners can use to assist clients with visual field deficits in being more independent. Anchoring techniques can be used to help cue clients about when they have reached the edge of the space they need to search (Figure 4-28). Anchors are especially helpful with reading and writing. For example, a client can use a bookmark placed vertically along the edge of the text on the side of impairment as an anchor. In this case, when the client sees the bookmark, they know that the end of the line has been reached. The client can also use a ruler or straightedge under each line of text to avoid losing track while reading (Scheiman, 2011). Markers can also be used in other ways, such as by adding color and contrast to door frames and furniture to help the client locate them and to aid in functional mobility (Warren, 2018).

Another compensatory strategy that can be used is to simply ensure that items that need to be located are placed in the intact visual field. This is especially important for items that are needed for safety, such as nurse call buttons or telephones. It is also a strategy that can be used for clients who lack awareness of their deficits. Another example of using this technique is when clients are taught to rotate reading material (e.g., books) 45 to 90 degrees so that the text is located in the intact visual field (Hellerstein et al., 2011; Kaldenberg, 2014).

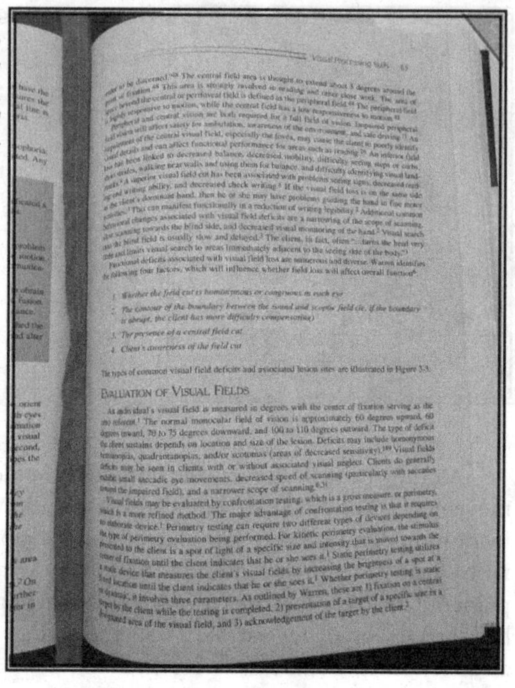

Visual Processing Skills 65

1. Whether the field cut is homonymous or congruous in each eye
2. The contour of the boundary between the sound and scoptic field (ie, if the boundary is abrupt, the client has more difficulty compensating)
3. The presence of a central field cut
4. Client's awareness of the field cut

The types of common visual field deficits and associated lesion sites are illustrated in Figure 3-3.

EVALUATION OF VISUAL FIELDS

Figure 4-28. Using an anchoring technique with a book. In this case, a bookmark is placed on the left side of the text. When the person sees the bookmark, they know that they have reached the beginning of the lines of text. (Reproduced from Zoltan, B. [2007]. *Vision, perception, and cognition: A manual for evaluation and treatment of the adult with acquired brain injury* [4th ed.]. SLACK Incorporated.)

Finally, as is the case with all types of visual deficits, it is essential to educate the client and their family about the field loss and how it will potentially affect function. Situations in which safety may be a problem should be covered in more detail. Examples include crossing intersections or maneuvering in busy environments, such as crowded stores.

Use of Optical Devices

Clients with visual field deficits can be referred to an eye care provider to assess for the use of prisms or other optical devices, such as mirror lenses and telescopes (Ajina & Kennard, 2012; Berryman et al., 2010; Grunda et al., 2013; Hellerstein et al., 2011; Kahn et al., 2008; Kaldenberg, 2014; Luu et al., 2010; Pollock et al., 2011b), with prisms being the most commonly used method. The rationale behind using these devices is that they can extend the visual field by directing information from the impaired field into the intact field (Ajina & Kennard, 2012; Berryman et al., 2010; Khan et al., 2008; Scheiman, 2011). Clients who respond best to this type of intervention are those who have awareness of their deficits, have good divided and alternating attention, and are willing and able to go through training to best use these devices (Berryman et al., 2010; Khan et al., 2008). The occupational therapy practitioner may be part of the training by assisting clients in using these devices in the context of functional activities (Scheiman, 2011).

There are different methods of using prisms with this population, including the use of prisms that are built into lenses and the use of prisms that are applied to lenses (called *Fresnel prisms*). Eye care practitioners who use Fresnel prisms typically will apply them by following a method called the *Peli system* in which Fresnel prisms are placed in strips on the top and bottom part of one lens of the client's glasses. This system helps to alert the client to objects that appear in the impaired field so that they can direct their gaze in that direction (Berryman et al., 2010; Scheiman, 2011). A Cochrane review of randomized controlled trials examining interventions for people with visual field cut concluded that there was insufficient evidence to determine the efficacy of prism use for people with visual field cut (Pollock et al., 2011b). Since the publication of that review, there was a randomized controlled trial completed that found that Peli prisms were more effective than placebo in helping people avoid obstacles while ambulating (Bowers et al., 2014). In addition, there are other studies that have used methods besides randomized controlled trials that have provided some evidence about the usefulness of this method (Bowers et al., 2008; Giorgi et al., 2009; Szlyk et al., 2005).

Another method is the Gottlieb system, in which a small round prism is built into one lens of the client's glasses. The client is taught to direct their gaze toward the prism, which will reflect information from the impaired field into the intact visual field. The placement of the prism is individually determined by the eye care provider (Berryman et al., 2010). There is less research on this type of prism placement, and the studies have been on a small scale, but those that have been performed indicate that this treatment method has potential (Gottlieb et al., 1992; Szlyk et al., 2005).

Restorative Training

Another approach that has been trialed with clients with visual field loss is restorative training (i.e., when clients receive repeated stimulation to the impaired visual field). The rationale behind this approach is that this stimulation can cause brain healing through neuroplasticity. The ideal outcome is one in which vision in the impaired visual field is restored. The training usually makes use of a computerized system and requires intensive treatment, with the client receiving intervention for approximately 1 hour each day, 6 days per week, for 6 months. The efficacy of this approach is inconclusive at this time, and this type of treatment remains controversial (Grunda et al., 2013; Hellerstein et al., 2011; Luu et al., 2010; Pollock et al., 2011b).

Treatment of Deficits in Oculomotor Control

As stated previously, if the occupational therapy practitioner's screening of oculomotor control, including convergence, visual pursuits, and saccades, indicates a problem, a referral should be made to an optometrist, ophthalmologist, or other vision specialist. When making the referral, the occupational therapy practitioner should be specific about what was observed during the screening process as well as how the oculomotor control issue is manifesting during functional activities (Warren, 2018). The eye care provider will then pursue different options depending on the individual client's presentation. The vision specialist may prescribe optics, such as prisms, partial or full occlusion, or visual training through a restorative exercise program, with the choice of intervention depending on the specific visual dysfunction (Greenwald et al., 2012; Hellerstein et al., 2011; Kahn et al., 2008; Kaldenberg, 2014; O'Dell et al., 1998; Scheiman, 2011; Suter, 2018).

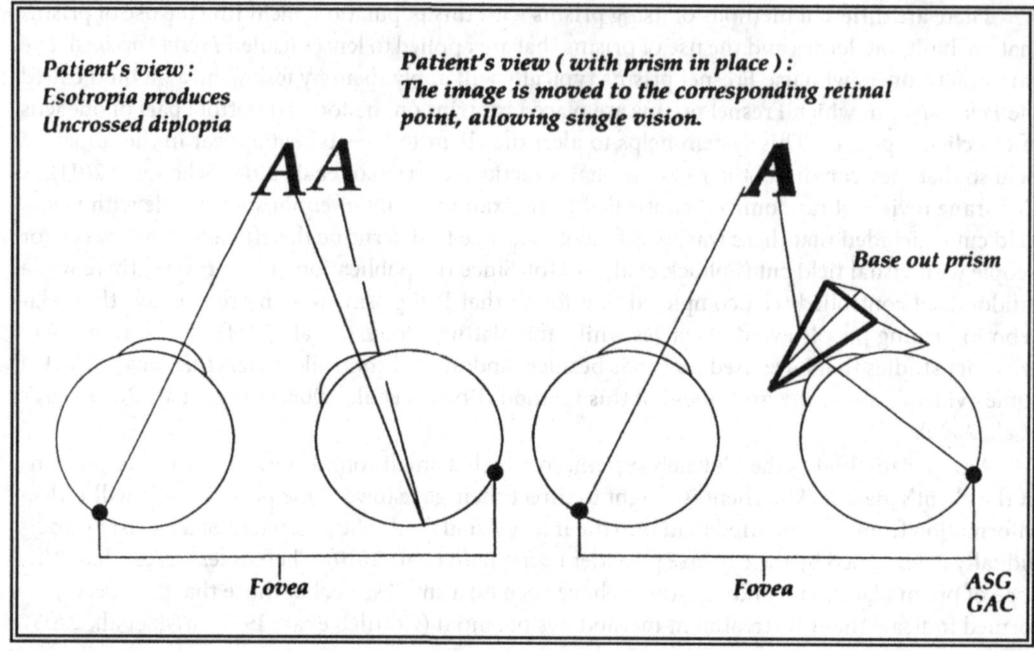

Figure 4-29. Prism use to eliminate diplopia in a client with impaired ocular alignment. (Reproduced with permission from Scheiman, S. [2011]. *Understanding and managing vision deficits: A guide for occupational therapists* [3rd ed.]. SLACK Incorporated.)

An eye care provider can prescribe glasses with prisms ground into the lens, which can be especially helpful in some cases when a client is experiencing diplopia (Greenwald et al., 2012; Hellerstein et al., 2011; Khan et al., 2008; Scheiman, 2011). The prisms will adjust the angle of the image entering the eye to help the visual system fuse the images into one (Figure 4-29). The occupational therapy practitioner's role may include working with the client to use the prisms during functional activity. The clinician should also maintain close communication with the optometrist relating to the effectiveness of the lenses or prisms, the client's comfort level or acceptance of their use, and whether symptoms of oculomotor deficits (e.g., diplopia) improve, remain the same, or worsen (Kaldenberg, 2014). Prisms have been shown to be effective for many clients with diplopia, especially those with vertical diplopia (Gunton & Brown, 2012).

If the client is experiencing diplopia that interferes with ADLs, occlusion may be used (Greenwald et al., 2012; Hellerstein et al., 2011; Khan et al., 2008; Scheiman, 2011; Warren, 2018). This can be accomplished through full occlusion by placing a patch over one eye (Figure 4-30). The patch should be worn on alternating eyes throughout the day to avoid potential weakening of the eye musculature on one eye (Khan et al., 2008). The treatment team should be aware that full occlusion can have a negative impact on the client's balance and orientation to space because it eliminates peripheral vision on one side (Warren, 2018). It can also interfere with depth perception, which is partly dependent on binocular vision (Khan et al., 2008). An alternative to full occlusion is to partially occlude vision. For example, a person with horizontal diplopia may benefit from opaque tape placed over the nasal field of one lens of their eyeglasses to eliminate the diplopia without impacting peripheral vision (Hellerstein et al., 2011; Khan et al., 2008; Warren, 2018). Typically, clients will find this method more comfortable if the occlusion is placed on the nondominant eye. In addition, it is best if the smallest area possible is occluded. In this case, the tape will be placed gradually over an increasingly larger area until the client reports that the diplopia has resolved. Another method for partial occlusion is to place a round disc of tape on one lens

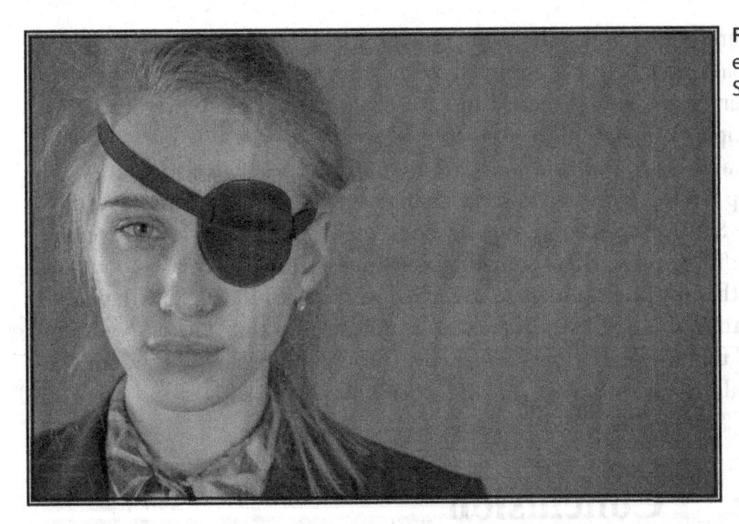

Figure 4-30. Full occlusion of one eye to eliminate diplopia. (galitsin/Shutterstock.com)

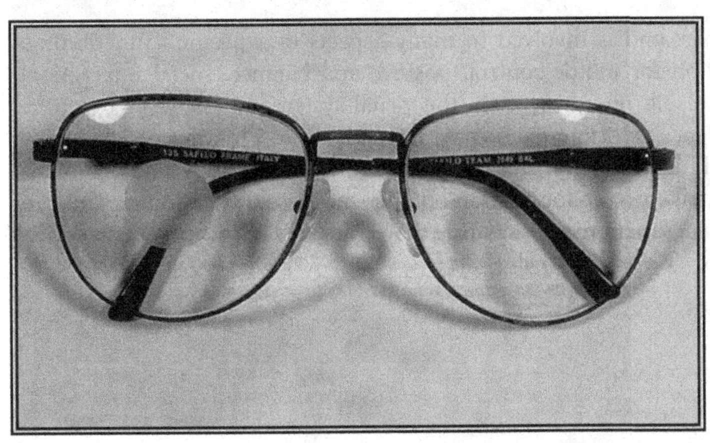

Figure 4-31. Partial occlusion accomplished by placing translucent tape over a portion of the lens on one eye. (Reproduced with permission from Scheiman, S. [2011]. *Understanding and managing vision deficits: A guide for occupational therapists* [3rd ed.]. SLACK Incorporated.)

of the client's glasses, positioning it in the location that best eliminates the diplopia as indicated by the client (Kaldenberg, 2014; Scheiman, 2011; Figure 4-31). As is the case for prisms, occlusion should be applied under the supervision of an eye care provider.

If it is established by the optometrist, ophthalmologist, or vision specialist that the client would benefit from strengthening of the eyes, eye exercises can be initiated. These exercises should be individualized for the client's specific needs and focused on improving functional performance. The occupational therapy practitioner may be involved in implementing these programs, although all exercises should be performed under the supervision of the eye care provider (Warren, 2018). Exercise programs can vary from relatively simple, such as is accomplished through patching one eye to strengthen the other, to complex with exercises that are designed to improve visual motion, such as saccades and/or visual tracking. Complex programs will include multiple exercises, including some that may be completed on a computer, and each treatment session will build on what was accomplished in the last session (Hellerstein et al., 2011; Scheiman, 2011). These exercises can be used to improve ocular alignment and reduce the effects of diplopia (Khan et al., 2008). Visual training has also been shown to improve issues related to convergence insufficiency (Scheiman et al., 2005), accommodative dysfunction (Thiagarajan & Ciuffreda, 2014), reading (Ciuffreda et al., 2006), and other oculomotor control issues (Daugherty et al., 2007). In 2020, an article was published describing a pilot randomized controlled trial examining the impact of 2 protocols for improving oculomotor control on 14 people with TBI who were being treated in inpatient rehabilitation (Berryman et al., 2020). One protocol (Six Eye Exercises) used a bottom-up approach in which participants ($n = 8$) completed 6 eye movement exercises 30 minutes per day 5 days/week. The other protocol (a standard of care protocol) used activity-based eye movement practice with participants ($n = 6$). Both protocols were administered by occupational therapy practitioners. The researchers found that both groups improved but in different ways, with the standard of care group having a greater average change on outcome measures examining oculomotor control and the Six Eye Exercises group having a greater reduction in the average number of symptoms. As a result, the researchers concluded that questions still remain about the best approach for occupational therapy practitioners to use when working with people with oculomotor control deficits (Berryman et al., 2020). More research is indicated for this type of treatment and the role of the occupational therapy practitioner, especially through high-quality randomized controlled trials (Berryman et al., 2020; Pollock et al., 2011a; Scheiman et al., 2011).

Conclusion

The visual system is complex and is involved in many aspects of a person's functioning, contributing essential information for motor control, posture and balance, social interaction, and cognitive processing. As a result, impairments in the visual system, on any level, can have a large negative impact on a client's ability to participate in occupation. This chapter discussed some aspects of a person's visual functioning, including visual acuity, visual fields, and oculomotor control. These visual skills make up the foundation of a person's visual functioning and can influence all other aspects of visual functioning, including the higher-level visual processing skills that are considered in Chapter 5.

References

Adams, E. (2009). *Visual problems in traumatic brain injury: A systematic review of sequelae and interventions for the veteran population*. VA Technology Assessment Program.

Ajina, S., & Kennard C. (2012). Rehabilitation of damage to the visual brain. *Revue Neurologique (Paris), 168*, 754-761. https://doi.org/10.1016/j.neurol.2012.07.015

Aloisio, L. (2004). Visual dysfunction. In G. Gillen & A. Burkhardt (Eds.), *Stroke rehabilitation: A function-based approach* (2nd ed., pp. 338-357). Mosby, Inc.

Anderson, A. J., Shuey, N. H., & Wall, M. (2009). Rapid confrontation screening for peripheral visual field defects and extinction. *Clinical and Experimental Optometry, 92*, 45-48. https://doi.org/10.1111/j.1444-0938.2008.00280.x

Arditi, A., & Cagenello, R. (1993). On the statistical reliability of letter-chart visual acuity measurements. *Investigative Ophthalmology & Visual Science, 34*, 120-129.

Azzam, D., & Ronquillo, Y. (2022, May 8). Snellen chart. StatPearls Publishing. https://ncbi.nlm.nih.gov/books/NBK558961/

Bass, S. J., Cooper, J., Feldman, J., & Horn, D. (2007). Comparison of an automated confrontation testing device versus finger counting in the detection of field loss. *Optometry, 78*, 390-395. https://doi.org/10.1016/j.optm.2006.06.019

Berryman, A., Rasavage, K., & Politzer, T. (2010). Practical clinical treatment strategies for evaluation and treatment of visual field loss and visual inattention. *NeuroRehabilitation, 27*, 261-268. https://doi.org/10.3233/NRE-2010-0607

Berryman, A., Rasavage, K., Politzer, T., & Gerber, D. (2020). Brief report—Oculomotor treatment in traumatic brain injury rehabilitation: A randomized controlled pilot trial. *American Journal of Occupational Therapy, 74*, 7401185050. https://doi.org/10.5014/ajot.2020.026880

Bowers, A. R., Keeney, K., & Peli, E. (2008). Community-based trial of a peripheral prism visual field expansion device for hemianopia. *Archives of Ophthalmology, 126*, 657-664. https://doi.org/10.1001/archopht.126.5.657

Bowers, A. R., Keeney, K., & Peli, E. (2014). Randomized crossover clinical trial of real and sham peripheral prism glasses for hemianopia. *JAMA Ophthalmology, 132*, 214-222. https://doi.org/10.1001/jamaophthalmol.2013.5636

Bryan, V. L., Harrington, D. W., & Elliott, M. G. (2018). Management of residual physical deficits. In M. J. Ashley & D. A. Hovda (Eds.), *Traumatic brain injury: Rehabilitation, treatment, and case management* (4th ed., pp. 541-575). CRC Press.

Bulson, R., Jun, W., & Hayes, J. (2012). Visual symptomatology and referral patterns for Operation Iraqi Freedom and Operation Enduring Freedom veterans with traumatic brain injury. *Journal of Rehabilitative Research and Development, 49*, 1075-1082. https://doi.org/10.1682/JRRD.2011.02.0017

Camparini, M., Cassinari, P., Ferrigno, L., & Macaluso, C. (2001). ETDRS-Fast: Implementing psychophysical adaptive methods to standardized visual acuity measurement with ETDRS charts. *Investigative Ophthalmology & Visual Science, 42*, 1226-1231.

Cate, Y., & Richards, L. (2000). Relationship between performance on tests of basic visual functions and visual-perceptual processing in persons after brain injury. *American Journal of Occupational Therapy, 54*, 326-334. https://doi.org/10.5014/ajot.54.3.326

Chaikitmongkol, V., Nanegrungsunk, O., Patikulsila, D., Ruamviboonsuk, P., & Bressler, N. M. (2018). Repeatability and agreement of visual acuity using the ETDRS number chart, Landolt C chart, or ETDRS alphabet chart in eyes with or without sight-threatening diseases. *JAMA Ophthalmology, 136*, 286-290. https://doi.org/10.1001/jamaophthalmol.2017.6290

Chusid, J. G. (1979). *Correlative neuroanatomy and functional neurology* (17th ed.). Lange Medical Publications.

Ciuffreda, K. J., Han, Y., Kapoor, N., & Suchoff, I. B. (2001). Oculomotor consequences of acquired brain injury. In I. B. Suchoff, K. J. Cuiffreda, & N. Kapoor (Eds.). *Visual and vestibular consequences of acquired brain injury*. Optometric Extension Program, Inc.

Ciuffreda, K. J., Han, Y., Kapoor, N., & Ficarra, A. P. (2006). Oculomotor rehabilitation for reading in acquired brain injury. *NeuroRehabilitation, 21*, 9-21. https://doi.org/10.3233/NRE-2006-21103

Cormican, D. (2004). Seeing the whole picture. *OT Practice, 9*, 14-17.

Daugherty, K. M., Frantz, K. A., Allison, C. L., & Gabriel, H. M. (2007). Evaluating changes in quality of life after vision therapy using the COVD Quality of Life Outcomes Assessment. *Optometry and Vision Development, 38*, 75-81.

Falk, N. S., & Askionoff, E. G. (1992). The primary care optometric evaluation of the traumatic brain injury patient. *Journal of the American Optometric Association*, 63, 547-553.

Felson, D. T., Anderson, J. J., Hannan, M. T., Milton, R. C., Wilson, P. W. F., & Kiel, D. P. (1989). Impaired vision and hip fracture: The Framingham study. *Journal of the American Geriatrics Society, 37*, 494-500. https://doi.org/10.1111/j.1532-5415.1989.tb05678.x

Gianutsos, R., Ramsey, G., & Perlin, R. R. (1988). Rehabilitative optometric services for survivors of acquired brain injury. *Archives of Physical Medicine and Rehabilitation*, 69, 573-579.

Gianutsos, R., & Suchoff, I. (2002). Visual fields after brain injury: Management issues for the occupational therapist. In M. Scheiman (Ed.), *Understanding and managing vision deficits* (2nd ed., pp. 248-262). SLACK Incorporated.

Giorgi, R. G., Woods, R. L., & Peli, E. (2009). Clinical and laboratory evaluation of peripheral prism glasses for hemianopia. *Optometry and Vision Science*, 86, 492-502. https://doi.org/10.1097/OPX.0b013e31819f9e4d

Goodrich, G. L., Flyg, H. M., Kirby, J. E., Chang, C. Y., & Martinsen, G. L. (2013). Mechanisms of TBI and visual consequences in military and veteran populations. *Optometry and Vision Science, 90*, 105-112. https://doi.org/10.1097/OPX.0b013e31827f15a1

Gottlieb, D. D., Freeman, P., & Williams, M. (1992). Clinical research and statistical analysis of a visual field awareness system. *Journal of the American Optometry Association, 63*, 581-588.

Greenwald, B. D., Kapoor, N., & Singh, A. D. (2012). Visual impairments in the first year after traumatic brain injury. *Brain Injury, 26*, 1338-1359. https://doi.org/10.3109/02699052.2012.706356

Grunda, T., Marsalek, P., & Sykorova, P. (2013). Homonymous hemianopia and related visual defects: Restoration of vision after a stroke. *Acta Neurobiologiae Experimentalis, 73*, 237-249.

Gunton, K. B., & Brown, A. (2012). Prism use in adult diplopia. *Current Opinions in Ophthalmology, 23*, 400-404. https://doi.org/10.1097/ICU.0b013e3283567276

Hellerstein, L., & Freed, S. (1994). Rehabilitative optometric management of a traumatic brain injury patient. *Journal of Behavioral Optometry, 5*, 143-147.

Hellerstein, L. F., Scheiman, M., Fishman, B. I., & Whittaker, S. G. (2011). Visual rehabilitation for patients with brain injury. In M. Scheiman (Ed.), *Understanding and managing vision deficits. A guide for occupational therapists* (3rd ed., pp. 201-232). SLACK Incorporated.

International Council of Ophthalmology. (1984). Visual acuity measurement standard. http://www.icoph.org/resources/47/visual-acuity-measurement-standard.html

Ivars, R. Q., Cumming, R. G., Mitchell, P., Simpson, J. M., & Peduto, A. J. (2003). Visual risk factors for hip fracture in older people. *Journal of the American Geriatric Society, 51*, 356-363. https://doi.org/10.1046/j.1532-5415.2003.51109.x

Jacobs, S. M., & Van Stavern, G. P. (2013). Neuro-ophthalmic deficits after head trauma. *Current Neurology and Neuroscience Reports, 13*, 389. https://doi.org/10.1007/s11910-013-0389-5

Kaldenberg, J. (2014). Optimizing vision and visual processing. In M. V. Radomski & C. A. Trombly Latham (Eds.), *Occupational therapy for physical dysfunction* (7th ed., pp. 699-724). Lippincott Williams & Wilkins.

Kapoor, N. (2012). *Photosensitivity following traumatic brain injury*. International Brain Injury Association.

Kerr, N. M., Chew, S. S. L., Eady, E. K., Gamble, G. D., & Danesh-Meyer, H. V. (2010). Diagnostic accuracy of confrontation visual field tests. *Neurology, 74*, 1184-1190. https://doi.org/10.1212/WNL.0b013e3181d90017

Khan, S., Leung, E., & Jay, W. M. (2008). Stroke and visual rehabilitation. *Topics in Stroke Rehabilitation, 15*, 27-36.

Luu, S., Lee, A. W., Daly, A., & Chen, C. S. (2010). Visual field defects after stroke. A practical guide for GPs. *Australian Family Physician, 39*, 499-503.

Magone, M. T., Kwon, E., & Shin, S. Y. (2014). Chronic visual dysfunction after blast-induced mild traumatic brain injury. *Journal of Rehabilitative Research and Development, 51*, 71-80. https://doi.org/10.1682/JRRD.2013.01.0008

Maples, W. C. (1995). *NSUCO oculomotor test manual.* Optometric Extension Program Foundation.

Maples, W. C. (2000). Test-retest reliability of the College of Optometrists in Vision Development Quality of Life Outcomes Assessment. *Optometry, 71*, 579-85.

Maples, W. C., Atchley, J., & Ficklin, T. (1992). Northeastern State University College of Optometry's oculomotor norms. *Journal of Behavioral Optometry, 3*, 143-150.

Maples, W. C., & Ficklin, T. W. (1988). Interrater and test-retest reliability of pursuits and saccades. *Journal of the American Optometric Association, 59*(7), 549-552.

Maples, W. C., & Ficklin, T. (1989). A preliminary study of the oculomotor skills of learning-disabled, gifted and normal children. *Journal of Optometry and Vision Development, 20*, 9-14.

Maples, W. C., & Ficklin, T. (1990). Comparison of eye movement skills between above and below average readers. *Journal of Behavioral Optometry, 1*, 87-91.

Morton, R. L. (2004). Visual dysfunction following traumatic brain injury. In M. J. Ashley (Ed.), *Traumatic brain injury rehabilitative treatment and case management* (pp. 183-207). CRC Press.

Niemeier, J. P. (2010). Neuropsychological assessment for visually impaired persons with traumatic brain injury. *NeuroRehabilitation, 27*, 275-283. https://doi.org/10.3233/NRE-2010-0609

O'Dell, M. W., Bell, K. R., & Sandel, M. E. (1998). Medical rehabilitation of brain injury AAPMR study guide in brain injury rehabilitation. *Archives of Physical Medicine and Rehabilitation, 79*, S10-S15. https://doi.org/10.1016/S0003-9993(98)90114-9

Padula, W. V., & Argyris, S. (1996). Post trauma vision syndrome and visual midline shift syndrome. *NeuroRehabiltation, 6*, 165-171. https://doi.org/10.3233/NRE-1996-6302

Padula, W. V., Argyris, S., & Ray, J. (1994). Visual evoked potentials: evaluating treatment for post-trauma vision syndrome in patients with traumatic brain injuries. *Brain Injury, 8*(2), 125-133.

Padula, W. V., & Shapiro, J. (1993). Head injury and the post-trauma vision syndrome. *Review: Rehabilitation and Education for Blindness and Visual Impairment, 24*, 153-158.

Pollock, A., Hazelton, C., Henderson, C. A., Angilley, J., Dhillon, B., Langhorne, P., Livingstone, K., Munro, F. A., Orr, H., Rowe, F. J., & Shahani, U. (2011a). Interventions for disorders of eye movement in patients with stroke. *Cochrane Database of Systematic Reviews, 2011*(10). https://doi.org/10.1002/14651858.CD008389.pub2

Pollock, A., Hazelton, C., Henderson, C.A., Angilley, J., Dhillon, B., Langhorne, P., Livingstone, K., Munro, F. A., Orr, H., Rowe, F. J., & Shahani, U. (2011b). Interventions for visual field defects in patients with stroke. *Cochrane Database of Systematic Reviews, 2011*(10). https://doi.org/10.1002/14651858.CD008388.pub2

Powell, J. M., Birk, K., Cummings, E. H., & Ciol, M. A. (2005). The need for adult norms on the Developmental Eye Movement Test (DEM). *Journal of Behavioral Optometry, 16*, 38-41.

Powell, J. M., Fan, M., Kiltz, P. J., Bergman, A. T., & Richman, J. (2006). A comparison of the Developmental Eye Movement Test (DEM) and the modified version of the Adult Developmental Eye Movement Test (A-DEM) with older adults. *Journal of Behavioral Optometry, 17*, 59-64.

Powell, J. M., & Togerson, N. G. (2011). Evaluation and treatment of vision and motor dysfunction following acquired brain injury from occupational and neuro-optometry perspectives. In P. S. Suter & L. H. Harvey (Eds.), *Vision rehabilitation: Multidisciplinary care of the patient following brain injury* (pp. 351-396). CRC Press.

Radomski, M. V., Finkelstein, M., Llanos, I., Scheiman, M., & Wagener, S. G. (2014). Composition of a vision screen for servicemembers with traumatic brain injury: Consensus using a modified nominal group technique. *American Journal of Occupational Therapy, 68*, 422-429. https://doi.org/10.5014/ajot.2014.011445

Richman, J. E. (2009). *The Developmental Eye Movement Test. Version 2.0 2009 manual.* Bernell Corporation.

Sampedro, A. G., Richman, J. E., & Pardo, M. S. (2003). The Adult Developmental Eye Movement Test (A-DEM). *Journal of Behavioral Optometry, 14*, 101-105.

Sanet, R. B., & Press, L. J. (2011). Spatial vision. In P. S. Suter & L. H. Harvey (Eds.), *Vision rehabilitation: Multidisciplinary care of the patient following brain injury* (pp. 77-151). CRC Press.

Scheiman, M. (2011). *Understanding and managing vision deficits A guide for occupational therapists* (3rd ed.). SLACK Incorporated.

Scheiman, M., Gwiazda, J., & Li, T. (2011). Non-surgical interventions for convergence insufficiency. *Cochrane Database of Systematic Reviews, 2011*(3). https://doi.org/10.1002/14651858.CD006768.pub2

Scheiman, M., Mitchell, G. L., Cotter, S., Kulp, M. T., Cooper, J. Rouse, M., Borsting, E., London, R., & Wensveen, J. (2005). A randomized clinical trial of vision therapy/orthoptics versus pencil pushups for the treatment of convergence insufficiency in young adults. *Optometry and Vision Science, 82*, E583-E595. https://doi.org/10.1097/01.opx.0000171331.36871.2f

Schlageter, K., Gray, B., Hall, K., Shaw, R., & Sammet, R. (1993). Incidence and treatment of visual dysfunction in traumatic brain injury. *Brain Injury, 7*, 439-448. https://doi.org/10.3109/02699059309029687

Schneck, M. E., Haegerstom-Portnoy, G., Lott, L. A. & Brabyn, J. A. (2010). Monocular vs. binocular measurement of spatial vision in elders. *Optometry and Vision Science, 87*, 526-531. https://doi.org/10.1097/OPX.0b013e3181e61a88

Stifter, E., König, F., Lang, T., Bauer, P., Richter-Müksch, S., Velikay-Parel, M., & Radner, W. (2004). Reliability of a standardized reaching chart system: Variance component analysis, test-retest and inter-chart reliability. *Graefe's Archive for Clinical and Experimental Ophthalmology, 242*, 31-39. https://doi.org/10.1007/s00417-003-0776-8

Suter, P. S. (2018). Rehabilitation and management of visual dysfunction following traumatic brain injury. In M. J. Ashley & D. A. Hovda (Eds.), *Traumatic brain injury: Rehabilitation, treatment, and case management* (4th ed., pp. 451-486). CRC Press.

Szlyk, J. P., Seiple, W., Stelmack, J., & McMahon, T. (2005). Use of prisms for navigation and driving in hemianopic patients. *Ophthalmic and Physiological Optics, 25*, 128-135. https://doi.org/10.1111/j.1475-1313.2004.00265.x

Teller, D. Y., McDonald, M. A., Preston, K., Sebris, S. L., & Dobson, V. (1986). Assessment of visual acuity in infants and children: The acuity card procedure. *Developmental Medicine and Child Neurology, 28*, 779-798. https://doi.org/10.1111/j.1469-8749.1986.tb03932.x

Thiagarajan, P., & Ciuffreda, K. J. (2014). Effect of oculomotor rehabilitation on accommodative responsivity in mild traumatic brain injury. *Journal of Rehabilitation Research and Development, 51*, 175-192. https://doi.org/10.1682/JRRD.2013.01.0027

Toglia, J. P. (1991). Generalization of treatment: A multicontext approach to cognitive perceptual impairment in adults with brain injury. *American Journal of Occupational Therapy, 45*, 505-516. https://doi.org/10.5014/ajot.45.6.505

Toglia, J. P. (2018). The dynamic interactional model and the multicontext approach. In N. Katz & J. Toglia (Eds.), *Cognition, occupation, and participation across the life span: Neuroscience, neurorehabilitation, and models of intervention in occupational therapy* (4th ed., pp. 355-385). AOTA Press.

Townend, B. S., Sturm, J. W., Petsoglou, C., O'Leary, B., Whyte, S., & Crimmins, D. (2007). Perimetric homonymous visual field loss post-stroke. *Journal of Clinical Neuroscience, 14*, 754-756. https://doi.org/10.1016/j.jocn.2006.02.022

Vision in Preschoolers Study Group. (2003). Visual acuity results in school-aged children and adults: Lea Symbols Chart versus Bailey-Lovie Chart. *Optometry and Vision Science, 80*, 650-654. https://doi.org/10.1097/00006324-200309000-00010

Wagener, S. G., Anheluk, M., Arulanantham, C., & Scheiman, M. (2015). Vision assessment and intervention. In M. Weightman, M. V. Radomski, P. A. Mashima, & C. R. Roth (Eds.), *Mild traumatic brain injury rehabilitation toolkit* (pp. 97-146). Borden Institute.

Warren, M. (1993a). A hierarchical model for evaluation and treatment of visual perceptual dysfunction in adult acquired brain injury, part 1. *American Journal of Occupational Therapy, 47*, 42-54. https://doi.org/10.5014/ajot.47.1.42

Warren, M. (1993b). A hierarchical model for evaluation and treatment of visual perceptual dysfunction in adult acquired brain injury, part 2. *American Journal of Occupational Therapy, 47*, 55-65. https://doi.org/10.5014/ajot.47.1.55

Warren, M. (1994). Visuospatial skills: Assessment and intervention strategies. In *AOTA Self Study Series: Cognitive Rehabilitation*. American Occupational Therapy Association.

Warren, M. (1998). *Brain Injury Assessment Battery for Adults: Test manual.* VisAbilities Rehab Services Inc.

Warren, M. (2018). Evaluation and treatment of visual deficits after brain injury. In H. M. Pendleton & W. Schultz-Krohn (Eds.), *Pedretti's occupational therapy: Practice skills for physical dysfunction* (8th ed., pp. 594-630). Elsevier.

Weisser-Pike, O. (2014). Assessing abilities and capacities: Vision and visual processing. In M. V. Radomski & C. A. Trombly Latham (Eds.), *Occupational therapy for physical dysfunction* (7th ed., pp. 103-120). Lippincott Williams & Wilkins.

Whyte, J., & DiPasquale, M. C. (1995). Assessment of vision and visual attention in minimally responsive brain injured patients. *Archives of Physical Medicine and Rehabilitation, 76*, 804-810. https://doi.org/10.1016/S0003-9993(95)80543-5

CHAPTER 5

Assessment and Treatment of Visual Perception

Perception is the process by which sensory information is analyzed and interpreted by the brain (Phipps, 2018). Perception of sensory information is influenced by numerous factors, including cognition, motor ability (which affects the way the person is able to gather and act on sensory input), and information from other sensory systems (Colarusso & Hammill, 2003; Warren, 2018). People with intact perception are able to analyze, interpret, and use sensory information to inform decision making and interactions with the world around them (Scheiman, 2011a). Using visual perception as an example, a person with intact visual perception is able to identify objects that are seen (even from multiple angles), pick out objects from their background, judge the distance between objects in space (including oneself), and more (Colarusso & Hammill, 2003; Phipps, 2018). As a result of these complex processes and the interconnection between numerous areas of the brain, damage to many places in the brain can result in a disruption in the ability to accurately process sensory information (Warren, 2018). Deficits in perception are correlated with less independence with activities of daily living (ADLs), decreased safety, and lessened quality of life (Brown & Elliott, 2011; Brown et al., 2013; Cate & Richards, 2000; Cooke et al., 2005; Phipps, 2018; Su et al., 2000). This chapter focuses primarily on visual perception, although the perception of other senses is included to some degree.

Visual Perception

Visual perceptual skills can be classified into three main categories: visual analysis, visuospatial, and visual motor integration (Scheiman, 2011b). The first category, visual analysis, includes skills needed for object identification. These skills include object constancy (i.e., the recognition of objects when seen from different angles); visual discrimination (i.e., the ability to identify different features of objects, such as shape, color, or texture); figure ground, which entails distinguishing an object from its background; and form closure, which is needed to identify an object when it is partially obscured (Scheiman, 2011b).

Kaminsky, T. A., & Powell, J. M.
Zoltan's Vision, Perception, and Cognition: Evaluation and Treatment of the Adult With Acquired Brain Injury, Fifth Edition (pp. 105-132).

The second category of visual perception includes visuospatial skills, which enable a person to judge position in space. Several skills are included in this category. One is the ability to determine the position of one's own body in space and one's distance from items in the environment. Another skill is the ability to identify different directions (e.g., right, left, up, down). The ability to judge the position of objects in relation to each other is also included in this category (Cooke et al., 2005; Phipps, 2018; Scheiman, 2011b).

The third major category of visual perception is visual motor integration. This aspect of visual perception "enables an individual to coordinate visual stimuli with the corresponding motor action in a timely and skillful manner" (Brown et al., 2013, p. 18). It is what enables people to use their vision to guide motor movement, as is needed for tasks requiring eye–hand coordination (Scheiman, 2011b). In this category is constructional ability, when the person is able to combine visual and motor skills to assemble parts into a whole, including in two dimensions (e.g., drawing or writing) and three dimensions (e.g., building a model; Cooke et al., 2005). The specific skills in these three categories are discussed in further detail later in this chapter.

Visual perceptual dysfunction has been reported to be relatively common after acquired brain injury (ABI) for both people with traumatic brain injury (TBI; McKenna et al., 2006) and a cerebrovascular accident (CVA; Paolucci et al., 2009). Incidence depends on the type of perceptual deficit being considered with inattention to a portion of visual space (discussed in Chapter 6), often the most frequently reported perceptual deficit after ABI (McKenna et al., 2006; Paolucci et al., 2009). One study found that body scheme disorders (described in more detail later in this chapter) and constructional skill deficits were also relatively common in a sample of people with severe TBI, with approximately 25% of the participants experiencing these issues (McKenna et al., 2006). Another group of researchers found similar prevalence of visual constructional deficits in a sample with CVAs (Paolucci et al., 2009), although body scheme disorders were rarer for these participants. Visual agnosia, which is an inability to identify objects through vision alone (Hellerstein & Scheiman, 2011), is reported to be rare for people with ABI, although survivors may have difficulty with some of the skills that contribute to object identification, such as form constancy, figure ground, or visual closure (Hellerstein & Scheiman, 2011; McKenna et al., 2006; Paolucci et al., 2009).

Visual perceptual deficits are reported to be more common if the parietal and/or occipital lobes are damaged by ABI (Hellerstein & Scheiman, 2011), although damage in the temporal lobe can also result in visual perceptual deficits, especially with reading ability (Laatsch & Krisky, 2006). The literature is mixed when reporting on the relationship between laterality (which side of the brain is affected) and visual perceptual deficits. Most researchers reported an increase in visual perceptual deficits when the right hemisphere was damaged (Cooke et al., 2005; McKenna et al., 2006; Phipps, 2018), although certain perceptual skills seem to be more commonly affected with damage to the left hemisphere. This includes figure ground (Colarusso & Hammill, 2003), but different research studies report varying results (McKenna et al., 2006; Su et al., 2000).

Although we know that damage to certain areas of the brain typically results in visual perceptual deficits, the brain processes that enable people to accurately understand visual input based on a two-dimensional image on the retina and respond effectively in the highly variable and complex three-dimensional world are not well understood. Our conscious experience leads us to believe that what we understand (perceive) is the same as what our eyes see, but that is not the case. For example, any object (e.g., a person) viewed from further away results in a smaller image on the retina; yet, our perception is that the person (or other object) is the same size whether they are next to us, across the room, or seen at a distance. Interestingly, these types of perceptual judgments break down in situations in which the viewing distance is much greater than that found in nature (e.g., when looking down at the street below from a tall building, we are often struck by how small the people and cars look). It is also possible for two (or more) objects of different sizes (e.g.,

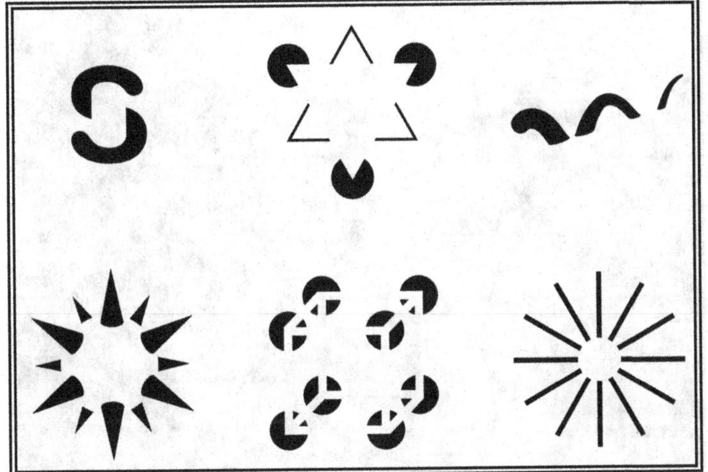

Figure 5-1. Figures illustrating the Gestalt idea that "the whole is something else than the sum of its parts" (Koffka, 1935, p. 176). In each of these images, we perceive forms that result from the arrangement of the individual segments or parts but are not actually present. (Peter Hermes Furian/shutterstock.com)

a chopstick and a vaulting pole) if positioned in just the right way and at just the right distance to result in a line of exactly the same length and diameter on the retina (Anderson & Stufflebeam, 2006); yet, we recognize one as a tool for a person to eat with and the other as a tool to propel a person through space. Furthermore, we are able to recognize objects even when the two-dimensional image on the retina is incomplete (i.e., ambiguous; Rust & Stocker, 2010). In everyday life, this might occur because another object is in the way and blocking part of our view, when the object is blurred as when seen through a fogged-up window, or when an object is too far away for the details to be seen clearly. We are also able to recognize objects as the same (i.e., invariant) when the two-dimensional image is different (e.g., when an object is viewed from two different angles).

Over the years, there have been multiple theories that have attempted to explain how visual perception works. None of the theories that have been proposed to date are viewed as fully explaining the process of visual perception. However, we briefly cover two key theories here to give the reader a basic understanding of some of the ways that vision scientists and others have attempted to better understand the complex process of visual perception.

The Gestalt theorists were a group of German psychologists who studied the question of perceptual organization in the early 1900s (Goldstein & Brockmole, 2017; Palmer, 1999; Wagemans, Elder, et al., 2012; Wagemans, Feldman, et al., 2012). Gestalt is a German word whose meaning in English in this context is often described as "whole form" or "configuration." An earlier theory of visual perception called *structuralism* proposed that the brain created perceptions by simply adding up and layering a series of sensations to result in a whole that was the sum of the individual parts. In contrast, the Gestalt theorists suggested that "the whole is something else than the sum of its parts" (Koffka, 1935, p. 176). Figure 5-1 contains several images that demonstrate this. Consider the top middle figure as an example. In this image, we perceive a white triangle in front of a triangle outlined in black and three black circles. However, the white triangle is not actually present in the drawing, and we can only see parts of the circles and the other triangle. It is only in our mind, in our perception, that the shapes exist. The photograph in Figure 5-2 of Drumheller Fountain on the University of Washington Seattle campus with Mount Rainier in the background is another example. There are many elements in this image that are only partially in view—the two people on the far left behind the bush, parts of the fountain spray behind some of the people, the light pole on the far right, most of the trees, and the mountain itself—and yet we do not see those as partial unrecognizable forms but rather as compete, familiar objects.

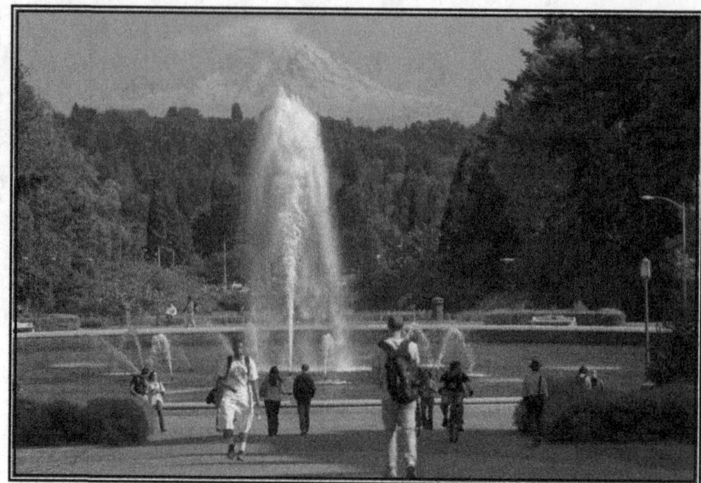

Figure 5-2. The many partial images that make up this campus scene are perceived as complete images in another example of "the whole is something more than the sum of its parts" (Koffka, 1935, p. 176) (Reproduced with permission from Doug Plummer for University of Washington.)

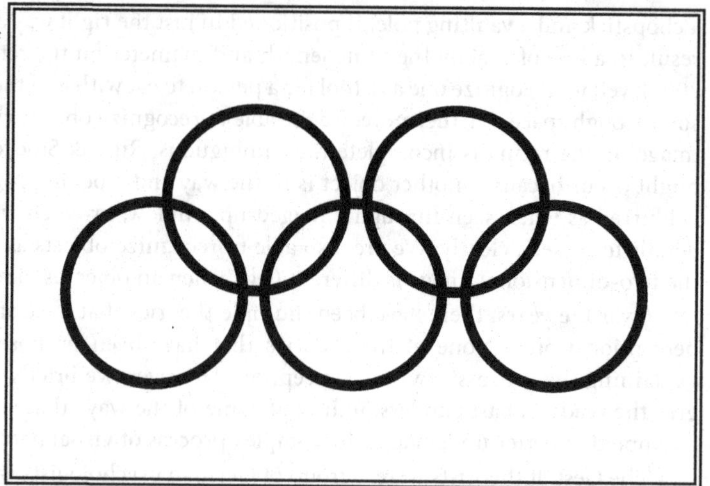

Figure 5-3. These overlapping rings are an example of the law of prägnanz, the overarching Gestalt principle that people perceive visual stimuli in as simple a way as possible.

The Gestalt theorists proposed a number of principles that they called the *laws of perceptual organization* to explain how humans perceive objects by grouping similar elements, recognizing patterns, and simplifying complex images (Goldstein & Brockmole, 2017). Although these principles were first identified using simple geometric designs and are often illustrated by those types of examples, the principles apply to experiences in our everyday lives as well.

One of the central Gestalt principles is the *law of prägnanz* (Goldstein & Brockmole, 2017). This principle states that visual stimuli are perceived in as simple a way as possible. For example, we perceive the image in Figure 5-3 as five overlapping circles rather than a set of nine more complex shapes.

A second Gestalt principle is the *law of similarity* (Goldstein & Brockmole, 2017). This principle says that similar things are perceived as being grouped together. For example, in Figure 5-4, people typically see three rows of filled circles and three rows of unfilled circles rather than six columns made up of alternating empty and filled circles.

Another Gestalt principle is the *law of good continuation* (Goldstein & Brockmole, 2017). As seen in Figure 5-5, this principle states that straight or smoothly curving lines are perceived as belonging together with the lines following the smoothest path. Other Gestalt principles include

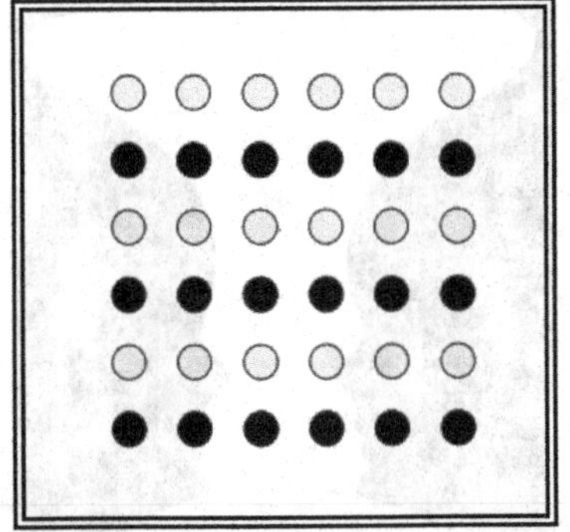

Figure 5-4. An example of the law of similarity. Per this Gestalt principle, similar visual stimuli (e.g., the filled and unfilled circles) are perceived as being grouped together.

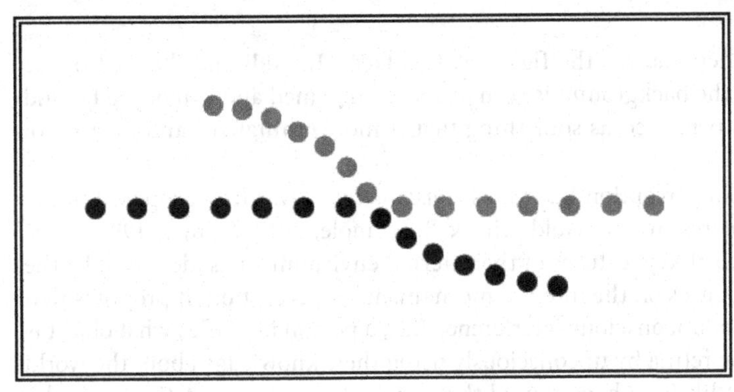

Figure 5-5. An example of the law of continuity. The gray and black dots that make up the curved line and the gray and black dots that make up the straight line are perceived as belonging together (i.e., continuing the curved and the straight lines) rather than as two combined curved and straight lines of the same color. (Courtesy of UserTesting, Inc.)

the law of proximity, *the law of common region*, *the law of synchrony*, and *the law of common fate*, which state, respectively, that things that are near each other, those within the same region of space, those that occur at the same time, and those that are moving in the same direction appear to be grouped together (Goldstein & Brockmole, 2017).

Although the Gestalt theorists first proposed their ideas more than 100 hundred years ago, the Gestalt principles are still seen as having an important contribution to our understanding of visual perception (Goldstein & Brockmole, 2017; Wagemans, Elder, et al., 2012; Wagemans, Feldman, et al., 2012). In recent years, scientists have been exploring ways to quantify the various Gestalt principles to address criticism that they only provide qualitative descriptions that are not specific enough to fully explain the process of visual perception (Jäkel et al., 2016; Wagemans, Elder, et al., 2012; Wagemans, Feldman, et al., 2012).

The Gestalt psychologists were also interested in how we perceive objects to be separate from one another. This is referred to as *figure–ground separation* because an object of interest is often perceived as a figure that is distinct from whatever is making up the background (Goldstein & Brockmole, 2017). Gestalt psychologists used reversible figure–ground patterns in which the figure and the background tend to alternate rather than stay stable as is typical in natural environments as one way to understand this category of perception. An example of this type of pattern is the reversible face–vase image in Figure 5-6, which can be perceived either as one vase or two faces. Studying these types of images helped the Gestalt psychologists clarify several key distinctions between what we tend to perceive as the figure, or object of interest, and what is seen as the background. One key feature is that the shared contour or border that separates the figure from the background is perceived as belonging to the figure. Thus, when you perceive the figure as a vase, the contour or border between the vase and the faces is seen as belonging to the vase rather

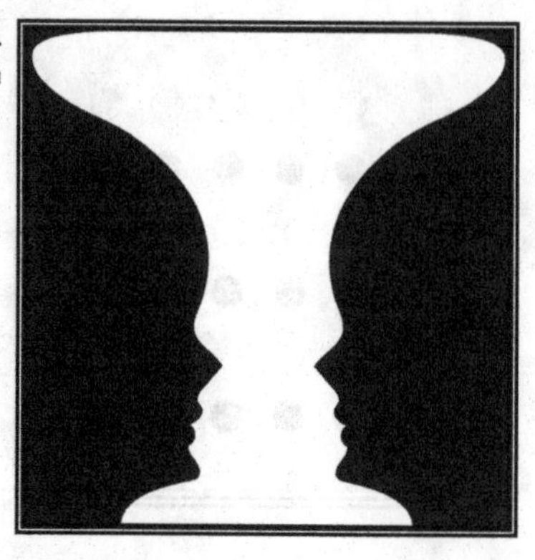

Figure 5-6. Rubin's vase, an example of a reversible figure–ground pattern. In this image, people are able to see either two faces or a vase, but not both at the same time. (Mochalu/shutterstock.com)

than the faces and vice versa when you see the figure as two faces. In addition, the part of the image that is being perceived as the background is seen as more unformed and extending behind the figure, whereas the figure is perceived as something that is more "thinglike" and in front of the background.

A second key theory of visual perception known as *constructivism* was first proposed in the 18th century and remains of interest today (Goldstein & Brockmole, 2017; Palmer, 1999). This theory recognizes the importance of key features of the external environment as identified by the Gestalt theorists but primarily focuses on the internal mechanisms of perception. It proposes that perception is based on a process of unconscious interference (i.e., a person identifies what object is causing a particular image on the retina by unconsciously using their knowledge about the world to figure out what object is most likely to have caused that particular pattern of retinal stimulation). In recent years, a statistical approach called the *Bayesian decision theory* has been used to explore how mathematical models could be used to determine the probability of a particular visual perceptual conclusion being accurate (Feldman, 2015; Mamassian et al., 2002; Wagemans, Feldman, et al., 2012).

Although our understanding of the process of visual perception is still evolving, one essential thing to remember in working with clients with visual perceptual impairments is that the basic visual skills of acuity, fields, and oculomotor control must be assessed first (Cate & Richards, 2000; Scheiman, 2011b). Deficits in these foundational visual skills are very common after ABI (Bulson et al., 2012; Goodrich et al., 2013; Khan et al., 2008; Magone et al., 2014) and can have a sizable impact on visual perception (Cate & Richards, 2000). Without intact functioning of these foundational skills, a person will not receive accurate visual information, which can lead to difficulty with accurately processing visual information (Cate & Richards, 2000; Scheiman, 2011b; Warren, 2018). The reader is referred to Chapters 3 and 4 for more details.

It is also important to consider a person's perceptual and cognitive abilities after ABI in relation to their preinjury capabilities. There is some normal variation among people without a brain injury on many of these skills. For example, many of you may know of someone (including, perhaps, yourself) who has difficulty telling right from left or who has difficulty finding their way even on frequently traveled routes. This information is best gathered through interviewing the client or close family and friends because there are rarely standardized test results available from before the brain injury.

Visual Analysis Skills and Deficits

Form, or Visual, Discrimination

The ability to distinguish different aspects of objects, which is called *form*, or *visual, discrimination*, is important for successful interaction with the environment and plays a primary role in human visual perception (Bryan, 2004). It is essential for visual recognition of objects, visually guided movement and interaction with objects (e.g., reaching for a cup), and navigation within the environment. There are many aspects of objects that need to be distinguished, including color, shape, size, weight, construction (what the object is made of), and texture, in addition to determining the object's function (Ashley et al., 2018). This is accomplished through interconnections with multiple visual areas in the brain (Ashley et al., 2018), but deficits appear most commonly after parietal and temporal lobe damage (Gulyas et al., 1994). A disorder in form perception involves an inability to attend to subtle variations in form. This, in turn, will affect the client's ability to recognize common objects. For example, the client may mistake a water pitcher for a plastic urinal or a button for a nickel.

Figure Ground

As described previously, figure–ground perception involves the ability to distinguish the foreground from the background, which is necessary to visually separate an object of interest from the items that surround it. That object of interest (i.e., the foreground) captures the individual's attention, with any other items in the visual scene forming a more vaguely perceived background (Bryan, 2004; Hellerstein & Scheiman, 2011). The separation of figures from their background is accomplished, in part, through differences in visual cues, such as color, luminance, depth, orientation, texture, motion, and perception of shadows, that assist in distinguishing edges (Fahle, 1993).

The assessments used by occupational therapy practitioners to identify figure–ground deficits often rely on paper/pencil tasks in which the person being assessed is asked to find a particular shape (e.g., a triangle) in an array of overlapping shapes. However, figure–ground perception is essential to effective everyday function. Figure ground enables people to locate objects that are not well defined from the background (Driver et al., 1992) and also contributes information on the layout of the visual scene (Bernspang et al., 1987). Therefore, a figure–ground deficit will negatively impact occupational performance. For example, the client with a figure–ground deficit may have difficulty finding desired items in a cluttered drawer (Figure 5-7).

Form Constancy

Form constancy refers to the ability to identify an object, even when it is not identical to prior viewings, such as can happen if the object is a different size or seen from another angle (Hellerstein & Scheiman, 2011; Phipps, 2018). For example, examine Figure 5-8. A person with intact form constancy will be able to recognize that the same car is illustrated in each picture even though it is shown from multiple viewpoints (i.e., from the front, back, each side, and above). However, someone with a deficit in form constancy will not be able to recognize an object unless it looks exactly the same as it has looked before, which makes object recognition difficult.

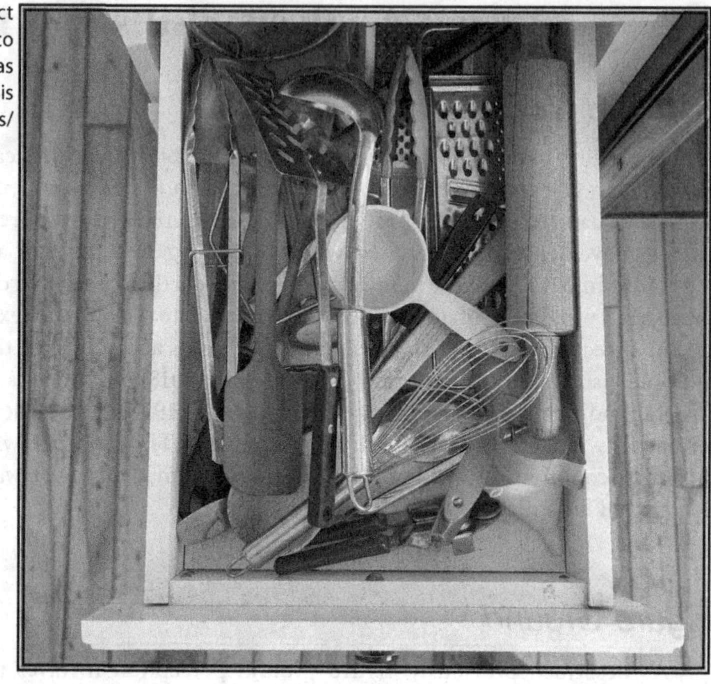

Figure 5-7. A person with intact figure ground would be able to locate individual objects, such as the ladle or the can opener, in this cluttered drawer. (Graham Hughes/shutterstock.com)

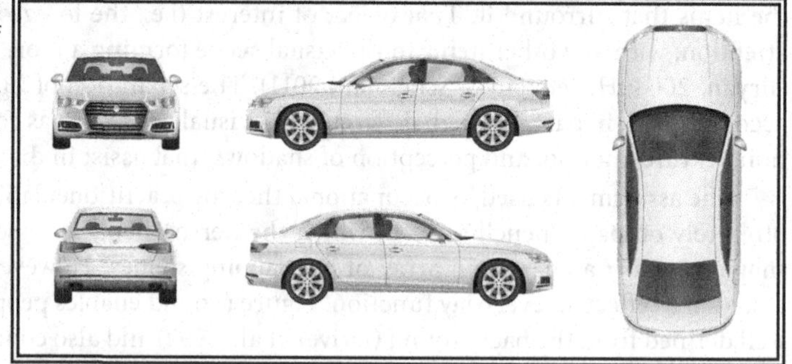

Figure 5-8. A person with intact form constancy would recognize that all of the images are of the same car even though they are taken from a variety of angles. (Yuri Schmidt/shutterstock.com)

Visual, or Perceptual, Closure

Visual, or perceptual, closure is a process that allows us to complete images when only some of the visual information is available (Wagemans, Elder, et al., 2012). This can include the ability to identify partially seen shapes as well as objects. A person with a deficit in this area will have difficulty with identifying an object that is partially obscured, such as if a spoon is partially covered by a napkin (Figure 5-9). Deficits of visual closure are more likely to occur with damage to the right cerebral hemisphere, especially the parietal lobe (Lezak et al., 2012), and appear to be less common than other perceptual deficits.

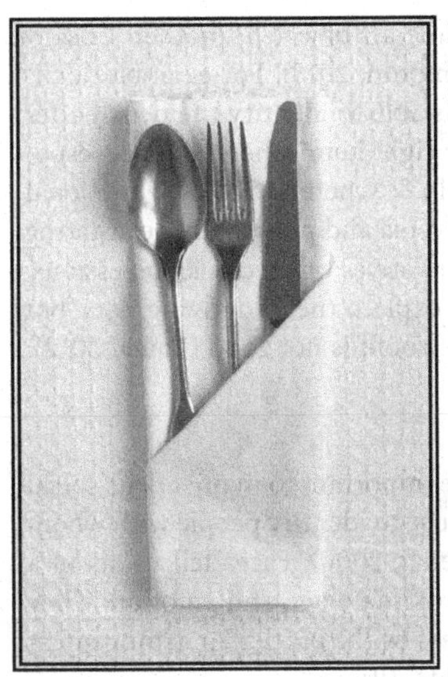

Figure 5-9. A person with intact visual closure would be able to identify the utensils even though they are partially covered by the napkin. (Ev Thomas/shutterstock.com)

Agnosia

Agnosia refers to a client's inability to recognize familiar objects perceived by the senses. Although relatively rare, agnosia can occur in clients who have sustained ABI. The brain damage that results in agnosia is usually diffuse and posterior (Devinsky & D'Esposito, 2004). Agnosia can occur in any sensory system and result in an inability to identify objects when information is only received through the impacted type of sensation. For example, a person with visual agnosia will be unable to recognize an object simply by looking at it. Object recognition and identification in this case will rely on information from other sensory systems (e.g., tactile, auditory, olfactory; De Renzi, 2000).

Agnosia is typically described as encompassing two types of deficits: associative and apperceptive agnosia (Banich & Compton, 2018; Bauer, 2012; De Renzi, 2000; Devinsky & D'Esposito, 2004), a distinction first made by Lissauer in 1890 (Lezak et al., 2012). In both of these types of agnosia, an individual is unable to recognize a stimulus as a whole despite being able to perceive various elements (e.g., shape, color, and texture in visual agnosia or frequency, pitch, and timbre in auditory agnosia; Lezak et al., 2012). However, there is a basic difference between these two types of agnosia in the underlying mechanism that results in impaired recognition. The lack of recognition in associative agnosia results from problems with retrieving knowledge about the stimulus from memory. In contrast, apperceptive agnosia is thought to be an issue with perceptual integration of the various aspects of the stimulus (Lezak et al., 2012).

Visual Agnosia

Visual agnosia refers to several different types of visual recognition and visual perception disorders. In general, visual agnosia refers to the inability to visually recognize items despite adequate functioning in visual skills, such as acuity, oculomotor function, and visual fields (Banich & Compton, 2018; Bauer, 2012; Devinsky & D'Esposito, 2004). Visual agnosia can be category specific with identification deficits for some categories of objects but not for others (Dixon, 2000). For example, prosopagnosia (described further later in this chapter) is a specific type of visual agnosia in which an individual is unable to visually identify faces.

The client with visual agnosia will typically be able to name an object if another sensory modality is used for identification (Aloisio, 2004; Banich & Compton, 2018). For example, a client may be unable to recognize a pencil when looking at it but is able to identify the pencil after touching and handling it. Visual agnosia is more common after right hemisphere damage, especially if the parietal and/or occipital lobes are involved (Hellerstein & Scheiman, 2011). Functional impairments that can occur as the result of visual agnosia are diverse and potentially devastating to the client. For example, the client can fail to recognize close relatives or precious possessions. When confronted with these deficits, clients may not be able to explain the underlying issue but instead say they need new glasses or complain the lighting in the room is not good (Bauer, 2012).

Prosopagnosia

The human face and our ability to read facial expressions are important to many of our social interactions and communication. Faces are the main method we use to identify people with whom we are familiar, either personally or through the media (De Renzi, 2000). Faces tell us about a number of things about people surrounding us, including approximate age and emotion. They also convey information about the individual's physical uniqueness by the particular arrangement of specific features. These features provide clues to the person's identity.

Prosopagnosia is a rare neurological deficit characterized by the inability to identify a known individual by facial recognition alone (Barton et al., 2021; Corrow et al., 2016). This inability is seen in the absence of severe sensory, intellectual, and visual impairments (Corrow et al., 2016; Damasio et al., 2000). Clients with prosopagnosia know that they are looking at a face but cannot say to whom the face belongs and are unable to match the whole image with stored memories (Bauer, 2012). Clients can usually point to or name the eyes, ears, nose, or mouth either on themselves or others and are able to categorically discriminate faces (e.g., by approximate age) or read their emotional expression (Banich & Compton, 2018; Damasio et al., 2000; De Renzi, 2000). In addition, semantic memory (i.e., general world knowledge) is intact in these clients, as demonstrated by the accurate retrieval of biographical information about the people these clients are attempting to identify (De Renzi, 2000). The severity of prosopagnosia can range from clients who cannot even identify themselves in a mirror to those who only fail to identify people met after the onset of ABI (De Renzi, 2000; Devinsky & D'Esposito, 2004). Often, staff or family members will mistakenly assume that the client has a memory deficit (Bauer, 2012).

Clients with acquired prosopagnosia may also have deficits in topographical orientation, visual field, and color vision (Barton et al., 2021; Moroz et al., 2016). Prosopagnosia has been associated with both CVAs involving the posterior cerebral arteries and head trauma (Barton et al., 2021). Although this condition is most often a result of bilateral damage to the medial occipitotemporal lobe, there are also instances in which the lesion is unilateral. With a unilateral lesion, it is more common for the right hemisphere to be involved than the left (Barton et al., 2021; Damasio, 2000). Imaging studies have also linked the anterior temporal cortex and the inferior frontal gyrus to prosopagnosia (Barton et al., 2021; Shah et al., 2001). The variety in the location of the lesions that can result in prosopagnosia indicate that face processing relies on a network that is more widely distributed throughout the brain than one dedicated area (Barton et al., 2021; Corrow et al., 2016).

Prosopagnosia typically becomes apparent to the clinician through personal experience with the client or through communication with a family member who has noticed that the client does not seem to recognize them (Bauer, 2012). Clients themselves may recognize that they have a problem and be upset by it. Many clients with sufficient cognitive abilities train themselves to use other types of cues to assist in recognition. For example, an individual may identify their spouse by the sound of their voice, the smell of their perfume, or their gait, height, or body shape (Bauer, 2012; Damasio et al., 2000; Devinsky & D'Esposito, 2004).

Tactile Agnosia/Astereognosis

Stereognosis, which is the ability to identify items through touch, requires the identification and integration of tactile features of an object, such as its temperature, texture, weight, and contour, followed by comparison to memories of objects encountered before and the name of the object being examined. Acquisition of tactile information through touch involves both the cutaneous and proprioceptive (muscle and joint receptors) sensory systems, in addition to sufficient motor control to manipulate objects (Dannenbaum & Jones, 1993). This process can be interrupted in various places, resulting in different deficits. The person may be able to distinguish tactile features of familiar objects but still be unable to identify them, a condition called *tactile agnosia,* or *astereognosis.*

As stated previously, agnosia can occur in any sensory system, although visual agnosia has been best described. Tactile agnosia, as compared with visual agnosia, is less understood, although it may be as common (Bauer, 2012). Tactile agnosia has traditionally been defined as an inability to recognize objects tactually even though tactile, thermal, and proprioceptive functions are still intact (Bauer, 2012; Platz et al., 2001). Clients with tactile agnosia cannot associate the retrieved tactile image with other sensory images, meaning that they cannot recognize objects through touch alone despite being able to recognize the tactile qualities. A person with tactile agnosia will be unable to do things such as select a specific object from inside a pocket or locate eyeglasses in a darkened room.

Auditory Agnosia

Auditory agnosia is the inability to recognize differences in sounds, including both word and nonword sounds. For example, a client may not be able to differentiate between the sound of a car engine running and the sound of a vacuum cleaner. The evaluation and treatment for auditory agnosia are usually managed by a speech-language pathologist.

Visuospatial Skills and Deficits

One of the major functions of visual perception is to provide a visual map of the space that surrounds the person (Sergent, 1991). Spatial relations, or visuospatial ability, allows people to localize objects in relation to each other and understand the location of objects with respect to themselves (Bryan, 2004; Manning, 2003). Through visuospatial skills, an individual can judge distances. Spatial relations are important for orienting in the environment, recognizing scenes, and setting the stage for the manipulation of objects with the hands (Sakata et al., 1997).

Damage to the parietal lobes, predominantly the right, has been associated with visuospatial deficits (Kerkhoff, 2003; Manning, 2003). Positron emission tomography studies have indicated that there is an occipitoparietal visual pathway for processing spatial location information. Therefore, damage in these areas of the brain is more likely to lead to spatial relations deficits (Petit et al., 1997). Functionally, spatial relations deficits can result in difficulties with tasks such as aligning buttons of a shirt, discerning which side of the shirt is the front and which is the back, perceiving whether the arm went through the armhole or the neck hole (Árnadóttir, 1999), and positioning oneself out of the way to open a cupboard door.

Body Scheme

The establishment of a good body scheme (i.e., a map of the self) is an important precursor to spatial relations because it allows a consistent point of origin from which to view the world. An accurate body scheme facilitates exploration and understanding of the environment, which leads, in turn, to the perception of objects and their relationship to the individual or to each other (Benton, 1959). It is important to mention that body scheme is dependent on more than just visual input. Prior and current sensory input (including proprioceptive, cutaneous, vestibular, tactile, visual, and auditory) form an awareness of the orientation of one's body and the spatial relations of its parts (Devinsky & D'Esposito, 2004). Attention, memory, and language also contribute to an individual's body scheme (Árnadóttir, 1999).

An individual's body scheme is a representation of the spatial relations among the parts of the body and is different from the psychodynamic sense of identity (Devinsky & D'Esposito, 2004). An intact body scheme allows the person to more easily identify where sensory input is coming from and is also involved in the triggering and guidance of movement (Newcombe & Ratcliff, 1989). It is the foundation for future skills in environmental perception (Maeshima et al., 1997). An intact body scheme allows the individual to know and understand the body's orientation in space, which is crucial for interacting with the environment. For example, information from multiple sensory systems (vestibular, somatosensory, and visual) gives the brain input that is necessary to recognize that the person is upright (as opposed to lying down). From there, the person can start to make determinations about what is located to the right, left, above, and below.

Many professionals think that there are multiple distinct yet interacting representations that contribute to an individual's body awareness or knowledge (Coslett, 1998). Sirigu et al. (1991) hypothesized that there are at least three kinds of representations that contribute to body knowledge processing. The first relates to semantic and lexical information about body parts, such as names; the functional relations that exist between body parts, such as the wrist and the ankle (e.g., that these body parts are joints and allow other body parts to move); and the functional purpose of the mouth, ear, and so forth. These representations are likely to be linked to the verbal systems. The second contains the visuospatial representations of both an individual's own body and bodies in general. Through this aspect of body scheme, the person is able to describe the body and specify in a detailed manner the position of individual parts on the body surface (e.g., the nose is in the middle of the face), the relationships that exist among body parts (e.g., the nose is near the eyes, the lower leg is between the ankle and the knee), and the boundaries that define each body part. These representations are necessary for part–whole analysis. They are likely to be linked to the nonverbal, visual, and somatosensory systems. The third gives information about the position and the changes in position of an individual's own body parts relative to each other and in relation to external space.

Body scheme disorders have been linked to damage of the parietal cortex (especially the right; Devinsky & D'Esposio, 2004). Clinically, the client may exhibit different types of problems. For example, the client may be able to localize body parts on themselves but not on others or be able to name body parts spatially but not functionally. In addition, the client's body alignment and positioning may influence the degree of body knowledge (Hansen, 1993). Autotopagnosia and right–left discrimination errors are examples of two different types of body scheme disorders.

Autotopagnosia

Autotopagnosia, a disturbance in body scheme, is the lack of awareness of body structure and the failure to recognize one's body parts and their relationship to each other. Clients can recognize body parts individually, indicating that the problem is not with knowledge of the parts themselves (Reed & Farah, 1995). In addition, they can move a body part when the examiner points to it, which indicates that the problem is not linguistic (Reed & Farah, 1995). A client who has such a deficit also has difficulties in their reference point to the outside world. A client with this difficulty may have trouble using their contralateral limbs, may confuse the sides of the body, and may not properly differentiate their own body parts and those of the examiner (Sirigu et al., 1991; Zoltan, 1992).

During evaluation, many clients with autotopagnosia will grope uncertainly along their body when asked to identify a body part (Denes et al., 2000). They may point to a body part near the target or point to one that has a similar function (Denes et al., 2000; Devinsky & D'Esposito, 2004). Denes and colleagues (2000) noted that body parts that are perceptually well defined, such as the nose, are more easily localized than those without specific boundaries, such as the cheek.

Right–Left Discrimination

Right–left discrimination is the ability to identify the right and left sides of one's body as well as that of others (Denburg & Tranel, 2012). Most people do not master right–left discrimination until late childhood (Newcombe & Ratcliff, 1989). Some degree of right–left disorientation is relatively common in people without a brain injury, and there is a tendency for worsening abilities in older age (Denburg & Tranel, 2012). In addition to spatial ability, successful right–left orientation requires many cognitive abilities, including mental rotation (Denburg & Tranel, 2012), and a somewhat high level of conceptualization (De Renzi, 1982).

The client who has sustained an ABI may exhibit difficulty with right–left discrimination, resulting in difficulty in identifying right from left, both on the client's own body as well as in space (Benton, 1959). Clients are usually able to identify other spatial concepts, such as up/down or front/back (Denburg & Tranel, 2012). Right–left disorientation is generally associated with left parietal lobe dysfunction when it occurs after ABI (Denburg & Tranel, 2012).

Depth Perception

Depth perception is the ability to see the world in three dimensions and to judge how far away an object is (Sakata et al., 1997). Depth perception is crucial to an individual's ability to locate objects in the visual environment, accurately reach for and use items, and function safely with tasks such as navigating stairs or driving (Cuiffreda et al., 2001). Impaired depth perception will affect almost all everyday activities because many tasks require the judgment of how far away one object is from another or from oneself. Just a few examples include threading a needle, putting toothpaste on a toothbrush, reaching for a straw, hammering, or catching a ball (Bryan, 2004). In severe cases, the client may completely lose the ability to see any differences in depth. This could result in dangerous situations, such as a flight of stairs being seen as a number of lines on the floor, an obvious safety hazard (Karnath & Zihl, 2003).

Depth perception is dependent on a number of different visual cues, one of which is stereopsis or retinal binocularity, the bringing together of the slightly different images from the two eyes. Other monocular cues include texture, shading (which gives information about the location of a light source), and linear perspective (with objects that are farther away appearing smaller), all of which contribute to the perception of three-dimensional shape and distance (Bruce et al., 2003; Cuiffreda et al., 2001; Devinsky & D'Esposito, 2004). Consider the image of the grove of trees shown in Figure 5-10. By using a variety of cues, you are able to tell that there are some trees that are close to you and others that are far away even though the image is two dimensional. As stated

Figure 5-10. A variety of visual cues enable you to interpret depth in this two-dimensional image of a grove of trees. (naTsumi/shutterstock.com)

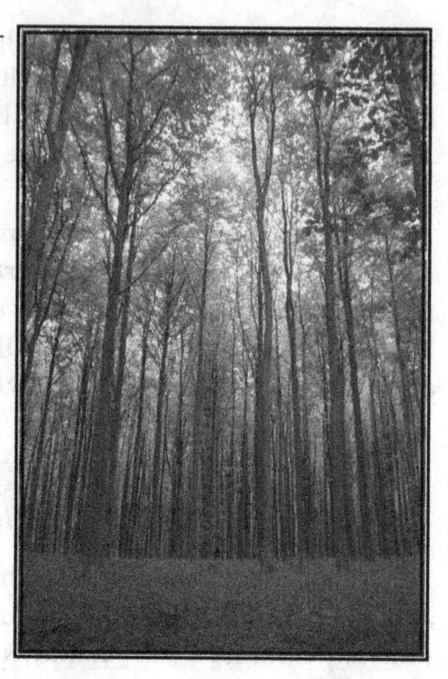

in Chapter 4, oculomotor control is commonly impacted after ABI, which can produce diplopia (i.e., double vision) and negatively affect stereopsis and depth perception. However, stereopsis may be impaired without an ocular misalignment leading to diplopia, so the absence of oculomotor deficits should not lead the occupational therapy practitioner to assume that stereopsis is intact (Rizzo, 1989).

Topographical Orientation

Topographical orientation is a complex behavior with many components. Topographical orientation allows people to follow a familiar route, locate a public building in a city, find the kitchen in their home, navigate through a grocery store or shopping mall, and describe how to get to a specific place (through written directions, verbal instruction, and/or with a map; Damasio et al., 2000). This ability requires knowledge of where one is currently, the target location, and the steps that need to be followed to get there (Wickens, 1998).

Topographical orientation requires specific skills related to specialized topographical orientation as well as general visuospatial abilities and memory (Farah & Epstein, 2012; Golisz & Toglia, 2003). For example, in order to interact effectively with the environment, individuals require information about the positions of objects relative to themselves. To establish this, people must have adequate processing of visual stimuli received from various parts of the visual field, adequate depth perception to determine distances between themselves and objects, and adequate integration of visual information (Riddoch & Humphreys, 1989). If these processes are impaired, there can be a decreased ability to recognize visual landmarks and routes. In addition to the visual processes, individuals require spatial working memory to hold information about where they are and to plan future movements. Adequate attentional processes and stored memories for previously experienced route features and landmarks are also required, as are executive functions that enable the person to create and follow a plan of action (Goulter et al., 2021).

Topographical disorientation is a disruption in the ability to orient oneself in one's surroundings and to navigate through the world (Goulter et al., 2021). This can be caused by a variety of factors. People may have difficulty using relevant environmental features, such as general views and specific landmarks, to identify where they are currently located (Devinsky & D'Esposito, 2004;

Goulter et al., 2021). They may have difficulty forming spatial relationships between themselves and objects in their environment and processing and remembering distances between key features (Devinsky & D'Esposito, 2004; Goulter et al., 2021). People may also have difficulty understanding and remembering how far they have moved (Goulter et al., 2021). People with right–left discrimination issues may also have difficulty with following directions. As a result of these types of deficits, clients with topographical disorientation can be severely impaired in navigating both familiar and unfamiliar environments (Farah & Epstein, 2012).

Visual Motor Integration Skills and Deficits

Visual motor integration encompasses the interrelationship between the visual and motor systems. These skills contribute to the process by which people can visually direct their bodies moving in space. This is essential for eye–hand coordination and is used in countless activities daily. For example, visual motor integration is necessary for writing a note, grasping a glass of water, inserting a key in a lock, and many other tasks. Visual motor integration is also essential for drawing or tracing patterns or images, in addition to construction or assembling objects (Brown et al., 2013; McKenna et al., 2006; Scheiman, 2011b).

Visual motor integration deficits can result from lesions in either cerebral hemisphere and limit the client's ability to perform purposeful acts while using objects in their environment (Fahle, 1993). Controversy exists about the frequency of occurrence of visual motor integration deficit among clients with right- versus left-sided brain damage. It is widely believed that clients with right-sided damage show a greater incidence of the deficit (Fisher, 1987); however, others hypothesize an equal distribution of the symptoms among those with right- and left-sided brain damage (Finlayson & Garner, 1994).

Visual motor integration deficit leads to difficulty in producing designs in two or three dimensions (copying, drawing, or constructing) whether on command or spontaneously (Brown et al., 2013; McKenna et al., 2006; Scheiman, 2011b). This failure cannot be attributed to primary motor or sensory impairments, including on the level of visual acuity, visual fields, or oculomotor control (Golisz & Toglia, 2003). Rather, these clients have lost the ability to assemble and organize an object from disarticulated pieces (Devinsky & D'Esposito, 2004). Functionally, visual motor integration deficits have been related to decreased independence and are correlated with lower functioning in ADLs (Bouska et al., 1990; Brown et al., 2013; Neistadt, 1990) and some instrumental activities of daily living (IADLs; Neistadt, 1990). Some researchers include this type of deficit as one manifestation of apraxia (Cooke et al., 2005), which is discussed further in Chapter 7.

Evaluation of Visual Perception

The evaluation of visual perceptual skills uses a number of the same principles that are followed when evaluating cognition. As a result, the approaches described in Chapter 8 are relevant when working with clients with these types of deficits. A number of assessment tools that are discussed in those sections will also consider the client's visual perceptual functioning.

Although assessments that provide information about specific deficits can be helpful in teasing out which impairments are present, it is essential that clinicians consider visual perception deficits in the context of activity because their impact on functioning can be understood best when skillfully observing clients' complete familiar occupations. In addition, a direct link between the presence of a deficit and the impact on function will be dependent on a number of factors (e.g., physical organization of the working environment, number of distractors present), so the evaluation of clients in the context of occupation is necessary (Cooke et al., 2005; Phipps, 2018; Warren, 2018). Assessment tools such as the ADL-focused Occupation-based Neurobehavioral Evaluation and the Assessment of Motor and Process Skills are standardized assessments of occupational performance that can be used to help uncover visual perceptual deficits in clients. These assessments are discussed further in Chapter 8.

Non-standardized observation of clients in the context of activity can also help occupational therapy practitioners uncover visual perceptual deficits and determine how much they impact functioning. For example, a client with difficulty locating a ladle in a drawer filled with many kitchen utensils may be experiencing a deficit with figure ground. Similarly, a client who is unable to identify a utensil solely with vision may have a deficit with visual discrimination. When considering visuospatial skills, a client with deficits in stereopsis may have difficulty judging distances, resulting in errors when reaching for objects while cooking or identifying edges of curbs or stairs. A client with topographical disorientation being seen for inpatient rehabilitation may display difficulty with navigating about a hospital, becoming confused and lost when attempting to locate the therapy gym and/or finding the way back to their room.

Dynamic assessment strategies (discussed in Chapter 8) can also be used during the completion of functional activities (Toglia, 2018). For example, if a client has a figure–ground deficit and is unable to find an item in a cluttered drawer, the occupational therapy practitioner can reduce the items one item at a time until the client is able to find the target item. This can serve as a baseline measure, providing the practitioner with a starting point for graded functional tasks. The practitioner can then alter the environment or task as the client improves.

There are some assessment tools that focus specifically on visual perceptual skills, which are discussed in the following sections. As stated earlier, these assessments should be administered after screening a client's visual acuity, visual fields, and oculomotor skills (described in Chapter 3) because deficits in those areas of visual functioning will negatively impact visual perception (Cate & Richards, 2000).

ADL-focused Occupation-based Neurobehavioral Evaluation (Árnadóttir, 1990)

Description

The ADL-focused Occupation-based Neurobehavioral Evaluation (A-ONE), which was originally titled Árnadóttir OT-ADL Neurobehavioral Evaluation, was designed as a top-down assessment for adults with cortical injury. Occupational therapy practitioners use the A-ONE to assess both the client's occupational performance in ADLs and to determine the underlying neurobehavioral impairments. Evaluators consider clients' performance in ADLs in five domains: dressing, grooming and hygiene, transfers and mobility, feeding, and communication. Evaluators report on the level of independence in ADLs, the type of assistance that is needed, and the types and severity of neurobehavioral impairment (Gardarsdóttir & Kaplan, 2002). The assessment is composed of two parts. In Part I , the client is rated on two scales: the Functional Independence Scale and the Neurobehavioral Impairment Scale. The Neurobehavioral Scale is further divided into two subscales: the Neurobehavioral Specific Impairment Subscale and the Neurobehavioral Pervasive Impairment Subscale. Part II is used to convert the results of Part I to reveal information pertaining to central nervous system (CNS) dysfunction. Figure 5-11 shows a sample (dressing) of the Neurobehavioral Specific Impairment Subscale.

Dressing Section of the Neurobehavioral Specific Impairment Subscale

Name ______________________ Date ______________________

ACTIVITIES OF DAILY LIVING FUNCTIONS	NEUROBEHAVIORAL IMPAIRMENT SCORE		
Dressing	**Present**	**Absent**	**Comment**
Motor apraxia			
1. Has difficulties related to motor planning. May grab a shirt or a sock, but has trouble adjusting the grasp according to needs.	☐	☐	
2. Difficulties with buttons or fastenings because of clumsy hand movements: R/L side?	☐	☐	
Ideational apraxia			
1. Does not know what to do with shirt, pants, or socks.	☐	☐	
2. Misuses clothes. Starts to put leg into armhole or arm into leg hole.	☐	☐	
(a) Other apraxia:	☐	☐	
Unilateral body neglect			
1. Does not dress the affected body side.	☐	☐	
2. Does not pull down shirt all the way on the affected side, or shirt gets stuck on the affected shoulder without the person trying to correct it or realizing what is wrong.	☐	☐	
Somatognosia			
1. Starts putting legs into armholes or arms into legholes.	☐	☐	
(b) Other body-scheme disorders:	☐	☐	
Spatial-relation disorders			
1. Unable to find armholes, legholes, or bottom of shirt.	☐	☐	
2. Pull sleeve in the wrong direction.	☐	☐	
3. Unable to differentiate front from back or inside from outside of clothes.	☐	☐	
4. Aims correctly at armholes but misses it without noticing.	☐	☐	
5. Matches buttons and buttonholes incorrectly.	☐	☐	
6. Puts hand into sleeve through distal instead of proximal opening.	☐	☐	
7. Legholes end up inside of pants at the top opening without the person realizing it or being able to correct it.	☐	☐	
8. Puts arm through neckhole.	☐	☐	

Figure 5-11. Dressing section of the Neurobehavioral Specific Impairment Subscale from the A-ONE. Note that the most recent version of this subscale includes two abnormal tone items (right and left) with scoring of all items on a 5-point scale (Árnadóttir, 2021). (Reproduced with permission from Árnadóttir G. [1990]. ***The brain and behavior: Assessing cortical dysfunction through activities of daily living.*** **CV Mosby: 234-236.)** ***(continued)***

Dressing Section of the Neurobehavioral Specific Impairment Subscale

ACTIVITIES OF DAILY LIVING FUNCTIONS	NEUROBEHAVIORAL IMPAIRMENT SCORE		
Dressing	**Present**	**Absent**	**Comment**
Spatial-relation disorders			
9. Unable to learn to tie lace one-handed when other hand is paralyzed. This may be the reason for refusing to try the method.	☐	☐	
10. Attempts to turn shirt front to back with the shirt on by pulling at the bottom of the shirt, not realizing that the shirt will not turn while arms are in the sleeves. Similarly, may try to turn pants front to back after placing one leg into leghole, by pulling at the waist opening.	☐	☐	
11. Places foot in the wrong leghole.	☐	☐	
Unilateral spatial neglect			
1. Does not pay attention to clothes	☐	☐	
(c) Other spatial-relations problems:	☐	☐	
Perseveration			
1. Repeats movements or acts and cannot stop them once initiated. Attempts, for example, to put on shirt without any progress. May pull the front edge of a long sleeve up arm way past the wrist.	☐	☐	
2. Attempts to button many buttonholes onto the same button.	☐	☐	
3. Attempts to put the same arm into both sleeves.	☐	☐	
4. Persists motorically in looking for the hole of a sock on the toe side, although the hole cannot be found there.	☐	☐	
(d) Other perserveration problems:	☐	☐	
Organization and sequencing			
1. Has difficulty sequencing the steps of the activity. Will, for example, dress the unaffected arm before the affected one, then run into trouble dressing the affected arm.	☐	☐	
2. Does not include all steps of the activity. Does not, for example, complete the fastenings (buttons, zippers, laces) as required by the nature of the activity.	☐	☐	
3. Will stop the activity after each step and will have to be "programmed" by the therapist to continue.	☐	☐	
4. Will put on the shoes before putting on the trousers.	☐	☐	
(e) Other organization problems:	☐	☐	

Figure 5-11 (continued). Dressing section of the Neurobehavioral Specific Impairment Subscale from the A-ONE. Note that the most recent version of this subscale includes two abnormal tone items (right and left) with scoring of all items on a 5-point scale (Árnadóttir, 2021). (Reproduced with permission from Árnadóttir G. [1990]. *The brain and behavior: Assessing cortical dysfunction through activities of daily living*. CV Mosby: 234-236.)

The Neurobehavioral Specific Impairment Subscale consists of 16 different impairments plus an other category (Árnadóttir, 2021). It includes impairments related to perception, hemi-inattention, and cognition, as well as items focused on motor function and communication. The specific impairments that relate to perception are spatial relations, topographic disorientation, and somatoagnosia. Somatoagnosia (or somatognosia), which is not covered in this text, is described by Árnadóttir (2021) as being related to both body image and spatial relations. According to Árnadóttir, a person with somatoagnosia would have difficulty knowing if a body part belongs to their own body or that of another person and difficulty relating objects to the correct body part. The Neurobehavioral Pervasive Impairment Subscale includes 30 different impairments plus an other category. This scale includes perceptual and cognitive impairments along with items related to emotions. The pervasive impairments related to perception include right–left discrimination, different types of visual agnosia, and astereognosis. See Chapters 6 and 8 for additional information on the hemi-inattention and cognitive impairments included in these two scales.

Test development efforts are currently underway (e.g., Árnadóttir & Fisher, 2008; Árnadóttir, Fisher, et al., 2009; Árnadóttir, Löfgren, et al., 2012) to determine if Rasch analysis can be used to convert the original ordinal scales of the A-ONE to interval scales. This change in measurement approach would allow for comparison of a client's performance over time, performance between clients, and performance among diagnostic groups.

Procedure

Training is required before clinicians can use the standardized A-ONE tool. To administer the A-ONE, the examiner observes clients while they perform ADLs, such as dressing, and rates their level of independence with the task by using the Functional Independence Scale. The examiner also makes note of errors that are made during task completion and connects the errors that are made to specific neurobehavioral impairments by using the Neurobehavioral Scale (Árnadóttir, 2021).

Scoring

The Functional Independence Scale focuses on the functional level of independence in the five categories described previously. The client's independence is scored on a 5-point scale from 0 (unable to perform) to 4 (independent and able to transfer activity to other environmental situations). Scores are given for each subtask within each domain. For example, the dressing domain includes shirt (or dress), pants, socks, shoes, fastenings, and an other category (Árnadóttir, 2021).

The Neurobehavioral Scale measures the number and type of neurobehavioral deficits that interfere with function. The presence and impact of each of the impairments on the Neurobehavioral Specific Impairment Subscale are scored on a 5-point scale from 4 (unable to perform due to neurobehavioral impairments/needs maximum physical assistance) to 0 (no neurobehavioral impairment observed). Not all of the 16 neurobehavioral impairments on the specific impairment portion of the scale are scored for each domain. For example, spatial relations is scored four times, once each for the dressing, grooming and hygiene, transfers and mobility, and feeding domains. On the other hand, topographic disorientation is only scored in the transfers and mobility domain. Each impairment on the Neurobehavioral Pervasive Impairment Subscale is scored once for presence or absence during the ADL observation. The test manual includes definitions and scoring criteria for each item (Árnadóttir, 2021).

Psychometric Properties

In order to ensure reliability with administration and scoring, it is necessary for evaluators to attend a 5-day training prior to using this assessment tool (http://www.a-one.is/index.html). Inter-rater reliability has been studied with the average Kappa coefficients for the degree of agreement between raters equal to 0.84, $p<.01$ (three items: $p<.05$; Árnadóttir, 1990). An additional study found that test–retest reliability was 0.85 for all items (Gardarsdóttir & Kaplan, 2002). Content validity was established through extensive literature review and expert opinion within the field. It has also been studied with 42 people with stroke and found to have some ability to distinguish between people with a left or right CVA (Gardarsdóttir & Kaplan, 2002). Additional normative psychometric studies have been performed and are summarized in *The Brain and Behavior: Assessing Cortical Dysfunction Through Activities of Daily Living* (Árnadóttir, 1990).

Motor-Free Visual Perception Test, Fourth Edition (Colarusso & Hammill, 2015)

Description

The Motor-Free Visual Perception Test, Fourth Edition (MVPT-4), is a standardized test battery that examines visual perception. Five types of visual perceptual skills (spatial relationships, visual discrimination, figure ground, visual closure, and visual memory) are considered, but the authors indicate that it is difficult to fully separate out the distinct skills. Instead, a single score is reported. Norms were generated from a sample of more than 2700 individuals who were representative of the demographics of the United States between 2012 and 2014. Detailed information pertaining to the sample is included in the manual. The test takes approximately 20 to 30 minutes to administer and approximately 5 minutes to score.

Procedure

The MVPT-4 uses simple black-and-white line drawings, and each item is presented in a multiple-choice format. No writing or drawing is needed to complete the test, which is often helpful to people with ABI due to the presence of motor control deficits that limit the ability to use writing instruments. The test manual includes additional details.

Scoring

MVPT-4 testing yields a single raw score that can be converted to a standard score, percentile ranks, and/or age equivalents. The final test result is reported as a single, overall visual perceptual score rather than reporting scores for each category of skill. The test authors' rationale for this type of scoring is that visual perceptual skills are not used in isolation but, rather, in conjunction with one another and are, therefore, correlated (Colarusso & Hammill, 2015). This assumption was tested by Brown and Elliott (2011) who completed a factor analysis of an earlier version of this test, the Motor-Free Visual Perception Test, Third Edition (MVPT-3), with data from 221 adults (49 of whom had neurological impairment). These researchers concluded that the MVPT-3 did not measure a single unidimensional construct. Instead, it loaded on 11 different factors, which may mean that reporting results of the MVPT-3 as a single score is not valid. These authors recommended that more research be performed.

Psychometric Properties

Internal consistency studies found Cronbach alpha equal to 0.70 to 0.87 with median reliability coefficient for age 4 and older of 0.80 (Colarusso & Hammill, 2015). According to the test developers, test–retest reliability had been found to be 0.92 (Colarusso & Hammill, 2015). However, others have found it to be lower, with one study reporting test–retest reliability as 0.71 (Brown et al., 2010). It should be noted that this study was conducted while using the third edition of the MVPT rather than the most recent version. The MVPT-4 was found to have a 0.66 correlation with the third edition of the Test of Visual Perceptual Skills (Colarusso & Hammill, 2015). Additional validity studies have been conducted and are described in the test manual.

Draw-A-Man (MacDonald, 1960; Maloney & Payne, 1969; Zoltan et al., 1983)

Description

This simple assessment can be used to screen for a variety of perceptual deficits, including issues with body scheme, right–left discrimination, visual motor integration, and hemi-inattention (discussed in Chapter 6).

Procedure

The client is given a blank piece of paper and a pencil and asked to draw a man.

Scoring

There are different ways to score this assessment described in the literature. Two of those are included here. The first scoring system is taken from MacDonald (1960); the second is from Zoltan et al. (1983).

Scoring System Number 1 (10 points are possible; a person who scores 10 points has intact performance on this task)

1. A total of four points are awarded for the presence of all body parts. One point each is given for the presence of the head; the trunk, two arms if the figure is facing forward or one arm if the figure is in profile, and two legs if the figure is facing forward or one leg if the figure is in profile.
2. A total of three points are awarded for the correct proportion of body parts to trunk. One point each is given if the area of the head is one-half the length of the trunk, the length of at least one arm is between one-half the length of the trunk and twice the length of the trunk, and the length of at least one leg is between one-half the length of the trunk and twice the length of the trunk.
3. One point is awarded for correct postural alignment (i.e., figure in normal standing or sitting position).
4. A total of two points are awarded for correct juxtaposition of the extremities with the trunk. One point each is given if the arms emerge from the upper one-half of the trunk and if the legs emerge from the lower one-half of the trunk.

Scoring System Number 2 (10 points are possible)

A person is scored based on the number of body parts that are present in the drawing. A total of 10 body parts are scored, with the client receiving one point for each of the following: head, trunk, right arm, left arm, right leg, left leg, right hand, left hand, right foot, left foot. Scores are reported as follows: intact, the client receives a score of 10; minimally impaired, the client scores between 6 and 9; and severely impaired, the client scores 5 or below.

Psychometric Properties

Research conducted on a sample of clients with TBI using this scoring system established good inter-rater reliability ($r = 0.86$; Baum, 1981) and 95.45% agreement (Chen-Sea, 2000). In addition, those who scored poorly on the assessment demonstrated poorer performance with ADLs, as assessed by the Klein-Bell ADL Scale (Chen-Sea, 2000).

Treatment of Visual Perception

As was the case with the evaluation of visual perceptual deficits, the treatment of people with these types of deficits overlaps greatly with the treatment for people with cognitive impairment. As a result, the general principles for treatment in these two areas will be similar. These treatment principles are discussed in more detail in Chapters 9 and 10, but are described briefly in the following sections with examples that are specific to visual perception deficits. The general approaches to take will be environmental modification and/or activity adaptation, awareness training, and strategy training. It is important to remember that the most effective approach is often one that uses a combination of treatments, with careful monitoring of what is most effective for the individual client.

Environmental or Task Modification

Environmental or task modification is performed in order to support the person's functioning in such a way that reliance on the lost visual perceptual skills is not needed. Instead, the task or environment is set up to best fit the person's capabilities (American Occupational Therapy Association, 2020; Radomski & Giles, 2018). The modifications can be made by the clients themselves or by others, such as caregivers. Clients with good awareness of their deficits and good problem-solving abilities can learn to modify their tasks and environments themselves. Patients without these skills will need the modifications performed by another person. In either situation, functioning can be improved, although it will likely be limited to the tasks and environments in which modifications were made. More details about environmental or task modification can be found in Chapter 10. Some of the modifications that were described in Chapter 4 will also be helpful for people with visual perceptual difficulties.

Examples of how environmental or task modification could be used specifically for people with visual perceptual deficits include the following:

- For a client with visual discrimination deficits, organize items and maintain this organization so the client can distinguish items by location rather than needing to rely on visual identification.
- For clients with figure–ground deficits, the visual environment could be simplified by keeping countertops and drawers clear of all but a few essential items. Wheelchair locks could be marked with red tape so that they are easier to distinguish from the wheels (Zoltan, 1990).

- For a client with stereopsis deficits, mark the edges of stairs with a contrasting color so that the client can safely locate them.
- For clients with topographical disorientation, signs can be placed in highly visible locations to help orient them to their spatial environment. In instances in which topographical disorientation occurs along with other visual perceptual impairments, it may be helpful to make the signs visually simple and use contrasting text and background.

Strategy Training and Awareness

Clients who are treated with this approach are taught to use strategies that are designed to work around the skills that are lost. Compensatory strategies include the use of other sensory systems to replace lost visual analysis skills, slowing down, and more consciously gathering information about the visual scene so that decisions can be made. Ideally, strategies that are learned by clients will be used in numerous situations, increasing independence in multiple occupations and contexts (Radomski & Giles, 2014).

Clients who use strategies need to have a good awareness of the nature of their deficits to be most successful. Without this awareness, clients are less likely to understand the need for and the utility of the strategies (Medley & Powell, 2010; Toglia & Maeir, 2018). Research has also shown that clients are unlikely to generalize these strategies for use in situations besides the one in which they are trained unless the occupational therapy practitioner is deliberate about helping with generalization (Geusgens et al., 2007). Information about treatment techniques that can be used to facilitate client awareness of deficits, learn and use strategies, and generalize strategy use are described further in Chapter 10.

Examples of how strategies can be used to help clients with visual perceptual deficits improve functioning include the following:

- A client with prosopagnosia could be taught to look for features besides the face that can help with the identification of people. For example, the client could use other characteristics of people, such as voice, manner of walk, and height.
- The occupational therapy practitioner could teach a client with stereopsis deficits to use other intact sensory systems rather than the visual system when completing activities. For example, the client could use tactile sensation in the fingers to identify the opening in a cup, glass, or pitcher when pouring water and could be taught to put their finger over the edge of the container to feel when they have poured a full glass of water.
- A client with topographical disorientation can be taught to use a global positioning device when navigating between locations in the community.

Conclusion

Perception is the process by which sensory information is interpreted and used by the brain in order to make decisions about and act on the environment that surrounds the person. After ABI, it is not uncommon for perceptual processes to be interrupted, which can have a sizable impact on a person's occupational performance. This chapter discussed some of the perceptual deficits that can be impacted after ABI along with some of the evaluations and treatments that should be considered with this population. The evaluation and treatment of visual perception deficits overlaps with the evaluation and treatment of cognitive deficits; this is discussed in more detail in Chapters 8, 9, and 10.

References

Aloisio, L. (2004). Visual dysfunction. In G. Gillen, & A. Burkhardt (Eds.), *Stroke rehabilitation: A function-based approach*. Mosby Inc.

American Occupational Therapy Association. (2020). Occupational therapy practice framework: Domain and process (4th ed.). *American Journal of Occupational Therapy, 74*(Suppl. 2), 7412410010. https://doi.org/10.5014/ajot.2020.74S2001

Anderson, D. L., & Stufflebeam, R. (2006). Introduction to the science of vision. Consortium on Cognitive Science Instruction. http://www.mind.ilstu.edu/curriculum/vision_science_intro/vision_science_intro.php

Árnadóttir, G. (1990). *The brain and behavior: Assessing cortical dysfunction through activities of daily living*. C. V. Mosby Company.

Árnadóttir, G. (1999). Evaluation and intervention with complex perceptual impairment. In C. Unsworth (Ed.), *Cognitive and perceptual dysfunction: A clinical reasoning approach to evaluation and treatment* (pp. 393-454). F.A. Davis.

Árnadóttir, G. (2021). Impact of neurobehavioral deficits on activities of daily living. In G. Gillen & D. M. Nilsen (Eds.). *Stroke rehabilitation: A function-based approach* (5th ed., pp. 556-592). Elsevier.

Árnadóttir, G., & Fisher, A. G. (2008). Rasch analysis of the ADL scale of the A-ONE. *American Journal of Occupational Therapy, 62*(1), 51-60. https://doi.org/10.5014/ajot.62.1.51

Árnadóttir, G., Fisher, A. G., & Löfgren, B. (2009). Dimensionality of nonmotor neurobehavioral impairments when observed in the natural context of ADL task performance. *Neurorehabilitation and Neural Repair, 23*(6), 579-586. http://dx.doi.org/10.1177/1545968308324223

Árnadóttir, G., Löfgren, B., & Fisher, A.G. (2012). Neurobehavioral functions evaluated in naturalistic contexts: Rasch analysis of the A-ONE Neurobehavioral Impact Scale. *Scandinavian Journal of Occupational Therapy 19*(5), 439-449. https://doi.org/10.3109/11038128.2011.638674

Ashley, M. J., Leal, R., Mehta, Z., Ashley, J. G., & Ashley, M. J. (2018). Remediative approaches for cognitive disorders after TBI. In M. J. Ashley & D. A. Hovda (Eds.), *Traumatic brain injury: Rehabilitation, treatment, and case management* (4th ed., pp. 487-511). CRC Press.

Banich, M. T., & Compton R. J. (2018). *Cognitive neuroscience* (4th ed.). Cambridge University Press.

Barton, J. J. S., Davies-Thompson, J., & Corrow, S. L. (2021). Prosopagnosia and disorders of face processing. In J. J. S. Barton & A. Leff (Eds.), *Handbook of clinical neurology* (pp. 175-193). Elsevier.

Bauer, R. M. (2012). Agnosia. In K. M. Heilman & E. Valenstein (Eds.), *Clinical neuropsychology* (5th ed., pp. 238-295). Oxford University Press.

Baum, B. (1981). *The establishment of reliability and validity of a perceptual evaluation on a sample of adult head trauma patients* [Unpublished master's thesis]. University of Southern California.

Benton, A. (1959). *Right-left discrimination and finger localization*. Harper Bros.

Bernspang, B., Asplung, K., Eriksson, S., & Fugl-Meyer, A. R. (1987). Motor and perceptual impairments in acute stroke patients: Effects on self-care ability. *Stroke, 18*, 1081-1086. https://doi.org/10.1161/01.STR.18.6.1081

Bouska, M. J., Kauffman, N. A., & Marcus, S. E. (1990). Disorders of the visual perceptual system. In D. A. Umphred (Ed.), *Neurological rehabilitation* (2nd ed., pp. 522-585). CV Mosby.

Brown, T., & Elliott, S. (2011). Factor structure of the Motor-Free Visual Perception Test–3rd edition (MVPT-3). *Canadian Journal of Occupational Therapy, 78*, 26-36. https://doi.org/10.2182/cjot.2011.78.1.4

Brown, T., Mapleston, J., Nairn, A., & Molloy, A. (2013). Relationship of cognitive and perceptual abilities to functional independence in adults who have had a stroke. *Occupational Therapy International, 20*, 11-22. https://doi.org/10.1002/oti.1334

Brown, T., Sutton, E., Burgess, D., Elliott, S., Bourne, R., Wigg, S., Glass, S., & Lalor, A. (2010). The reliability of three visual perception tests used to assess adults. *Perceptual and Motor Skills, 111*, 45-59. https://doi.org/10.2466/03.24.27.PMS.111.4.45-59

Bruce, V., Green, P. R., & Georgeson, M. A. (2003). *Visual perception: Physiology, psychology and ecology* (4th ed.). Psychology Press.

Bryan, V. L. (2004). Management of residual physical deficits. In M. J. Ashley & D. K. Krych (Eds.), *Traumatic brain injury: Rehabilitative treatment and case management* (2nd ed., pp. 455-508). CRC Press.

Bulson, R., Jun, W., & Hayes, J. (2012). Visual symptomatology and referral patterns for Operation Iraqi Freedom and Operation Enduring Freedom veterans with traumatic brain injury. *Journal of Rehabilitative Research and Development, 49*, 1075-1082. https://doi.org/10.1682/JRRD.2011.02.0017

Cate, Y., & Richards, L. (2000). Relationship between performance on tests of basic visual functions and visual-perceptual processing in persons after brain injury. *American Journal of Occupational Therapy, 54*, 326-334. https://doi.org/10.5014/ajot.54.3.326

Chen-Sea, M.-J. (2000). Validating the Draw-A-Man test as a personal neglect test. *American Journal of Occupational Therapy, 54*(4), 391-397. https://doi.org/10.5014/ajot.54.4.391

Colarusso, R. P., & Hammill, D. D. (2003). *Motor-Free Visual Perception Test* (3rd ed.). Academic Therapy Publications.

Colarusso, R. P., & Hammill, D. D. (2015). *MVPT-4: Motor-Free Visual Perception Test-4*. ATP Assessments.

Cooke, D. M., McKenna, K., & Fleming, J. (2005). Development of a standardized occupational therapy screening for visual perception in adults. *Scandinavian Journal of Occupational Therapy, 12*, 59-71. https://doi.org/10.1080/11038120410020683-1

Corrow, S. L., Dalrymple, K. A., & Barton, J. S. (2016). Prosopagnosia: Current perspectives. *Eye and Brain, 8*, 165-175. https://doi.org/10.2147/EB.S92838

Coslett, H. B. (1998). Evidence for a disturbance of the body schema in neglect. *Brain and Cognition, 37*(3), 527-544. https://doi.org/10.1006/brcg.1998.1011

Cuiffreda, K. J., Suchoff, I. B., Kapoor, N., Jackowski, M. M., Wainapel, S. F., Gonzalez, E. G., Myers, S. J., Edelstein, J. F., Lieberman, J. S., & Downey, J. A. (2001). Normal vision function. In E. G. Gonzales, S. J. Myers, J. E. Edelstein, J. Lieberman, & J. A. Downey (Eds.), *Downey and Darling's physiological basis of rehabilitation medicine* (3rd ed., pp. 241-216). Butterworth Heimann.

Damasio, A. R., Tranel, D., & Rizzo, M. (2000). Disorders of complex visual processing. In M. M. Mesulam (Ed.), *Principles of behavioral and cognitive neurology* (2nd ed., pp. 332-372). Oxford University Press.

Dannenbaum, R. M., & Jones, L. A. (1993). The assessment and treatment of patients who have sensory loss following cortical lesions. *Journal of Hand Therapy, 6*, 130-138. https://doi.org/10.1016/S0894-1130(12)80294-8

De Renzi, E. (1982). *Disorders of space exploration and cognition*. Wiley.

De Renzi, E. (2000). Disorders of visual recognition. *Seminars in Neurology, 20*, 479-485. https://doi.org/10.1055/s-2000-13181

Denburg, N., & Tranel, D. (2012). Acalculia and disturbances of the body schema. In K. M. Heilman & E. Valenstein (Eds.), *Clinical neuropsychology* (5th ed., pp. 169-197). Oxford University Press.

Denes, G., Cappelletti, J. Y., Zilli, T., Dalla Porta, F., & Gallana, A. (2000). A category-specific deficit of spatial representation: The case of autotopagnosia. *Neuropsychologia, 38*, 345-350. https://doi.org/10.1016/S0028-3932(99)00101-3

Devinsky, O., & D'Esposito, M. (2004). *Neurology of cognitive and behavioral disorders*. Oxford University Press.

Dixon, M. J. (2000). A new paradigm for investigating category-specific agnosia in the new millennium. *Brain and Cognition, 42*, 142-145. https://doi.org/10.1006/brcg.1999.1185

Driver, J., Baylis, G. C., & Rafal, R. D. (1992). Preserved figure-ground segregation and symmetry perception in visual neglect. *Nature, 360*, 73-75. https://doi.org/10.1038/360073a0

Fahle, M. (1993). Figure-ground discrimination from temporal information. *Proceedings of the Royal Society: Biological Sciences, 254*, 199-302. https://doi.org/10.1098/rspb.1993.0146

Farah, M. J., & Epstein, R. A. (2012). Disorders of visual-spatial perception and cognition. In K. M. Heilman & E. Valenstein (Eds.), *Clinical neuropsychology* (5th ed., pp. 152-168). Oxford University Press.

Feldman, J. (2015). Bayesian models of perceptual organization. In J. Wagemans (Ed.), *Oxford handbook of perceptual organization* (pp. 1008-1026). Oxford University Press.

Finlayson, M. A. J., & Garner, S. H. (Eds.). (1994). *Brain injury rehabilitation: Clinical considerations*. Williams and Wilkins.

Fisher, B. (1987). Effect of trunk control and alignment on limb function. *Journal of Head Trauma Rehabilitation, 2*(2), 72-79. https://doi.org/10.1097/00001199-198706000-00011

Gardarsdóttir, S., & Kaplan, S. (2002). Validity of the Árnadóttir OT-ADL Neurobehavioral Evaluation (A-ONE): Performance in activities of daily living and neurobehavioral impairments of persons with left and right hemisphere damage. *American Journal of Occupational Therapy, 56*, 499-508. https://doi.org/10.5014/ajot.56.5.499

Geusgens, C. A. V., Winkens, I., van Heugten, C. M., Josses, J., & van den Heuvel, W. J. A. (2007). Occurrence and measurement of transfer in cognitive rehabilitation: A critical review. *Journal of Rehabilitation Medicine, 39*, 425-439. https://doi.org/10.2340/16501977-0092

Goldstein, E. B., & Brockmole, J. (2017). *Sensation and perception* (10th ed.). Cengage Learning.

Golisz, K., & Toglia, J. (2003). Perception and cognition. In E. Crepeau, E. S. Cohn, & B. A. B. Schell (Eds.), *Willard & Spackman's occupational therapy* (10th ed., 395-416). Lippincott Williams and Wilkins.

Goodrich, G. L., Flyg, H. M., Kirby, J. E., Chang, C. Y., & Martinsen, G. L. (2013). Mechanisms of TBI and visual consequences in military and veteran populations. *Optometry and Vision Science, 90*, 105-112. https://doi.org/10.1097/OPX.0b013e31827f15a1

Goulter, J. R., Fitzpatrick, L. E., & Crowe, S. F. (2021). An analysis of distinct navigational domains and topographical disorientation syndromes in ABI: A meta-analysis. *Journal of Experimental Neuropsychology, 43*, 449-468. https://doi.org/10.1080/13803395.2021.1926933

Gulyas, B., Heywood, C. A., Popplewell, D. A., Roland, P. E., & Cowey, A. (1994). Visual form discrimination from color or motion cues: Functional anatomy by positron emission tomography. *Proceedings of the National Academy of Sciences, USA, 91*, 9965-9969. https://doi.org/10.1073/pnas.91.21.9965

Hansen, C. S. (1993). Traumatic brain injury. In J. Van Deusen (Ed.), *Body image and perceptual dysfunction in adults* (pp. 39-63). WB Saunders.

Hellerstein, L. F., & Scheiman, M. (2011). Visual problems associated with acquired brain injury. In M. Scheiman (Ed.), *Understanding and managing vision deficits: A guide for occupational therapists* (3rd ed., pp. 189-200). SLACK Incorporated.

Jäkel, F., Singh, M., Wichmann, F. A., & Herzog, M. H. (2016). An overview of quantitative approaches in Gestalt perception. *Vision Research, 126*, 3-8. https://doi.org/10.1016/j.visres.2016.06.004

Karnath, H. O., & Zihl, J. (2003). Disorders of spatial orientation. In T. Brandt, L. R. Caplan, J. Dichgans, C. H. Diener, & C. Kennard (Eds.), *Neurological disorders: Course and treatment* (pp. 277-286). Academic Press.

Kerkhoff, G. (2003). Multimodal spatial orientation deficits in left-sided visual neglect. *Neuropsychologia, 37*, 1387-1405. https://doi.org/10.1016/S0028-3932(99)00031-7

Khan, S., Leung, E., & Jay, W. M. (2008). Stroke and visual rehabilitation. *Topics in Stroke Rehabilitation, 15*, 27-36. https://doi.org/10.1310/tsr1501-27

Koffka, K. (1935). *Principles of Gestalt psychology*. Harcourt, Brace, and Company.

Laatsch, L., & Krisky, C. (2006). Changes in fMRI activation following rehabilitation of reading and visual processing deficits in subjects with traumatic brain injury. *Brain Injury, 20*, 1367-1375. https://doi.org/10.1080/02699050600983743

Lezak, M. D., Howieson, D. B., Bigler, E. D., & Tranel, D. (2012). *Neuropsychological assessment* (5th ed.). Oxford University Press.

MacDonald, J. (1960). An investigation of body scheme in adults with cerebral vascular accident. *American Journal of Occupational Therapy, 14*, 72-79.

Maeshima, S., Dohi, N., Funahashi, K., Nakai, K., Itakura, T., & Komai, N. (1997). Rehabilitation of patients with anosognosia for hemiplegia due to intracerebral haemorrhage. *Brain Injury, 11*, 691-697. https://doi.org/10.1080/026990597123232

Magone, M. T., Kwon, E., & Shin, S. Y. (2014). Chronic visual dysfunction after blast-induced mild traumatic brain injury. *Journal of Rehabilitative Research and Development, 51*, 71-80. https://doi.org/10.1682/JRRD.2013.01.0008

Maloney, M. P., & Payne L. (1969). Validity of the Draw-a-Person test as a measure of body image. *Perceptual and Motor Skills, 29*, 119-122. https://doi.org/10.2466/pms.1969.29.1.119

Mamassian, P., Landy, M. & Maloney, L. (2002). Bayesian modeling of visual perception. In R. P. N. Rao, B. A. Olshausen, & M. S. Lewicki (Eds.), *Probabilistic models of the brain* (pp. 13-36). MIT Press.

Manning, L. (2003). Assessment and treatment of disorders of visuospatial, imaginal, and constructional processes. In P. Halligan, U. Kischka, & J. C. Marshall (Eds.), *Handbook of clinical neuropsychology* (pp. 190-193). Oxford University Press.

McKenna, K., Cooke, D. M., Fleming, J., Jefferson, A., & Ogden, S. (2006). The incidence of visual perceptual impairment in patients with severe traumatic brain injury. *Brain Injury, 20*, 507-518. https://doi.org/10.1080/02699050600664368

Medley, A. R., & Powell, T. (2010). Motivational interviewing to promote self-awareness and engagement in rehabilitation following acquired brain injury: A conceptual review. *Neuropsychological Rehabilitation, 20*, 481-508. https://doi.org/10.1080/09602010903529610

Moroz, D., Corrow, S. L., Corrow, J. C., Barton, A. R., Duchaine, B., & Barton, J. J. (2016). Localization and patterns of cerebral dyschromatopsia: A study of subjects with prospagnosia. *Neuropsychologia, 89*, 153-160. https://doi.org/10.1016/j.neuropsychologia.2016.06.012

Neistadt, M. E. (1990). A critical analysis of occupational therapy approach for perceptual deficits in adults with brain injury. *American Journal of Occupational Therapy, 44*, 299-304. https://doi.org/10.5014/ajot.44.4.299

Newcombe, F., & Ratcliff, G. (1989). Disorders of visuospatial analysis. In F. Boller & J. Grafman (Eds.), *Handbook of neuropsychology* (Vol. 2, pp. 333-356). Elsevier.

Palmer, S. E. (1999). *Vision science: Photons to phenomenology*. MIT Press.

Paolucci, A., McKenna, K., & Cooke, D. M. (2009). Factors affecting the number and type of impairments of visual perception and praxis following stroke. *Australian Occupational Therapy Journal, 56*, 350-360. https://doi.org/10.1111/j.1440-1630.2008.00743.x

Petit, L., Orssaud, C., Tzourio, N., Mazoyer, B., & Berthoz, A. (1997). Superior parietal involvement in the representation of visual space: A PET review. In P. Tier & H. O. Karnath (Eds.), *Parietal lobe contributions to orientation in 3D space* (pp. 77-91). Springer Verlag.

Phipps, S. C. (2018). Evaluation and treatment for perceptual dysfunction. In H. M. Pendleton & W. Schultz-Krohn (Eds.), *Pedretti's occupational therapy: Practice skills for physical dysfunction* (8th ed., pp. 631-644). Elsevier.

Platz, T., Winter, T., Müller, N., Pinkowski, C., Eickhof, C., & Mauritz, K. H. (2001). Arm ability training for stroke and traumatic brain injury patients with mild arm paresis: A single-blind, randomized, controlled trial. *Archives of Physical Medicine and Rehabilitation, 82*, 961-968. https://doi.org/10.1053/apmr.2001.23982

Radomski, M. V., & Giles, G. M. (2014). Optimizing cognitive performance. In M. V. Radomski & C. A. Trombly Latham (Eds.), *Occupational therapy for physical dysfunction* (7th ed., pp. 725-752). Lippincott Williams & Wilkins.

Radomski, M. V., & Giles, G. M. (2018). Cognitive intervention. In D. P. Dirette & S. A. Gutman (Eds.), *Occupational therapy for physical dysfunction* (8th ed., pp. 161-175). Wolters Kluwer.

Reed, C. L., & Farah, M. J. (1995). The psychological reality of the body schema: A test with normal participants. *Journal of Experimental Psychology: Human Perception and Performance, 21*, 334-343. https://doi.org/10.1037/0096-1523.21.2.334

Riddoch, M. J., & Humphreys, G. W. (1989). Finding the way around topographical impairments. In W. Brown (Ed.), *Neuropsychology of visual impairments* (pp. 79-103). Lawrence Erlbaum Assoc.

Rizzo, M. (1989). Astereopsis. In F. Boller & J. Grafman (Eds.), *Handbook of neuropsychology* (Vol. 2, pp. 415-427). Elsevier.

Rust, N. C., & Stocker, A. A. (2010). Ambiguity and invariance: Two fundamental challenges for visual processing. *Current Opinion in Neurobiology, 20*, 382-388. https://doi.org/10.1016/j.conb.2010.04.013

Sakata, H., Taira, M., Kusunoki, M., Murata, A, & Tanaka, Y. (1997). The TINS lecture: The parietal association cortex in depth perception and visual control of hand action. *Trends in Neuroscience, 20*, 350-357. https://doi.org/10.1016/S0166-2236(97)01067-9

Scheiman, M. (2011a). Three component model of vision, part three: Visual information processing skills. In M. Scheiman (Ed.), *Understanding and managing vision deficits: A guide for occupational therapists* (3rd ed., pp. 79-94). SLACK Incorporated.

Scheiman, M. (2011b). Management of refractive, visual efficiency, and visual information processing disorders. In M. Scheiman (Ed.), *Understanding and managing vision deficits: A guide for occupational therapists* (3rd ed., pp. 119-176). SLACK Incorporated.

Sergent, J. (1991). Judgements of relative position and distance on representations of spatial relations. *Journal of Experimental Psychology: Human Perception and Performance, 20*, 762-780. https://doi.org/10.1037/0096-1523.17.3.762

Shah, N. J., Marshall, J. C., Zafiris, O., Schwab, A., Zilles, K., Markowitsch, H. J., & Fink, G. R. (2001). The neural correlates of person familiarity. A functional magnetic resonance imaging study with clinical implications. *Brain, 124*, 804-815. https://doi.org/10.1093/brain/124.4.804

Sirigu, A., Grafman, J., Bressler, K., & Sunderland, T. (1991). Multiple representations contribute to body knowledge processing: Evidence from a case of autotopagnosia. *Brain, 114*(1B), 629-642. https://doi.org/10.1093/brain/114.1.629

Su, C.-Y., Chang, J.-J., Chen, H.-M., Su, C.-J., Chien, T.-H., & Huang, M.-H. (2000). Perceptual differences between stroke patients with cerebral infarction and intracerebral hemorrhage. *Archives of Physical Medicine and Rehabilitation, 81*, 706-714. https://doi.org/10.1016/S0003-9993(00)90097-2

Toglia, J. P. (2018). The dynamic interactional model and the multicontext approach. In N. Katz & J. Toglia (Eds.), *Cognition, occupation, and participation across the life span: Neuroscience, neurorehabilitation, and models of intervention in occupational therapy* (4th ed., pp. 355-385). AOTA Press.

Toglia, J., & Maeir, A. (2018). Self-awareness and metacognition: Effect on occupational performance and outcome across the lifespan. In N. Katz & J. Toglia (Eds.), *Cognition, occupation, and participation across the life span: Neuroscience, neurorehabilitation, and models of intervention in occupational therapy* (4th ed., pp. 143-162). AOTA Press.

Wagemans, J., Elder, J. H., Kubovy, M., Palmer, S. E., Peterson, M. A., Singh, M., & von der Heydt, R. (2012). A century of Gestalt psychology in visual perception I: Perceptual grouping and figure-ground organization. *Psychological Bulletin, 138*, 1172-1217. https://doi.org/10.1037/a0029333

Wagemans, J., Feldman, J., Gepshtein, S., Kimchi, R., Pamerantz, J. R., van der Helm, P. A., & van Leeuwen, C. (2012). A century of Gestalt psychology in visual perception II: Conceptual and theoretical foundations. *Psychological Bulletin, 138*, 1218-1252. https://doi.org/10.1037/a0029334

Warren, M. (2018). Evaluation and treatment of visual deficits after brain injury. In H. M. Pendleton & W. Schultz-Krohn (Eds.), *Pedretti's occupational therapy: Practice skills for physical dysfunction* (8th ed., pp. 594-630). Elsevier.

Wickens, C. (1998). Frames of reference for navigation. In D. Gopher & A. Koriat (Eds.), *Attention and performance XVII* (pp. 113-144). MIT Press.

Zoltan, B. (1990). Remediation of visual-perceptual and perceptual-motor deficits. In M. Rosenthal, E. R. Griffith, M. R. Bond, & J. D. Miller (Eds.), *Rehabilitation of the adult and child with traumatic brain injury*. F. A. Davis.

Zoltan, B. (1992). Visual, visual perceptual and perceptual-motor deficits in brain injured adults: Evaluation, treatment and functional implications. In G. H. Kraft & S. Berrol (Eds.), *Physical medicine and rehabilitation clinics of North America*. WB Saunders.

Zoltan, B., Jabri, J., Panikoff, L., & Rychman, D. (1983). *Perceptual motor evaluation for head injured and other neurologically impaired adults*. Santa Clara Valley Medical Center.

CHAPTER 6

Assessment and Treatment of Hemi-Inattention

Before discussing the evaluation and treatment of hemi-inattention, we briefly discuss our rationale for describing this phenomenon in its own chapter and for our use of terminology. Many other texts house information about hemi-inattention within chapters that discuss visual functioning, perhaps because this phenomenon is most frequently and readily observed as clients visually search their surroundings. As a result of the way that clients with hemi-inattention typically interact with visual space, clinicians frequently confuse visual hemi-inattention with visual field cut. In an attempt to help alleviate this confusion and more accurately describe the phenomenon, we have deliberately separated hemi-inattention from the chapters detailing visual processing for two reasons. The first reason is because the condition can manifest through multiple sensory systems and motorically, not just through visual searching. The second reason is that it is important to understand that although hemi-inattention is frequently observed as the client with acquired brain injury (ABI) visually searches the environment, it is not a result of a disruption with primary visual functioning. It is better, instead, to think of this issue as based in perception and cognition. As Mesulam (1981) stated, "The deficit is not one of seeing, hearing, feeling, or moving, but one of looking, listening, touching, and exploring" (p. 318).

Another point of confusion with this condition is that it is referred to by many different names in the literature. In addition to the term hemi-inattention, authors have used visual neglect, hemispatial neglect, unilateral spatial neglect, unilateral neglect, spatial neglect, visuospatial hemineglect, unilateral visual neglect, visuospatial neglect, left or right neglect, hemineglect, and simply neglect. This book uses the term hemi-inattention for manifestations of this phenomenon. We believe that this term is more descriptive of what is happening for these clients and avoids the judgment implied in the term *neglect* that there is some sort of purposeful avoidance or negligence on the part of the individual.

This chapter is organized with the background and what is understood about hemi-inattention first, followed by common assessment and treatment approaches that can be used by occupational therapy practitioners in their treatment of these clients.

Kaminsky, T. A., & Powell, J. M.
Zoltan's Vision, Perception, and Cognition: Evaluation and Treatment of the Adult With Acquired Brain Injury, Fifth Edition (pp. 133-175).

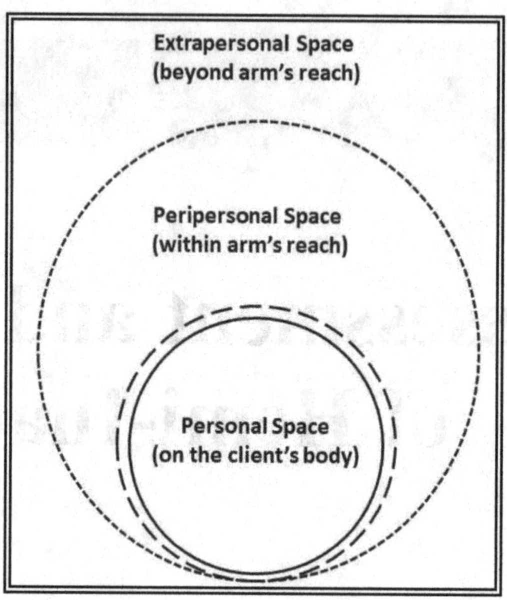

Figure 6-1. Types of space that can be affected for people with hemi-inattention. Personal space is on the person's body. Peripersonal space is the area surrounding the person that is within arm's reach. Extrapersonal space is the area that is beyond arm's reach.

Hemi-Inattention Described

Individuals with hemi-inattention do not orient to, register, respond to, or interact with sensory information that is located contralesionally or do so to a lesser degree, more slowly, and/or less automatically than is typical. These responses to stimuli are beyond what can be accounted for solely by sensory and/or motor loss after ABI (Kaldenberg, 2014; Pierce & Buxbaum, 2002; Shinsha & Ishigami, 1999; Stein et al., 2009; Tham et al., 1999). Hemi-inattention is a complex and heterogenous disorder, manifesting differently depending on the specific region or regions of the brain that are damaged. It is often observed as an inattention to visual information but can also be seen as an inattention to tactile or auditory stimuli, as well as a decrease in the use of contralesional limbs despite the motor ability to use them and difficulty using the ipsilesional limbs when crossing midline. Hemi-inattention can present in different types of spaces, specifically personal space (on the person's body), peripersonal space (within arm's reach), and extrapersonal space (beyond arm's reach), with any or all of these spaces impacted for different individuals with this condition (Bailey et al., 2000; Castiello et al., 2004; Chan & Man, 2013; Christy & Huffine, 2021; Halligan & Marshall, 1991; Klinke, Zahavi et al., 2015; Mesulam, 1994; Pierce & Buxbaum, 2002; Proto et al., 2009; Tham et al., 1999; Tham & Kielhofner, 2003; Figure 6-1). Differences have also been noted in the location of the reference point that divides attended and unattended space. In some instances, the reference point is the self with people attending to stimuli on one side of their midline but not the other. This is called *egocentric hemi-inattention*. In contrast, in *allocentric hemi-inattention*, the reference point is in relation to the object itself. In this case, attention to one side of an individual item will be affected regardless of the position of the object in relation to a person's midline (Marsh & Hillis, 2008). For example, someone with egocentric hemi-inattention may not attend to and eat all of the food on the left side of their plate when it is placed at midline but may do a little better when it is placed to the right of midline (although they will likely still miss some of the food). A person with allocentric hemi-inattention will not attend to food on the left side of the plate no matter where it is placed on the table.

Hemi-inattention can be observed after damage to either hemisphere, although it is widely agreed that hemi-inattention is more prevalent, more severe, and longer lasting after damage to the right hemisphere (Bailey et al., 2000; Barrett et al., 2006; Chan & Man, 2013; Christy & Huffine, 2021; Mapstone et al., 2003; Mesulam, 1981, 1990, 1994, 1999; Pierce & Buxbaum, 2002; Shinsha & Ishigami, 1999; Stein et al., 2009). Hemi-inattention appears to be a common deficit after a cerebrovascular accident (CVA), although the exact incidence varies widely depending on how hemi-inattention is defined or measured and how much time has elapsed since the onset of the stroke for the studied population. The prevalence of hemi-inattention has been reported from 10% to 82% of people with infarcts in the right hemisphere and 15% to 65% of people with infarcts in the left hemisphere (Chan & Man, 2013; Proto et al., 2009). There is also some evidence that even those without clinically observed hemi-inattention may have impairments in visual search of contralesional space after right-sided cerebral damage, so these numbers may underestimate the incidence of milder forms of this condition for client populations (Mapstone et al., 2003).

Some people spontaneously recover from hemi-inattention, although the exact numbers are not clear. One study reported that as many as 43% of people with hemi-inattention recovered completely, with the majority of them recovering within the first 3 months after infarct (Proto et al., 2009). However, clients who experience long-lasting hemi-inattention, especially those for whom it is severe, have been reported to have longer hospital stays, poorer rehabilitation potential, and decreased independence (Barrett et al., 2006; Chan & Man, 2013; Kaldenberg, 2014; Niemeier et al., 2001; Parton et al., 2004; Pierce & Buxbaum, 2002; Proto et al., 2009; Shinsha & Ishigami, 1999; Stein et al., 2009).

Neurological Basis of Attention to Sensory Stimulation

Attention to sensory stimulation is needed to gather information about the environment, a precursor to appropriate interaction with objects and others. By attending to sensory stimulation, a person is able to identify relevant object and environmental features and disregard irrelevant ones. The person is then able to interpret sensory information, recognize what has meaning for the task at hand and what does not, and make motor adjustments to allow the gathering of more information (e.g., moving the body, head, and/or eyes in the direction of a stimulus of interest). For visual attention, a person needs to be able to focus on different aspects of the visual scene, disengage and shift focus, and systematically examine the visual scene in order to ensure that complete and accurate information has been obtained (Warren, 2018; Weisser-Pike, 2014). Gathering visual information is a complex process, and it appears that there are multiple parts of the brain that are involved, with each responsible for different aspects of attending. The major areas that have been identified thus far are the postcentral gyrus in the parietal lobe, the frontal eye fields in the frontal lobe, the cingulate gyrus, and some subcortical structures, including portions of the thalamus and basal ganglia (Mesulam, 1994, 1999).

The postcentral gyrus in the dorsolateral posterior parietal cortex appears to be heavily involved with the ability to perceive sensory stimulation. It receives information from numerous areas of the brain, although not directly from the primary sensory areas. This means that the parietal lobe gathers information that has already begun to be processed by other areas of the brain (the unimodal and polymodal areas) and that it gets input from multiple sensory systems (Mesulam, 1981, 1990, 1999). The postcentral gyrus also receives information from the cingulate gyrus, which is part of the limbic system. The cingulate gyrus appears to be the part of the attentional network that is responsible for determining whether or not sensory stimulation is relevant to the person (Mesulam, 1981, 1990, 1999). The postcentral gyrus has efferent projections as well, some of which go to the frontal eye fields in the dorsolateral premotor-prefrontal cortex and the

Figure 6-2. Hemisphere differences in attention.

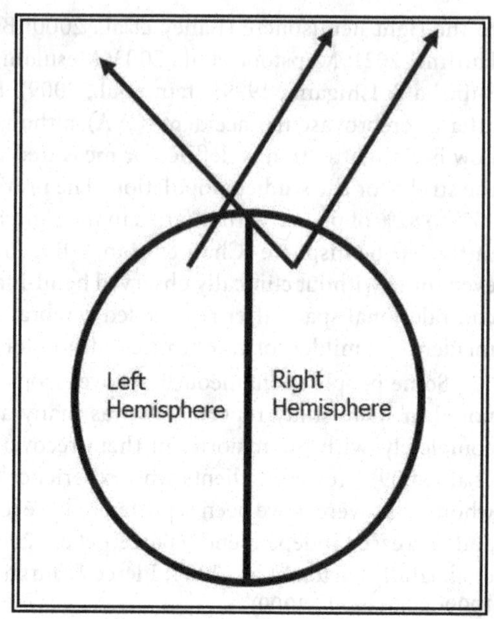

superior colliculus. The frontal eye fields also receive input from the cingulate gyrus. The frontal eye fields and the superior colliculus are essential for directing head and eye movement, which are necessary for exploration, specifically for searching the environment and changing focus to new portions of the visual scene (Mesulam, 1981, 1990, 1999). Damage to any of these areas (i.e., the postcentral gyrus, cingulate gyrus, and frontal eye fields) can cause hemi-inattention, as can damage to some subcortical structures, including portions of the thalamus and the basal ganglia (Mesulam, 1994, 1999).

As stated previously, hemi-inattention is more common, more severe, and longer lasting when it occurs after right hemisphere damage (Bailey et al., 2000; Barrett et al., 2006; Chan & Man, 2013; Mapstone et al., 2003; Mesulam, 1981, 1990, 1994, 1999; Pierce & Buxbaum, 2002; Shinsha & Ishigami, 1999; Stein et al., 2009; Weisser-Pike, 2014). This is believed to be because of the way that the two hemispheres attend to the environment in a normally functioning brain. The right hemisphere is thought to be responsible for attending more globally to both the right and left space, whereas the left hemisphere is thought to attend almost entirely to the right side of space (Figure 6-2). As a result, when there is damage to the right hemisphere that impacts its ability to direct attention, the left hemisphere does not focus attention to the left, resulting in difficulties in perceiving and interacting with the side left of midline. On the other hand, when the left hemisphere is damaged, it is more likely that the right hemisphere will be successful in directing attention to both sides of space given its function under normal conditions (Mapstone et al., 2003; Mesulam, 1981, 1990; Proto et al., 2009; Warren, 2018). However, this relationship is not perfect. It is commonly thought that those with right hemisphere damage are only inattentive to the left, but research has found that participants with right brain lesions and confirmed left hemi-inattention also had reductions in attention to the far right, approximately 60 degrees to the right of midline and beyond (Ellis et al., 2006). The authors of this study theorized that the decrease in responsiveness to the ipsilesional side of space was caused by transhemispheric diaschisis, which happens when damage in one hemisphere leads to a reduction in activation and functioning in similar locations in the opposite hemisphere. As a result of these findings, clinicians are encouraged to consider clients' attention to both sides of space rather than focusing solely on interactions with contralesional space.

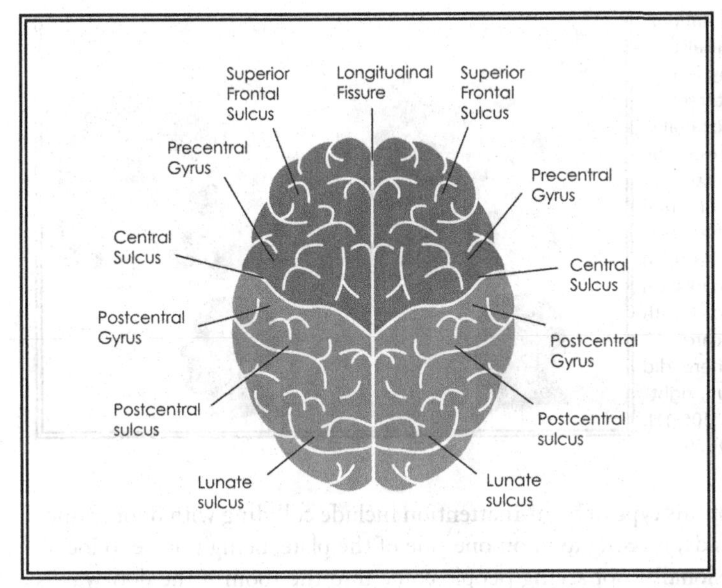

Figure 6-3. The cerebral cortex. Damage to the postcentral gyrus, especially on the right, is linked to perceptual/representational hemi-inattention. (BigMouse/shutterstock.com)

Types of Hemi-Inattention and Symptoms

The symptoms of hemi-inattention can be quite variable for different people depending on which portions of the brain are damaged and the extent of the damage. Hemi-inattention can be very subtle (with people only missing some information in some situations) or extremely severe (with a complete inability to interact with contralesional space and the contralesional side of the body), and anywhere in between. There are three components of hemi-inattention (perceptual/representational, motor/exploratory, and motivational) that can be present to a greater or lesser extent in clients with a brain injury (Mesulam, 1981, 1990, 1994, 1999). It is also important to understand that the portions of the brain that help to direct attention are strongly associated with each other. As a result, damage to one area of the brain can lead to disruption in the functioning of other areas of the brain, thus resulting in multiple types of hemi-inattention. Therefore, it is rare to see people with only one type of hemi-inattention (Mesulam, 1981).

Perceptual/Representational Hemi-Inattention

Perceptual/representational hemi-inattention manifests through impairment in sensory perception, primarily vision, in addition to difficulties in forming an internal representation of the external world. This issue usually follows damage to the postcentral gyrus in the parietal cortex (Mesulam, 1981, 1990, 1994, 1999; Figure 6-3). People with this type of hemi-inattention have difficulty perceiving the contralesional side of the world. The amount of difficulty people have will vary depending on the severity of the hemi-inattention. Those with severe cases may not attend to any input from the contralesional side. Those with mild cases may respond but more slowly than

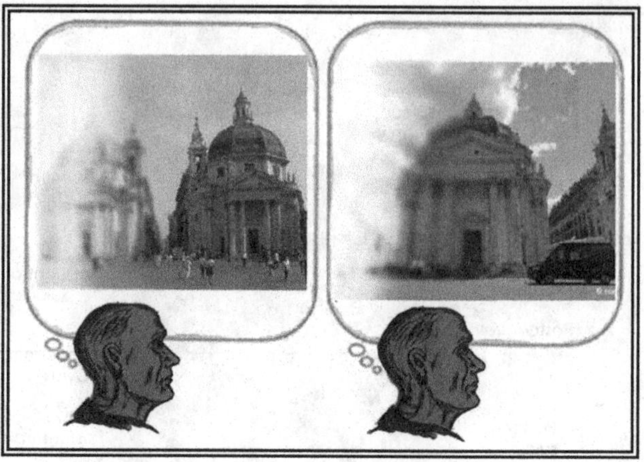

Figure 6-4. For people with representational hemi-inattention, visualizing a space will also be negatively affected. In a 1978 study by Bisiach and Luzzatti, two people with hemi-inattention were asked to describe plazas that were familiar to them. At first, they were asked to describe what they saw when standing on one side of the plaza. Then, they were asked to describe what they saw when standing on the other side of the plaza. In both situations, research participants failed to mention landmarks on the left side of the plaza. (Reproduced with permission from Committeri, G., Piccardi, L., Galati, G., & Guariglia, C. [2015]. Where did you "left" Piazza del Popolo? At your "right" temporo-parietal junction. *Cortex, 73*, 106-111. https://doi.org/10.1016/j.cortex.2015.08.009)

would be expected. Other signs of this type of hemi-inattention include colliding with door frames or objects on the contralesional side, missing food on one side of the plate, being unable to locate objects that are located contralesionally, not seeing people come into the room if the doorway is located on the contralesional side, and feeling that objects appear or disappear unexpectedly. This type of hemi-inattention can happen for objects that are within arm's reach (peripersonal space), objects that are beyond arm's reach (extrapersonal space), or both (Mesulam, 1981, 1990, 1994, 1999). People can also feel like the affected side of their body no longer belongs to them, which is a problem with perception of within-body (personal) space (Klinke, Zahavi et al., 2015). In addition, clients can exhibit hemi-inattention for auditory and tactile stimulation by not responding to these types of input from the contralesional side or responding as if the input were coming from the ipsilesional side, such as by responding to people on the right when the speaker was on the left (Barrett et al., 2006). One of the challenges for this population is that the world appears complete for them, so it can be very difficult for them to understand that they are missing information from a portion of space (Tham et al., 1999; Weisser-Pike, 2014).

In addition to having difficulty perceiving the external world, people with perceptual/representational hemi-inattention have deficits with the internal representation of space (Mesulam, 1999; Pierce & Buxbaum, 2002). In one landmark study (Bisiach & Luzzatti, 1978), two clients with hemi-inattention were asked to imagine themselves standing on one side of a plaza near their homes, a space with which they were very familiar. They were then asked to describe the plaza. They described everything that would have been to their right, which was their ipsilesional side. They were then asked to imagine themselves standing on the opposite side of the plaza and describe what they saw. They again described everything that was on their right. What they described the second time, however, were the portions of space they had not reported in the first version of the exercise because they were imagining themselves facing a different direction (Figure 6-4). This difficulty with internal representation of space leads to challenges with navigation. For people with this condition, it is easy for them to become disoriented because the path that they followed going in one direction appears very different from the path they follow going in the opposite direction. They attend to different stimulation depending on which way they are going so that going to and returning from a location, even along the same path, is perceived as two different routes (Klinke, Zahavi et al., 2015).

It is important to remember that this type of hemi-inattention is not caused by a primary sensory deficit but, instead, is an issue of not attending to contralesional space. One way to illustrate this point is through the observation that some people with left hemi-inattention (from damage to the right hemisphere) present with decreased tactile sensation on their left limbs when those limbs are positioned to the left of midline. If the left limb is positioned to the right of midline, however, tactile sensation improves. In this case, the only change is that the limb was moved from the left (unattended) side of space to the right (attended) side (Barrett et al., 2006).

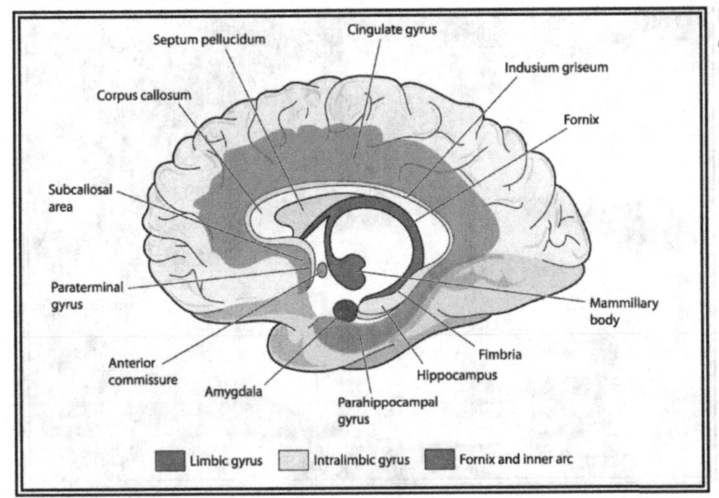

Figure 6-5. Damage to the cingulate gyrus can result in motivational hemi-inattention. (Blamb/shutterstock.com)

Motor/Exploratory Hemi-Inattention

People with motor/exploratory hemi-inattention show deficits with physically exploring the contralesional side of space. This type of hemi-inattention is most common after damage to the premotor-prefrontal cortex (including the frontal eye fields) and/or the superior colliculus. Those with motor/exploratory hemi-inattention have difficulty in turning their eyes, head, and body beyond midline to focus on and search the contralesional space. They can also have difficulty with reaching into the contralesional space (Mesulam, 1981, 1990, 1994, 1999). This can occur with the involved upper extremity and is beyond what would be expected based on motor deficits alone (Bailey et al., 2000; Parton et al., 2004). Deficits with reaching can also occur when the client is crossing midline with the uninvolved upper extremity, which provides more evidence that this deficit is not due to a primary motor lesion (Bailey et al., 2000; Barrett et al., 2006; Mesulam, 1999).

Motivational Hemi-Inattention

The final type of hemi-inattention is motivational. This is most common after damage to the cingulate gyrus, which is part of the limbic system (Figure 6-5). Individuals with motivational hemi-inattention seem to find information from the contralesional part of space irrelevant or of little value. As a result, they do not have the internal drive to explore the contralesional environment (Mesulam, 1981, 1990, 1999).

Presentation of People With Hemi-Inattention

Because of the different ways that hemi-inattention can manifest, there is variability in how people with hemi-inattention appear. However, there are some commonalities for clients with this condition, most notably an impairment in visual search, which leads to missing important details on the contralesional (usually the left) side of space. Figure 6-6 provides an example of how a client with hemi-inattention may miss information on the left. Other features that can be present for people with hemi-inattention are extinction and a decrease or lack of attention to the contralesional part of the body.

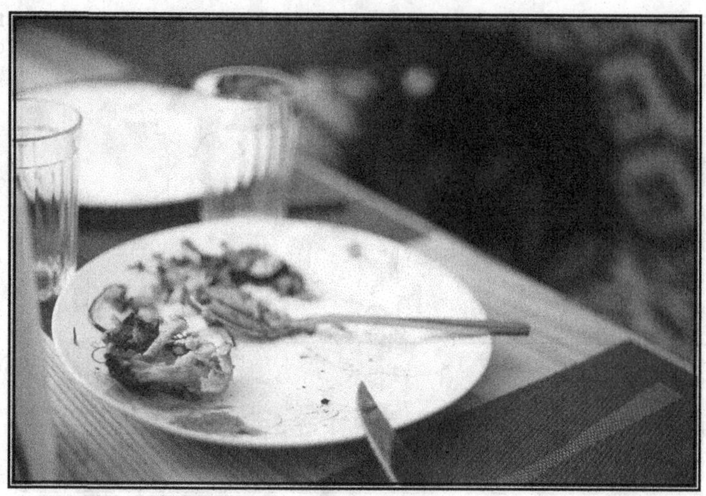

Figure 6-6. People with hemi-inattention often fail to perceive objects in the contralesional visual space. This is often observed during functional activity, such as with a client who is not able to locate food on the contralesional side of the plate. (Konstantin Savusia/shutterstock.com)

Visual Search

People without a brain injury will look for and locate information in the environment in a systematic and predictable way. They can implement this searching consciously and deliberately (e.g., when looking for your favorite cereal brand in an unfamiliar grocery store), but visual searching can also be done automatically without much conscious thought. For people with hemi-inattention, both types of visual search can be disrupted. In fact, according to some authors, impaired visual searching is a major way that hemi-inattention is observed (Warren, 2018; Weisser-Pike, 2014). Rather than using a thorough, organized, and systematic search strategy, people with hemi-inattention often demonstrate an incomplete, disorganized, and random search strategy (Warren, 2018). For example, people with left hemi-inattention will often start their search on the right instead of the left, and they can show enormous difficulty disengaging their attention from the right side, which is referred to as a *magnetic attraction to the right* (Klinke, Zahavi et al., 2015; Mesulam, 1990, 1999; Parton et al., 2004; Proto et al., 2009). Even when they are able to disengage their attention from the right, that disengagement can be brief, and their focus will be drawn to the right side again. In more extreme cases of left hemi-inattention, people will physically orient themselves to the right, turning their bodies, heads, and eyes in that direction (Mesulam, 1990; Parton et al., 2004). They can even feel as if the left side of space is a void, as was stated by one participant in a qualitative study by Klinke, Zahavi et al. (2015): "They asked me to turn [left]—but I literally feel it as if I am expecting to enter a free fall" (p. 6).

People with hemi-inattention will also often display a search pattern that is incomplete. This population tends to spend much more time searching the ipsilesional side of space as opposed to the contralesional side, sometimes never exploring the contralesional side of space at all. They also tend to miss details in their search. They often are reluctant to re-search the environment or repeatedly search the same area (usually ipsilesional). The time they spend in their visual search is also different from those without hemi-inattention. They may either search for a very short time, terminating their search early, or search for an inordinately long time, continuing to use an inefficient search strategy to attempt to locate missing objects or information (Cicek et al., 2007; Mesulam, 1999; Warren, 2018; Weisser-Pike, 2014).

Although visual search is almost always negatively impacted for this population, it is important to remember that it can occur differently in different types of space, specifically in peripersonal and extrapersonal space (Bailey et al., 2000; Castiello et al., 2004; Chan & Man, 2013; Christy & Huffine, 2021; Mesulam, 1994; Pierce & Buxbaum, 2002; Proto et al., 2009; Tham et al., 1999; Tham & Kielhofner, 2003). Individuals with impairments in visual search for peripersonal space have difficulty locating objects within arm's reach on the nonattended (or less attended) side, such as grooming items on a sink counter, food on a plate, or words on a page when reading. For people who have hemi-inattention issues in extrapersonal space, visual search is impaired when looking for objects beyond arm's reach, which can include looking for information on grocery store signs or scanning for traffic to determine whether it is safe to cross the street. People with hemi-inattention can demonstrate visual searching deficits in peripersonal space, extrapersonal space, or both (Bailey et al., 2000; Castiello et al., 2004; Chan & Man, 2013; Christy & Huffine, 2021; Mesulam, 1994; Pierce & Buxbaum, 2002; Proto et al., 2009; Tham et al., 1999; Tham & Kielhofner, 2003).

Visual searching can also be disrupted for different reasons. As stated previously, an infarct involving the parietal cortex can cause sensory/representational hemi-inattention, which can result in people not being aware that they are only searching one portion of space. Damage to the premotor cortex, including the frontal eye fields, can result in motor/exploratory hemi-inattention with a disruption in the motor ability to execute a systematic and complete visual search. Finally, damage to the cingulate gyrus can cause motivational hemi-inattention, resulting in disinterest in searching the contralesional visual field. For many clients, the visual search is likely disrupted as a result of more than one type of hemi-inattention (Mesulam, 1981, 1990, 1994, 1999).

Extinction

Another common sign of hemi-inattention is extinction, which can occur in more than one sensory modality (Cicek et al., 2007; Kaldenberg, 2014; Klinke, Zahavi et al., 2015; Mesulam, 1981; Parton et al., 2004). Visual extinction is demonstrated when the client is able to identify and report on a single visual stimulus, even when it is presented in the contralesional visual space, but has an inability or severe limitation in perceiving two objects displayed simultaneously in the ipsilesional and contralesional space (DiPellegrino et al., 1997; Mattingley et al., 1997). People with extinction ignore one of two objects held in intact visual fields on either side of the midline when presented simultaneously. This may occur not only for midline opposite stimuli but also for contralateral upper and lower quadrants. For example, a lower right quadrant stimulus can cause a simultaneous stimulus in the upper left quadrant to be ignored. Similarly, extinction can be observed for tactile stimuli (when a client is touched on both sides of the body but only reports the stimulus on the ipsilesional side even in the absence of sensory loss) and auditory input (Parton et al., 2004).

There are many theories as to why extinction occurs. The main hypotheses are that (a) impaired attentional orienting to contralesional targets, (b) a problem disengaging attention from ipsilateral stimuli, or (c) an abnormal attraction of attention toward the spared side of space exists (DiPelligrino et al., 1997). Research in the field supports the hypothesis that extinction is the result of a weaker competitive weight that is assigned to contralesional items than to ipsilateral ones (DiPelligrino et al., 1997). A study conducted by Mattingley et al. (1997) not only supported this hypothesis but also took it one step further when the researchers observed that a variance in competitive weight occurred from stimuli from different modalities or senses. For example, when the participant was given tactile and visual stimuli at the same time, the client still extinguished the stimulus contralateral to the lesion, whether that stimulus was visual or tactile. These researchers found that extinction could manifest within any of the primary senses and could occur within several senses in a given client (Mattingley et al., 1997).

Personal Inattention

Some people with hemi-inattention can demonstrate an inability to attend to the contralesional part of their body. This can be severe, resulting in people neglecting to dress their contralesional arm or leg, not shaving half of their face, or not brushing half of their hair (Parton et al., 2004; Pierce & Buxbaum, 2002). It can also result in feeling like the contralesional part of their bodies do not belong to them. Over time, many people can learn to attend to all of their body parts, although the feeling of being estranged from one half of their body may never fully resolve (Tham et al., 1999; Tham & Kielhofner, 2003). One participant in the study by Klinke, Zahavi, et al. (2015) described this feeling well when she said the following:

> I often try ... imagining that my body is like the body of inseparable [conjoined] twins—accordingly, when I move, I simultaneously need to pay attention to my twin—we are part of the same body even though we are different ... I find that producing this kind of mental picture ... somehow makes [my left side] more real, more a part of me. (p. 8)

Conditions That Co-Occur With Hemi-Inattention

Hemi-inattention occurs with damage to the brain. As a result, the person with hemi-inattention almost certainly presents with other deficits, including but not limited to contralesional hemiparesis, contralesional sensory loss including visual field deficit, reduction in arousal and general attention, and anosognosia (i.e., a lack of awareness of deficits; Barrett et al., 2006; Shinsha & Ishigami, 1999). Information about treating hemiparesis and tactile loss is beyond the scope of this text, but other common co-occurring conditions are discussed in this chapter.

Visual Field Cut

A disruption in the visual pathway can occur after ABI, which can result in a visual field cut, meaning that the link between the eye and the brain is damaged and the person will be unable to see a portion of the visual field (Lundy-Ekman, 2018; Warren, 2018). It is important for the clinician to consider the impact of a visual field deficit on the client with hemi-inattention because visual field deficits exacerbate the issues that people with hemi-inattention can have. As stated in Chapter 4, to accurately determine the presence and scope of visual field deficits, an evaluation by an ophthalmologist or optometrist is recommended, although the occupational therapy practitioner can administer a screening test as a preliminary step in determining the nature and extent of the impairment.

Visual field deficits can result in clients having an abbreviated visual search and missing information from the contralesional visual field, symptoms that can also be present for people with hemi-inattention. As a result, it is not uncommon for occupational therapy practitioners to have difficulty deciding if a client has a visual field cut, hemi-inattention, or both. According to some authors, there are differences in how patients with a visual field cut alone versus patients with hemi-inattention search and interact with the world that can assist clinicians in determining the underlying issues for clients (Warren, 2018; Weisser-Pike, 2014). People with a visual field deficit without hemi-inattention may show a shortened visual search and miss information from the contralesional visual field but are more likely to conduct their visual search in an organized way. They are also more likely to search for missing information, and their search time will be similar to people without visual search deficits (Warren, 2018; Weisser-Pike, 2014). Table 6-1 provides a comparison between people with visual field cut and those with hemi-inattention.

Table 6-1

Comparison of Search Patterns: Persons With Visual Field Deficit Versus Persons With Hemi-Inattention

VISUAL FIELD DEFICIT	HEMI-INATTENTION
• Search pattern is abbreviated toward blind field	• Search pattern is asymmetrical (initiated/confined to the right side)
• Client attempts to direct search toward blind side	• Client makes no attempt to direct search toward left side
• Search pattern is organized and generally efficient	• Search pattern is random and generally inefficient
• Client rescans to check accuracy of performance	• Client does not rescan to check accuracy of performance
• Time spent on task is appropriate to level of difficulty	• Client completes task quickly; level of effort applied is not consistent with difficulty of task

Reproduced with permission from Warren, M. (1998). *Brain Injury Visual Assessment Battery for Adults: Test manual* (pp. 4-43). VisAbilities Rehab Services Inc.

In addition to differences in the visual search itself, there will often be distinctions noted between the two client populations over time. People with visual field cut alone usually show better adaptation to their deficits with an improved ability to find objects even when those objects are located in the impaired portion of the visual field. One group of researchers studied people with hemi-inattention and/or homonymous hemianopsia (i.e., a visual field cut affecting the contralesional visual field in each eye; see Chapter 3 for a further description of this condition). Four groups of clients were included: (a) people with severe hemi-inattention and hemianopsia, (b) people with severe hemi-inattention without hemianopsia, (c) people with no hemi-inattention and no hemianopsia, and (d) people with hemianopsia and no hemi-inattention. The researchers found that people with hemianopsia alone initially missed information contralesionally but then adapted, missing no information within a few weeks after the infarct. People with hemi-inattention, with or without hemianopsia, continued to miss information contralesionally even weeks later (Saj et al., 2012).

Reduced Arousal and General Inattention

Hemi-inattention appears to be a deficit associated with problems with the attentional system, and, increasingly, the role of attention in hemi-inattention is being recognized and examined. People with hemi-inattention have been observed having an impairment in alertness and different types of attention, including sustained and selective attention (Barrett et al., 2006; Christy & Huffine, 2021; Klinke, Zahavi et al., 2015; Parton et al., 2004; Pierce & Buxbaum, 2002; Proto et al., 2009). In addition, clients typically show worsening hemi-inattention when general attentional demands increase (Barrett et al., 2006). Some have theorized that this reduction in arousal and general attention may be partly caused by deficits with the reticular system (Mesulam, 1981).

In their research of clients with hemi-inattention, Robertson and colleagues (1995) found that sustained attention was an important modulation variable that influenced the pattern of hemi-inattention. These researchers hypothesized that impaired sustained attention may be an underlying cause of persistent hemi-inattention and that clients with hemi-inattention in acute stages who then recover spontaneously may not show the same sustained attention deficits that people without spontaneous recovery show (Robertson et al., 1995).

Anosognosia

Anosognosia is defined as an unawareness of one's deficit and is common for this population, although the exact incidence is not known. One review found that an estimated 20% to 58% of people with hemi-inattention also had anosognosia (Pierce & Buxbaum, 2002), whereas another study reported incidence as high as 74% in the population with hemi-inattention (Proto et al., 2009). In some cases, anosognosia is severe, with the client completely denying that there is an issue in all situations; in other cases, it is less severe, resulting in the need for reminders but not constant cueing. Anosognosia is also variable depending on the task, with people more easily able to identify errors in some situations (e.g., those in which they are actively performing tasks) than others, indicating that anosognosia, like hemi-inattention itself, is a heterogenous phenomenon (Ronchi et al., 2014). Those with anosognosia have worse outcomes than those without and will be less likely to be able to overcome their deficits. This is partly because of the fact that people are unlikely to use compensatory strategies if they do not understand the reason for their use (Barrett et al., 2006; Pierce & Buxbaum, 2002; Ronchi et al., 2014; Tham et al., 1999).

The awareness of deficits can change over time for some individuals as they get feedback from others and experience the impact of the deficit. This has been illustrated in qualitative studies in which researchers have interviewed and observed people with hemi-inattention in the acute stages of recovery (Klinke, Zahavi et al., 2015; Tham et al., 1999; Tham & Kielhofner, 2003). These studies showed evolution of the participants' awareness of their hemi-inattention. In the early stages of recovery, the study participants experienced the world as chaotic and bewildering and did not understand why they were told that they were missing objects on the contralesional side of space. Over time, they had increasing understanding of the nature of their hemi-inattention, although even in the later stages of recovery in these studies, participants still needed to consciously, rather than automatically, apply compensatory strategies to search to the left (Klinke, Zahavi et al., 2015; Tham et al., 1999; Tham & Kielhofner, 2003). However, for many people, especially in more severe cases, awareness can remain limited or nonexistent.

Functional Impact of Hemi-Inattention

Functional implications for the client with visuospatial inattention are varied and often severe. Clients have difficulty not just with specific tasks involving reading, writing, and drawing but also any or all areas of occupation, including activities of daily living (ADLs), instrumental activities of daily living (IADLs),, work, leisure, and social participation depending on the severity of deficit (Chen Sea et al., 1993; Heilman et al., 2000). Hemi-inattention generally causes clients to be more prone to accidents than those without this deficit because they are most often not aware of the deficit and less likely to implement strategies that enable them to avoid obstacles and dangers in the environment (Suter, 2018). Hemi-inattention is associated with lower scores not only for ADLs but also with sensorimotor and cognitive measures (Kelly, 1985). The most impacted areas are those that increase demands during visual search, such as visually complex or dynamic environments (Warren, 2018). These can include driving, shopping, and, in general, all community mobility. For example, imagine Deion, a 56-year-old man who had a right middle cerebral artery stroke 4 years ago. Deion lives in his own home with a family caregiver. At home, he is independent with his ADLs and some simple meal preparation (e.g., making a sandwich). This environment is largely static and predictable, and Deion does not have difficulty with locating objects. However, when he goes into the community, he needs more assistance from his caregiver because the environment is dynamic and unpredictable. Without the extra help, Deion is more likely to miss obstacles or other information. Even with assistance, Deion has had falls in the community, including sustaining a humeral fracture after tripping over a curb he had not noticed on his left.

Assessment of Hemi-Inattention

Because hemi-inattention is a heterogenous disorder, clients often show differential results on different screening tools, demonstrating hemi-inattention with some assessments and not with others (Azouvi et al., 1996, 2003; Bailey et al., 2000, 2004; Barrett et al., 2006; Maeshima et al., 2001; Parton et al., 2004). Researchers have conducted studies to determine the most sensitive combination of tests to administer to clients (Maeshima et al., 2001). Included in these studies have been a variety of what are often called *conventional pen-and-paper tests*, such as cancellation tests (i.e., when clients need to cross off a target stimulus and disregard distractors), line bisection tests (i.e., when clients are asked to mark the center of one or more lines), reading tests, figure copy tests (i.e., when clients are asked to copy a drawing or shape), and representational drawing tests (i.e., when clients draw an object, such as a clock or a person, from memory), in addition to tools involving observation of simulated or naturalistic functional tasks. According to some authors, the most sensitive test battery appears to be one that includes multiple types of tests (e.g., a line bisection test, a cancellation test, and the Baking Tray Task [BTT; described later]; Bailey et al., 2000, 2004). Additional information about representational hemi-inattention may be acquired from administering a representational drawing test (Maeshima et al., 2001). In addition, it is essential to consider hemi-inattention in the context of function. This can be accomplished through skilled observation during occupation and through the use of instruments such as the Catherine Bergego Scale (Azouvi et al., 1996, 2003; Barrett et al., 2006) or the Kessler Foundation Neglect Assessment Process (KF-NAP; Chen, Chen, et al., 2015; Chen, Hreah, et al., 2012; Chen & Hreha, 2015), which are described later in this chapter. This final recommendation is in keeping with the findings of Donoso-Brown and Powell (2017), who found that the performance of clients with hemi-inattention was substantially better in a structured test environment than with similar tasks in a more naturalistic environment.

Skilled Observation During Occupation

It is essential for the treating practitioner to look for hemi-inattention in the context of functional activity. Hemi-inattention is most likely to present itself as an impairment in visual search, resulting in missing details contralesionally, including difficulty locating items during activities and colliding with obstacles, such as doorways, during functional mobility. In addition to impairments in visual search, clinicians may notice that clients are reluctant to direct their gaze contralesionally, orient their head and/or bodies ipsilesionally, have difficulty crossing midline with their unaffected limbs, or do not attend (or attend less) to body parts on one side (e.g., brushing hair on only one part of their head, washing only one half of their body, or performing those tasks with poorer quality on the affected side; Parton et al., 2004). As stated previously, it can be difficult to distinguish when an impairment in visual search is caused by hemianopsia or another visual field cut, hemi-inattention, or both. Signs that hemi-inattention is present are if the person visually searches in a disorganized and/or random manner, misses searching areas of the visual scene, searches either faster or slower than expected, and does not re-search areas to find missed information (Warren, 2018; Weisser-Pike, 2014).

Other questions to ask during observation of the client in functional activity include the following:

- What is the client's posture and head position? Is there any head turning/tilt? Is the client oriented to the ipsilesional side with reluctance or decreased ability to orient to midline or contralesionally (Parton et al., 2004)?
- What is the level of the client's sustained attention? Is the client easily distracted (Barrett et al., 2006)? (We recommend assessing this in different environments; clients with more mild deficits are more likely to demonstrate difficulties in complex or dynamic environments.)
- Where does the client start their visual search? For example, with left hemi-inattention, does the search start on the right (a sign of hemi-inattention) or on the left (Warren, 2018; Weisser-Pike, 2014)?
- Does the client perform visual search in an organized manner within the intact visual fields? Refer to Table 6-1 for a description of search patterns of the client with hemianopsia versus the client with visual inattention. Is the speed of the search decreased or increased (Warren, 2018; Weisser-Pike, 2014)?
- Does the client's performance improve if the visual array is set up in an organized and structured manner (Warren, 2018)?
- Does hemi-inattention become apparent in personal space (on the person's body), peripersonal space (within arm's reach), or extrapersonal space (beyond arm's reach)? In more than one type of space? Under what conditions? What specific functional activities appear to be affected by the hemi-inattention? Does hemi-inattention mostly appear during activities such as eating, reading, or hygiene? Or is it more prevalent during mobility (e.g., decreased awareness of doorways or turning wheelchair only in one direction; Aloiso, 2004)?
- Does increasing the complexity of the visual array decrease performance? For example, does performance worsen when looking for an object in a crowded refrigerator versus one with only a few items (Warren, 2018)?
- Does verbal cueing help performance? Does tactile, auditory, proprioceptive, or kinesthetic cueing help (Toglia & Cermak, 2009)?
- Does the client show the ability to identify and correct errors (Rochi et al., 2014)?
- How does altering the task and/or the environment affect performance (Toglia & Cermak, 2009)?

Catherine Bergego Scale (Azouvi et al., 1996)

Description

The Catherine Bergego Scale (Figure 6-7) was developed to standardize observations of left hemi-inattention in the context of functional activity. It was also designed to address the concern that the majority of conventional assessment tools for hemi-inattention only consider peripersonal space and could, therefore, miss people with hemi-inattention in other areas of space. As a result, the test designers sought a way to consider the impact of hemi-inattention in extrapersonal and personal space as well. In addition, the developers were concerned that conventional tests are less likely to require people to use attention in a more automatic manner because clients are focusing their attention on the hemi-inattention assessment task. The Catherine Bergego Scale considers performance during engagement in occupation, which is more likely to require automatic spatial attention.

	0	1	2	3
1. Forgets to groom or shave the left part of his/her face	❑	❑	❑	❑
2. Experiences difficulty in adjusting his/her left sleeve or slipper	❑	❑	❑	❑
3. Forgets to eat food on the left side of his/her plate	❑	❑	❑	❑
4. Forgets to clean the left side of his/her mouth after eating	❑	❑	❑	❑
5. Experiences difficulty in looking towards the left	❑	❑	❑	❑
6. Forgets about a left part of his/her body (eg, forgets to put his/her upper limb on the armrest, or his/her left foot on the wheelchair rest, or forgets to use his/her left arm when he/she needs to)	❑	❑	❑	❑
7. Has difficulty in paying attention to noise or people addressing him/her from the left	❑	❑	❑	❑
8. Collides with people or objects on the left side, such as doors or furniture (either while walking or driving a wheelchair)	❑	❑	❑	❑
9. Experiences difficulty in finding his/her way towards the left when traveling in familiar places or in the rehabilitation unit	❑	❑	❑	❑
10. Experiences difficulty finding his/her personal belongings in the room or bathroom when they are on the left side	❑	❑	❑	❑
Total score (/30)				

0=no neglect; 1=mild neglect; 2=moderate neglect; 3=severe neglect

Figure 6-7. The Catherine Bergego Scale. (Reproduced with permission from Bergego, C., Azouvi, P., Samuel, C., Marchal, F., Louis-Dreyfus, A., Jokic, C., Morin, L., Renard, C., Pradat-Diehl, P., & Deloche, G. [1995]. Validation d'une échelle d'évaluation fonctionnelle del'héminégligence dans la vie quotidienne: l'échelle CB. *Annales de Readaptation et de Medecine Physique, 38*[4], 183-189.)

Procedure

Practitioners observe the client's performance in 10 areas: (a) grooming and shaving, (b) wearing the left sleeve or slipper, (c) eating food on the left side of the plate, (d) cleaning the left side of the mouth after eating, (e) directing gaze to the left spontaneously, (f) attending to the left side of the body, (g) attending to noise or people on the left, (h) avoiding collisions with objects on the left, (i) traveling toward the left in familiar places, and (j) finding belongings located on the left.

Scoring

The practitioner uses a 4-point scale to rate the impact of left hemi-inattention on the client's performance in each of the 10 areas with 0 indicating no issues with hemi-inattention, 1 indicating mild issues, 2 indicating moderate issues, and 3 indicating severe issues. As a result, a higher score indicates more severe hemi-inattention. In addition to the rating scale that is completed by practitioners, a companion scale is completed by the clients themselves. Comparison of the two scores allows clinicians to assess the presence and extent of anosognosia related to hemi-inattention.

Psychometric Properties

Several studies have examined the reliability and validity of the Catherine Bergego Scale. One study found inter-rater reliability of $r = 0.96$ when the scale was used with 18 people with hemi-inattention (Bergego et al., 1995 as cited in Azouvi et al., 1996). A subsequent study with 50 people with a right CVA examined the internal and external validity of the scale when compared to conventional tests (i.e., drawing tasks, cancellation tasks, and a reading task; Azouvi et al., 1996). The researchers also considered the scale's relationship with functional performance and deficit awareness. Spearman's rho for internal consistency was found to range from 0.58 to 0.88, indicating that the questions were highly correlated with each other. In addition, Spearman's rho ranged from 0.50 to 0.74 for correlations with conventional hemi-inattention tests, demonstrating that the Catherine Bergego Scale was able to differentiate between people with no or mild hemi-inattention and those with more severe hemi-inattention. The Catherine Bergego Scale was also found to be correlated (Spearman's rho = 0.63) with the Barthel Index, a test of ADL functioning, and helped to quantify the extent of anosognosia for the study population. The researchers also found that more people were found to have hemi-inattention on the Catherine Bergego Scale than on conventional tests, demonstrating that it may be a more sensitive assessment tool (Azouvi et al., 1996).

A more recent study, conducted with 83 people with right CVA, also considered the validity and sensitivity of the scale (Azouvi et al., 2003). These researchers found that the Catherine Bergego Scale was correlated (Spearman's rho = 0.54 to 0.76) with a cancellation test, a figure copy test, and a reading test. In addition, more people were judged to have hemi-inattention when rated with the Catherine Bergego Scale than with the conventional tests, supporting the previous finding that the scale may be a more sensitive measure of hemi-inattention.

Kessler Foundation Neglect Assessment Process (Chen & Hreha, 2015)

Description

In 2012, a group of researchers described a tool they had developed based on the Catherine Bergego Scale (Chen et al., 2012). These researchers had noted some limitations when using the scale. These included insufficient context for clinician observations (e.g., whether clients should be assessed once or over several sessions) and lack of information about standardization of tasks (e.g., how items were placed in relation to the client's midline). The researchers also thought that scoring would benefit from expansion and clarification, especially distinguishing between mild and moderate hemi-inattention deficits (Chen et al., 2012). The authors created the Kessler Foundation Neglect Assessment Process (KF-NAP) to overcome these limitations.

Procedure

A manual for the KF-NAP was published in 2014 with a revised manual published 1 year later (Chen & Hreha, 2015). The authors recommend that the test be administered only after training. A video tutorial can be found online (https://www.kflearn.org/courses/KF-NAP). The manual contains instructions for administering each of the 10 items. It takes approximately 20 to 40 minutes to administer the entire assessment, with the meals task needing the most time. The assessment can be administered over the course of more than one session. The authors recommend that any re-assessment with the KF-NAP be completed at the same time of the day and in the same order as initial assessment to minimize the influence of factors such as fatigue (Chen & Hreha, 2015).

Scoring

The manual includes instructions for scoring each of the 10 items.

Psychometric Properties

One study has been published examining the psychometric properties of the KF-NAP (Chen et al., 2015). The researchers found that the KF-NAP had internal consistency of $\alpha = 0.96$. It was correlated with the Functional Independence Measure ($r(82) = -0.62$, $p < .00001$) and the Barthel Index ($r(82) = -0.56$, $p < .00001$), two assessments looking at general functioning in ADLs, although the KF-NAP provided unique information about the presence, severity, and client awareness of hemi-inattention (Chen et al., 2015).

ADL-focused Occupation-based Neurobehavioral Evaluation (Árnadóttir, 1990)

Description

The ADL-focused Occupation-based Neurobehavioral Evaluation (A-ONE), which was originally titled Árnadóttir OT-ADL Neurobehavioral Evaluation, is described in detail in Chapter 5. The A-ONE is used by occupational therapy practitioners to assess both the client's occupational performance in activities of daily living (ADLs) and to determine the underlying neurobehavioral impairments. Evaluators consider clients' performance in ADLs in five domains: dressing, grooming and hygiene, transfers and mobility, feeding, and communication. Evaluators report on the level of independence in ADLs, the type of assistance that is needed, and the types and severity of neurobehavioral impairment (Gardarsdóttir & Kaplan, 2002).

In addition to the impairments related to perception and cognition, 2 of the 16 impairments on the Neurobehavioral Specific Impairment Scale relate to hemi-inattention: unilateral body neglect and unilateral spatial neglect (Árnadóttir, 2021). There is one item on the Neurobehavioral Pervasive Impairment Subscale that directly relates to hemi-inattention. This impairment is anosognosia (i.e., lack of awareness of deficits).

Procedure

As noted in Chapter 5, training is required before clinicians can use the standardized A-ONE tool. To administer the A-ONE, the examiner observes clients while they perform ADLs, such as dressing, and rates their level of independence with the task by using the Functional Independence Scale. The examiner also makes note of errors that are made during task completion and connects the errors that are made to specific neurobehavioral impairments by using the Neurobehavioral Scale (Árnadóttir, 2021).

Scoring

The general scoring strategy for the A-ONE is described in Chapter 5. The two impairments related to hemi-inattention (i.e., unilateral body neglect and unilateral spatial neglect) are both scored for the ADL domains of dressing, grooming and hygiene, transfers and mobility, and feeding on the Specific Impairment Scale. Communication is the only domain that is not scored for the hemi-inattention specific impairments. As per the other items on the Pervasive Impairment Scale, anosognosia is scored once for presence or absence during the ADL observation (Árnadóttir, 2021).

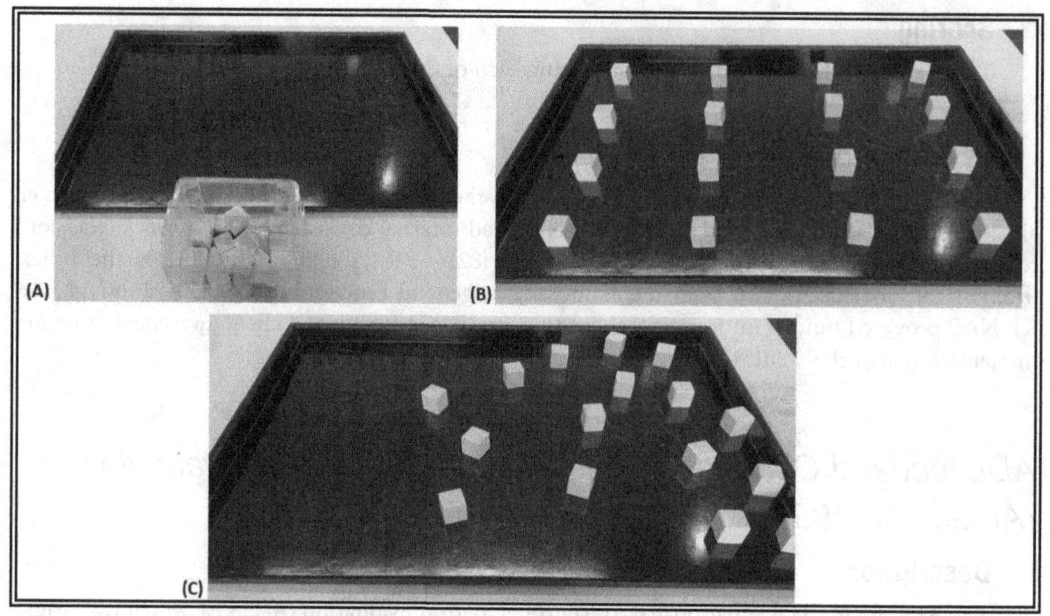

Figure 6-8. The Baking Tray Task. (A) The setup of the assessment. (B) The result that would be expected from someone without hemi-inattention. (C) A person with left hemi-inattention may have a result similar to this.

Psychometric Properties

There are no psychometric studies of the A-ONE that are specific to the impairments related to hemi-inattention. See Chapter 5 for additional information on research examining the tool as a whole.

Baking Tray Task (Tham & Tegner, 1996)

Description

The Baking Tray Task (BTT) was designed as a quick and sensitive tool of hemi-inattention. It is not commercially available but can be constructed from the description given by Tham and Tegner (1996; Figure 6-8.) One advantage of this measure is that it makes use of a wider space than conventional tabletop tasks so is able to assess hemi-inattention in distant peripersonal space. Research has indicated that tests that use a wider space are more likely to identify people with hemi-inattention (Barrett et al., 2006; Ellis et al., 2006). The test uses a tray that is 75 cm by 100 cm with a 3.5-cm high rim on three sides and 16 cubes in a contrasting color. The cubes measure 3.5 cm on each side. The BTT was administered to 52 people with a CVA and 30 age-matched healthy controls to determine normative data (Tham & Tegner, 1996).

Procedure

The tray is placed in front of the client with the midpoint of the tray lined up with the client's midline. The cubes are placed in a box in front of the client, and the client is instructed to place the cubes on the tray spread out "as evenly as possible all over the board as if they were buns on a tray that was to be put in the oven." (Note that this test was created in the United Kingdom. Clients in the United States may understand the instructions better if "buns" are referred to as "cookies" and the "baking tray" is called a "cookie sheet." However, this adjustment in wording has not been tested for any potential impact on the reliability and/or validity of the assessment tool.) The test is not timed, and the client is asked to inform the clinician when the test has been completed. All cubes must be used. If the client does not use all of the cubes, the clinician gives reminders until they are used (Tham & Tegner, 1996).

Scoring

Upon completion of the test, the number of cubes on the left and right of the center of the tray are recorded as a ratio (such as 8:8 if the cubes are equally distributed). If a cube straddles the midline, 0.5 is recorded on each side. The cutoff score is 7:9, indicating seven cubes on the left and nine on the right, or 9:7, indicating nine cubes on the left and seven on the right (Bailey et al., 2000; Tham & Tegner, 1996). The clinician can also make notes about the client's approach to the task, such as whether cubes are initially placed on the left or the right and whether the client approaches the task systematically or in a disorganized fashion.

Psychometric Properties

Participants in the normative study were also administered line cancellation, letter cancellation, representational drawing, cube copying, and line bisection tasks. The researchers found that the BTT was more sensitive than conventional tests in identifying hemi-inattention (Tham & Tegner, 1996). These findings were supported by a subsequent study that compared numerous assessment tools, including star cancellation, line bisection, figure copy, and representational drawing. The findings from this study indicated that the most sensitive assessment tools were star cancellation, line bisection, and the BTT (Bailey et al., 2000).

Behavioural Inattention Test (Wilson et al., 1987)

Description

The Behavioural Inattention Test (BIT) is a standardized test of skills relevant to hemi-inattention. (This test was developed in England and uses the standard United Kingdom spelling of behavioral in the title.) The BIT has six conventional pencil-and-paper subtests and nine behavioral subtests. The conventional subtests include line crossing, letter cancellation, star cancellation, figure and shape copying, line bisection, and representational drawing. The behavioral subtests consist of simulated functional tasks (i.e., performed within the testing environment with simulated test materials rather than a naturalistic setting). These subtests include photograph scanning, telephone dialing, menu reading, article reading, telling and setting the time, coin sorting, address and sentence copying, map navigation, and card sorting. Research has indicated that the line bisection and star cancellation subtests are some of the most sensitive tools for detecting hemi-inattention (Bailey et al., 2000, 2004).

Procedure

All of the subtests are performed with the examiner and client sitting at a table. The test manual includes additional details for administering the assessment.

Scoring

In each subtest, the number of omissions is recorded. In addition, errors of commission (i.e., when the client makes a mistake that involves incorrectly adding something, such as crossing out a distractor on the star cancellation test) are noted, but these types of errors are not incorporated into the score. The total score from the conventional subtests determines the presence of visual hemi-inattention. Behavioral subtests are then used to identify how the hemi-inattention is causing everyday problems and as a guide in treatment strategy (Wilson et al., 1987). Detailed information on scoring is contained in the test manual.

Psychometric Properties

The test developers completed a study with 80 people with a CVA and 50 control participants to establish reliability and validity of the BIT (Wilson et al., 1987). The behavioral tests were compared to the conventional tests and were found to be highly correlated (0.92; $p<.001$). Behavioral scores were also compared with a short questionnaire completed by the practitioner at the time of assessment. The correlation was 0.67 ($p<.001$). This same study established inter-rater reliability at 0.99 ($p<.001$), parallel form reliability between two test versions at 0.91 ($p<.001$), and test–retest reliability at 0.99 ($p<.001$). A later study assessed 40 participants with a CVA with the BIT, performance tasks, and a checklist of ADLs (Hartman-Maeir & Katz, 1995). The results supported the construct and predictive validity of most of the BIT subtest as functional measures of unilateral hemi-inattention. A more recent study was conducted to assess the inter-rater reliability of the BIT focusing on the star cancellation, line bisection, line crossing, figure and shape copying, and representational drawing subtests. These researchers found the intraclass correlation coefficient (ICC) for inter-rater reliability for the test battery to be 0.994 (Hannaford et al., 2003).

Line Bisection Test

Description

In line bisection tests, the client attempts to mark the midpoint of each of a series of horizontal lines presented on a piece of paper (Figure 6-9). Clients with hemi-inattention have been shown to have difficulty marking the center of the lines and instead make marks that are to the ipsilesional side of the line's midpoint (Schenkenberg et al., 1980). For example, clients with left hemi-inattention will make marks to the right of the midpoint of the lines. Various forms of the line bisection test are available including one of the BIT subtests. Another version of the line bisection test can be downloaded through Stroke Engine (https://www.strokengine.ca/en/assess/lbt/).

Procedure

The client and the clinician sit at a table. The clinician places the page with a series of horizontal lines at the client's midline. The client is then instructed to make a mark at the midpoint of each of the lines.

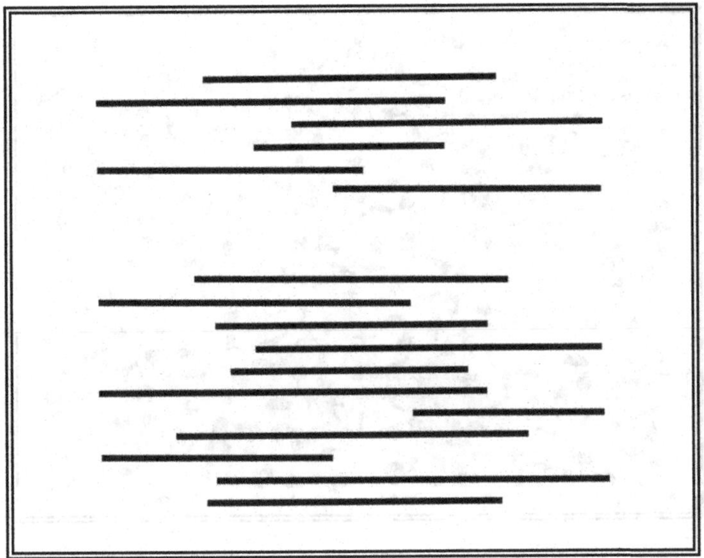

Figure 6-9. The line bisection test. The assessment is placed at the client's midline, and they are instructed to make a mark at the center of each line. Clients with hemi-inattention will often make marks ipsilesionally from center (e.g., clients with left hemi-inattention will make marks to the right of the center of the lines). (Reproduced with permission from Schenkenberg, T., Bradford, D. C., & Ajax, E. T. [1980]. Line bisection and unilateral visual neglect in patients with neurologic impairment. *Neurology, 30*[5], 509-517.)

Scoring

Although many versions of the line bisection test are readily available, few are standardized with clear guidelines for scoring and interpretation. An exception is the BIT line bisection, which, as part of the standardized test battery, has clear guidelines for scoring (Wilson et al., 1997). Since most line bisection tests are not standardized and have inconsistent recommendations for scoring and interpretation, it is recommended that they be used for screening rather than diagnosing (Plummer et al., 2003).

Psychometric Properties

The line bisection test has been shown to be a good screening tool for people with hemi-inattention, with psychometric testing showing test–retest reliability ranging from $r = 0.64$ (Kinsella et al., 1995) to $r = 0.93$ (Chen-Sea & Henderson, 1994; Schenkenberg et al., 1980). Another study reported an ICC of 0.97 for test–retest reliability (Bailey et al., 2004). The line bisection test has also been found to have good construct validity, correlating significantly with the star cancellation test (Marsh & Kersel, 1993). People with hemi-inattention have also scored differently on the measure than people without (Bailey et al., 2000), showing that the screening tool is able to identify those with hemi-inattention.

Bells Test (Gauthier et al., 1989)

Description

Various cancellation tasks are available to use when assessing clients for possible hemi-inattention. With all cancellation tests, the client is asked to attend to one specific item while ignoring distractors. One example is the star cancellation task in the BIT. Another option is the Bells Test (Figure 6-10), which is described in more detail later (Gauthier et al., 1989).

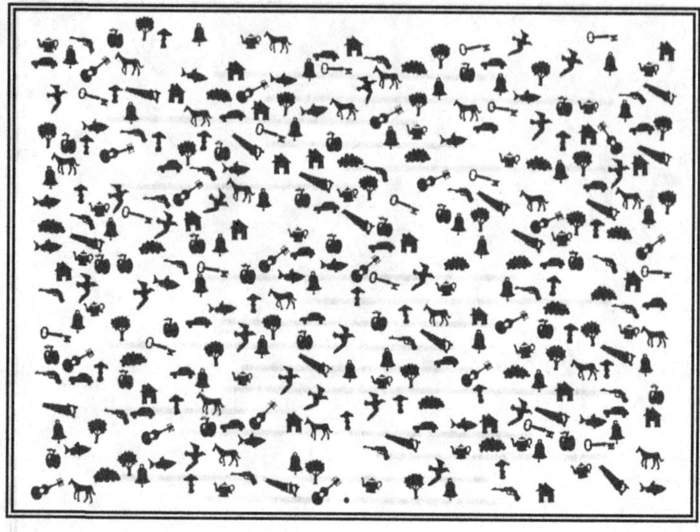

Figure 6-10. The Bells Test. With this assessment, the sheet is placed at the client's midline, and they are instructed to circle all of the bells. (The Bells Test was created under the leadership of Pr. Yves Joanette and Ms. Louise Gauthier, University of Montreal, Quebec, Canada.)

Procedure

All cancellation tests follow the same general procedure. A page with a variety of symbols and/or letters is placed on a table in front of the client at their midline. The person is then directed to cross out or circle one of the symbols but not the others. When the Bells Test is administered, the client is instructed to circle all of the bells on the page.

Scoring

The clinician records the number of bells located (out of 35) and the time it takes the client to complete the task. A client who misses more than three bells has a suspected attention deficit. A client who misses six or more bells on one half of the page has suspected hemi-inattention (left hemi-inattention if the missed bells are on the left and right hemi-inattention if the missed bells are on the right). In addition to recording the number of targets that are missed and the time taken to complete the task, clinicians can make note of the search strategy used by clients. Individuals with hemi-inattention are more likely to demonstrate a disorganized search (Gauthier et al., 1989).

Psychometric Properties

Test–retest reliability research with the Bells Test has shown that scores between the first and second administration are not significantly different from each other ($p > .05$; Wong et al., 2018). The Bells Test has also been shown to be a sensitive test, identifying more people with hemi-inattention than other pencil-and-paper tests, such as the line bisection test (Azouvi et al., 2002; Ferber & Karnath, 2001).

Figure Copying and Representational Drawing

Description

Two of the subtests in the BIT are a figure/shape copying task and representational drawing. These tests can be conducted on their own as well, with clients asked to copy simple line drawings or to draw objects without models (Figure 6-11).

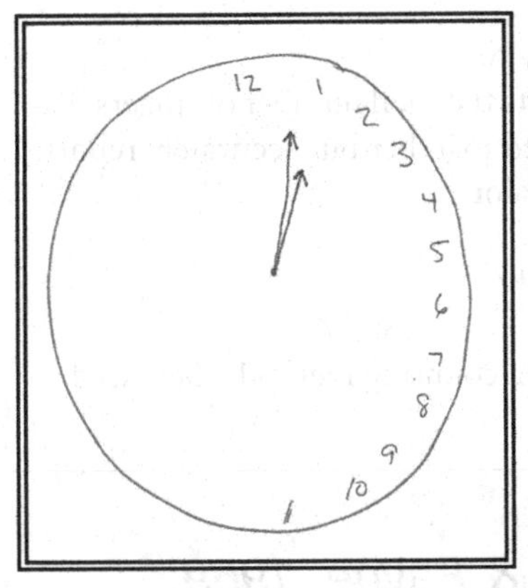

Figure 6-11. Many clients with hemi-inattention will show errors in figure copying (when they copy a picture) and with representational drawing (when they create a picture without a physical model). This is an example of what a client with hemi-inattention may produce when asked to draw a clock from memory.

Procedure

In figure/shape copying, the client is shown line drawings and is asked to draw what they see. In the representation drawing task, the person is given a blank sheet of paper centered at midline and asked to draw a clock, a person, and a butterfly (Wilson et al., 1997).

Scoring

The scoring of these activities is based on completion of the picture, with a note made of omission of components of the images. A rating scale used by Bailey et al. (2000) can be used to assess performance on representational drawing and figure copying tasks. It is a 4-point scale that rates clients' performance as follows: 4 is awarded for a complete drawing, 3 is awarded for a drawing that has some omissions but is not clearly lateralized, 2 is awarded for more omissions on one side of the drawing than the other, and 1 is awarded if there are major omissions on one side of the drawing (e.g., numbers on a clock only being drawn on one side). These researchers studied 107 people with a CVA and compared their performance to 43 age-matched controls without a CVA and found that a score of 3 or lower was considered atypical (Bailey et al., 2000).

Psychometric Properties

No research was found examining the psychometric properties of figure copying and representational drawing.

Confrontation Screening and Extinction: Finger Counting Method (Anderson et al., 2009)

Description

The finger counting method of confrontation screening is described in Chapter 4 because it is often used to screen for visual field cuts. It can also be used to screen for the presence of visual extinction, which is an issue seen in many people with hemi-inattention.

Procedure

The procedure is the same as that described for the finger counting method of confrontation screening for visual field cuts in Chapter 4.

Scoring

Extinction should be suspected if a client inaccurately reports the total number of fingers displayed when both superior fields or both inferior fields are tested together but accurately reports the correct number of fingers when displayed in each quadrant alone.

Psychometric Properties

No information about psychometric properties for the finger-counting method when used as a tool to assess extinction could be found in the literature.

Draw-A-Man (MacDonald, 1960; Maloney & Payne, 1969; Zoltan et al., 1983)

Description

The Draw-A Man test is described in detail in Chapter 5. This simple assessment can be used to screen for hemi-inattention in addition to a variety of other perceptual deficits.

Procedure

The procedure was described in Chapter 5 with the client being given a blank piece of paper and a pencil and asked to draw a man.

Scoring

Either one of the two scoring systems described in Chapter 5 (MacDonald, 1960; Zoltan et al., 1983) is appropriate for screening for hemi-inattention. The focus, however, shifts to identifying body parts that are missing or abbreviated on one side of the client's drawing versus the other. These types of errors are most typically seen on the left side after a right-sided infarct, but errors may also be on the right for some clients.

Psychometric Properties

Chen-Sea (2000) examined the validity of the tool using the scoring system developed by Zoltan et al. (1983). This study found that the Draw-A-Man test differentiated between people with hemi-inattention and those without.

ScanBoard and ScanCourse From the Brain Injury Visual Assessment Battery for Adults (Warren, 1998)

The Brain Injury Visual Assessment Battery for Adults (biVABA) is an assessment kit with a collection of screening tools that are intended for use with adults with suspected visual impairment, either due to eye disease or to damage to the nervous system. Two of the subtests, the ScanBoard and ScanCourse, are designed to observe the client's visual search strategies. According to Warren (1998), the quality and style of the client's search pattern can provide information that may help differentiate between a client with hemianopsia and one with hemi-inattention (see Table 6-1).

These subtests are conducted in far peripersonal and extrapersonal space so may help to identify clients with hemi-inattention in those areas of the environment.

ScanBoard Test (Warren, 1998)

Description

This subtest uses a large board (approximately 20 in. by 30 in.) with 10 numbers (0 to 9) that are arranged in a rough butterfly shape in a nonsequential order. The board is placed in such a way that the client is able to touch it. The client is instructed to point out numbers as they see them. The clinician makes note of the search pattern that is used during the test. According to Warren (1998), adults without brain injury will employ an organized sequential search pattern to identify the numbers on the board using one of three patterns: clockwise, counterclockwise, or rectilinear (as with reading left to right). An advantage of this test is that it asks clients to view an area that is larger than a single sheet of paper.

Procedure

The ScanBoard is placed vertically in front of the client. It should be close enough for the client to be able to touch each number. The client is told that there are 10 numbers on the board. They are instructed to point to and read the numbers aloud as they see each number. They are asked to go slowly so that the test administrator can record the numbers. The test manual provides additional details.

Scoring

The clinician writes down the numbers that the client reads in the order they are read. Following test administration, the clinician should make note of any numbers that are missed or repeated and where they are located (e.g., left vs. right side of the board). The clinician should also make note of the search pattern that is used. According to Warren (1998), clients without hemi-inattention will use a search pattern that is predictable, organized, and initiated from the left. Examples of effective versus ineffective search patterns are included in the test manual.

Psychometric Properties

One study was conducted with 46 people (23 with a CVA and 23 healthy controls) to examine the psychometric properties of the ScanBoard. The researcher found that the ScanBoard had an inter-rater reliability rating of $r = 1.0$ and a test–retest reliability rating of $r = 0.68$. There were also differences between the search strategies used by people with and without neurological impairments. Control participants in the study used an organized search strategy 91% of the time and people with a CVA used an organized search strategy 52% of the time (Warren, 1990).

ScanCourse Test (Warren, 1998)

Description

The ScanCourse is an informal test to observe the client's skill in combining visual search of extrapersonal space with ambulation. The client is asked to walk down a hallway in which the practitioner has placed 10 cards on each wall. The client is asked to point to and read each card during ambulation. The practitioner makes note of any cards that are missed and their location (e.g., to the left vs. the right of the client).

Procedure

The test administrator places 10 cards with letters or numbers on each side of a hallway and then asks the client to walk down the hallway while searching for the cards. The client is instructed to point out each card and read the number or letter aloud as they walk without stopping down the hallway. The task is completed twice, with the client walking down the hallway on the first trial and then turning around to walk down the same hallway on the second trial. Additional details can be found in the test manual.

Scoring

The clinician should make note of the number of cards missed on each trial, specifying the number of cards missed on the right and how many were missed on the left. Additional observations should be noted, including if there are patterns to what is missed and if the client is able to simultaneously search for the cards and ambulate.

Psychometric Properties

No information about the psychometric properties of the ScanCourse could be found.

Treatment of Hemi-Inattention

There are a variety of treatment strategies for hemi-inattention that have been described in the literature. The most commonly reported treatment strategy involves teaching a client to use a systematic and organized visual search pattern to increase the likelihood that all of the important features in the environment will be attended to (Barrett et al., 2006; Cicerone et al., 2000; Pierce & Buxbaum, 2002; Proto et al., 2009; Shinsha & Ishigami, 1999). This, along with other treatment strategies, has shown promise in generalizing to certain situations, often ones that are most similar to the training sessions and ones in which a client can focus more conscious attention on the task (such as occurs during much conventional assessment approaches such as paper/pencil tasks). However, a continuing challenge is assisting people in generalizing strategies to other situations, especially those that are more complex, such as those with added task demands (e.g., preparing a multicourse meal) or increased environmental demands (e.g., navigating in crowded or busy locations; Longley et al., 2021; Proto et al., 2009). There are likely numerous reasons why the treatment of this population has only been partly successful. One potential reason is that many of the treatment strategies require a client to have insight into the extent and impact of hemi-inattention. As stated earlier, anosognosia is a common problem faced by this population, which may lead to clients having difficulty in understanding the need for compensatory strategies (Parton et al., 2004). Another potential reason that treatment has only been partly successful is that hemi-inattention is a heterogenous disorder. As a result, different treatment strategies may work better for clients with some forms of hemi-inattention than others (Barrett et al., 2006). Clinicians may find that a combination of treatments is most effective (Lisa et al., 2013) or that a treatment strategy that works well with one client will work less well for another. Finally, clients who have motivational hemi-inattention (described previously) lack the drive to search the contralesional space, which is a difficult deficit to overcome (Mesulam, 1981, 1990, 1999).

Anosognosia Considerations in Treatment Planning and Implementation

Anosognosia can have a sizable impact on the rehabilitation outcome for people with hemi-inattention. Without insight into deficits, a person is less likely to use compensatory strategies, including spontaneous use of a visual search technique (Tham et al., 1999). As a result, a good understanding of the client's awareness into the scope of hemi-inattention is essential when treatment planning. If clients do not have insight into their deficits, treatment strategies that are designed to improve awareness are a good place to start (Kaldenberg, 2014), in addition to using environmental modification to ensure safety (Tham & Kielhofner, 2003). Some research has indicated that awareness training with clients with hemi-inattention resulted not only in increased awareness but also in improved ability to perform various ADL tasks, although the studies were small and more research in this area needs to be completed (Chen Sea et al., 1993; Tham et al., 2001).

Many of the treatment strategies described in the following sections can be used to improve clients' awareness of their deficits. In addition, it is important to allow clients to make mistakes when it is safe for them to do so in order for them to learn about their own limits (Klinke, Zahavi et al., 2015; Tham et al., 1999; Tham & Kielhofner, 2003). Strategies such as having a client predict performance on an activity followed by reflection on both the outcome and the strategies used can also be helpful in assisting some clients to understand what is and is not working for them (Ronchi et al., 2014; Warren, 2006). Others, especially those with more severe deficits, may not benefit from making errors or reflecting on their errors because they may not be able to recognize when errors are being made (Kessels & de Haan, 2003).

Another strategy that may assist in helping clients develop insight into their condition is the use of video recordings. Utilizing this technique, the practitioner records a client with hemi-inattention completing an activity. The client then watches the recording and critiques their performance. This can enable the client to observe and recognize their errors. This approach has the added benefit of allowing the client to view their performance with the portion of unattended visual space located ipsilesionally. Research has indicated that recording clients and having them view their performance can improve client function in some instances (Luauté et al., 2006; Tham et al., 2001; Yoon et al., 2012).

Environmental Modification

Environmental modification can be used for all clients with hemi-inattention whether or not they have insight into the nature and scope of their disorder. An important piece of environmental modification includes education of the client and the family about the hemi-inattention and how it will affect the client functionally. Families need to know that the client is not willfully ignoring information on one side and that asking the client to try harder to pay attention is rarely, if ever, enough (Tham & Kielhofner, 2003). Activities in which safety is an issue should be highlighted in order to reduce the risk of injury for the client. In order to draw attention to items of importance, several strategies can be used. Techniques can be used to simplify the visual environment and structure it in such a way that items of importance are more easily noticed. These techniques include increasing lighting, reducing glare, improving contrast, and simplifying patterns and visual complexity (Warren, 2018). These strategies are also used for clients with reduced visual acuity and are described in more detail in Chapter 4. Other environmental modification strategies are essential to consider for the client's safety. Items that are necessary for safety, such as call buttons, should be placed within the visual space most readily perceived by the client, typically from midline to 60 degrees on the ipsilesional side (Figure 6-12); this way the environment can be

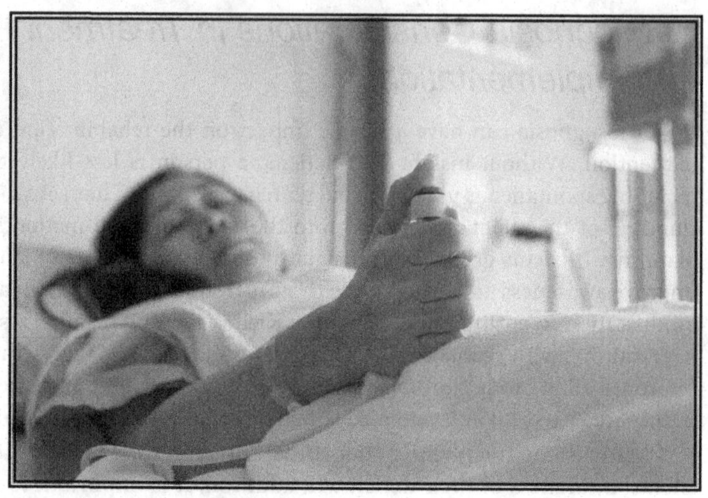

Figure 6-12. When modifying the environment for people with hemi-inattention, objects needed for safety, such as call buttons in the hospital, should be placed on the ipsilesional side so that clients are better able to locate them. (sbw18/shutterstock.com)

designed to reduce the risk of injury and increase the potential for successful interaction with the environment (Heilman et al., 2000). Placing needed items on the ipsilesional side may also give comfort to clients who are bewildered by the changes they are experiencing, especially in the more acute stage of recovery (Tham & Kielhofner, 2003).

Environmental modification can also be used to help clients attend to the contralesional visual space. One strategy includes anchoring or cueing the client as to where to begin the visual search. For example, red tape or another anchor marker can be placed to the left at the beginning of all lines to be read to provide a target so that clients know they have scanned all the way to the left. Items can be placed on the contralesional side of the environment during therapy or family members can sit on the contralesional side of the client when visiting in order to encourage interaction with objects and people on that side (Warren, 2018).

Visual Searching

Teaching clients with hemi-inattention to visually search their environment with an organized and systematic search pattern is a primary intervention method with this population. Many studies have been conducted to examine the impact of teaching visual searching to clients with hemi-inattention, and most show that this strategy is effective, at least for some people for certain tasks within the therapy context. The generalizability and sustainability of this treatment strategy are less clear, and many clients reportedly fail to use techniques in situations different from those practiced in training sessions (Christy & Huffine, 2021; Parton et al., 2004; Pierce & Buxbaum, 2002; Proto et al., 2009). Some studies and reviews have found that training with searching can improve performance on conventional assessment tools, including cancellation and line bisection tests, and may improve performance with ADLs (Chan & Man, 2013; Cicerone et al., 2000; Gillen et al., 2015; Luauté et al., 2006). A Cochrane review of randomized controlled trials did not find convincing evidence that improvements made in therapy translate to increased and long-lasting independence with ADLs, and the reviewers recommended that more research be completed in order to determine when and how this approach should be used (Longley et al., 2021).

Different authors approach teaching visual searching to clients with hemi-inattention in different ways, although the goal is always spontaneous, independent utilization of a systematic, thorough, and organized search pattern in order to improve occupational performance. In general, it is important to provide activities that stimulate the reorganization of the patient's searching

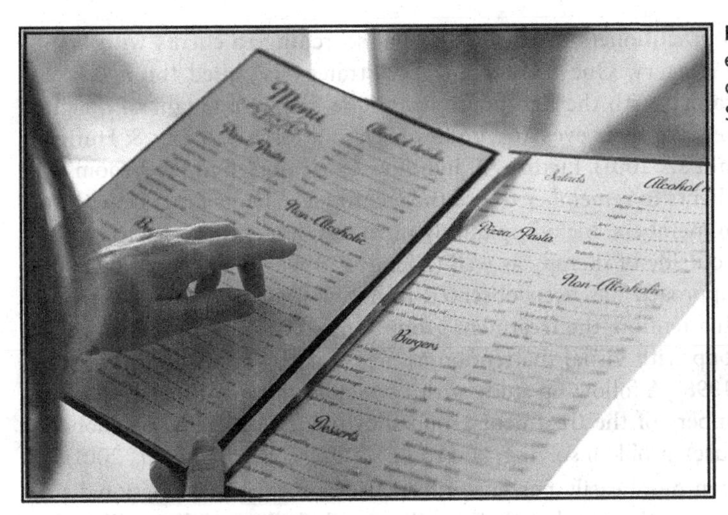

Figure 6-13. Reading a menu is an example of a task that relies on an organized visual search. (Aquarius Studio/shutterstock.com)

patterns (Warren, 2018). According to Warren (2018), activities should be arranged to first teach a left-to-right rectilinear pattern for reading and searching for small visual details and second a left-to-right clockwise or counterclockwise pattern for viewing unstructured visual arrays in the extrapersonal environment (e.g., rooms in a home or the grocery store).

Warren (2006) recommended following several principles when working on activities to reorganize the client's searching. She stated that treatment activities (a) should require the client to search as broad a visual space as possible, (b) will be more effective if the client is required to interact physically with the target once it is located, and (c) should emphasize conscious attention to visual detail and careful inspection and comparison of targets. According to Warren (2006), it is important to remember to set up the environment to support these treatment principles. For example, during therapy, when speaking to the client, occupational therapy practitioners should sit or stand in the contralesional space to encourage clients to turn and to make eye contact. Practitioners may also add a motor component to activities, such as by asking clients to hand something to a person standing contralesionally or manipulating objects on that side. For example, the practitioner may have the client place a piece of a puzzle in its appropriate spot in contralesional space.

Several researchers have found that clients are more likely to attend to items in contralesional space if those items are emotionally laden (e.g., photographs of loved ones) or meaningful in some other way (Grabowska et al., 2011; Klinke, Zahavi et al., 2015; Lucas & Vuilleumier, 2008). Clients with hemi-inattention may also have an easier time attending to contralesional space in the context of relevant and familiar tasks. As a result, it is recommended that the client perform functional activities for which effective visual searching is required to complete the activity (Tham & Kielhofner, 2003). The choice of activities should reflect input from the client regarding functional goals in order to make the activities relevant and meaningful (Gordon et al., 1985).

The following are examples of functionally oriented tasks that incorporate visual searching:

- ADL and IADL tasks that require visual searching for successful completion, such as locating grooming items on a sink counter or in a medicine cabinet, locating clothing in closets or drawers, locating food on a plate, looking for salad ingredients in a refrigerator, and sorting laundry items by color
- Going to a community setting, such as a grocery, department, drug, or hardware store, and retrieving a set of prespecified items
- Locating names and prices of food items on a menu (Figure 6-13)
- Completing paper mazes, puzzles, or other activities that require visual searching

Other strategies may help practitioners in teaching visual searching to clients with hemi-inattention, including mental imagery. One mental imagery strategy is called the *lighthouse technique*. When clients are trained with the lighthouse technique, they are taught to imagine themselves as a lighthouse, sweeping their eyes and bodies back and forth (Christy & Huffine, 2021; Niemeier, 1998; Niemeier et al., 2001). Pictures of lighthouses are posted in their room and treatment areas to encourage clients to remember to use the technique. Clients practice with the technique in therapy, and team members, including family members, are encouraged to remind the clients to use this strategy outside of therapy as well (Niemeier, 1998; Niemeier et al., 2001). Preliminary support for this approach has been observed in a couple of smaller studies. In a study of 16 clients with hemi-inattention, the treatment group showed significant improvement compared with the control group with visual inattention as measured by a facility rating scale and family reports (Niemeier, 1998). A follow-up study with 19 people with hemi-inattention had similar findings, with the members of the treatment group showing greater gains on mobility (both walking and wheelchair use), problem solving, and route finding (Niemeier et al., 2001).

Another way that clients can more easily perceive information on their contralesional side is by adjusting their physical orientation so that their midline is shifted contralesionally. This is accomplished by physically turning their eyes, head, and trunk toward the unattended space. There is some evidence that shows that clients who are taught to combine visual searching with trunk rotation have improved function compared with those who are not taught about voluntary trunk rotation as a supplement to visual searching (Parton et al., 2004; Wiart et al., 1997).

Prisms

Another treatment that has been tried with people with hemi-inattention involves the use of prisms to widen the attended visual space by causing a midline shift in what the client is perceiving. The prism adaptation treatment consists of the client reaching for objects while wearing goggles fitted with binocular unidirectional prismatic lenses. The lenses cause a contralesional shift in the client's perception of midline (i.e., information to the contralesional side of midline is perceived as located in the ipsilesional, or attended, space; Luauté et al., 2006). Initially, the client will undershoot in the direction of the perceptual midline shift when reaching. With repeated attempts, the brain adapts to the perceived midline shift, and the accuracy of the person's reach improves. If the treatment is successful, the client experiences a shift in the opposite direction after the goggles are removed, which improves the processing of information in the contralesional space (Rich, 2020).

Research into the effects of prism use for those with hemi-inattention indicated that there is some promise in this treatment approach. Participants in these studies who received treatment with prisms showed improvement, including in some aspects of occupation, such as functional mobility, reading, and writing (Barrett et al., 2006; Goedert et al., 2013; Gillen et al., 2015; Kaldenberg, 2014; Luauté et al., 2006; Parton et al., 2004; Proto et al., 2009; Shinsha & Ishigami, 1999). There also has been some preliminary evidence showing that prism use results in longer-lasting change, although more research is indicated (Frassinetti et al., 2002; Luauté et al., 2006; Parton et al., 2004; Pierce & Buxbaum, 2002). One of the potential advantages of using prisms is that they can result in improvements even when clients do not have awareness of their deficits, which is difficult to achieve with other treatments, such as visual search training (Parton et al., 2004).

As with the use of prisms for the treatment of diplopia, we recommend that the occupational therapy practitioner work in collaboration with a qualified vision provider for the evaluation and treatment of hemi-inattention using prisms. This is a critical step in ensuring that any co-occurring foundational visual impairments or conditions of the eye are accurately identified and appropriately treated as well as the identification of any contraindications to the use of prisms for a particular individual. The occupational therapy practitioner may then work collaboratively with the vision provider by having the client wear the prescribed prisms during therapy. An essential part of the collaboration is for the occupational therapy practitioner to provide feedback to the vision provider about what is and is not helping to improve functional outcomes for the client.

Patching

Patching is another treatment that has been tried with people with hemi-inattention. This treatment consists of either complete monocular occlusion of the ipsilesional eye or partial binocular occlusion of the ipsilesional half of each eye. In the case of the latter approach, tape is placed on the client's eyeglasses or on a set of safety glasses such that the occlusion covers the visual space starting at midline and extending ipsilesionally. The theory is that by removing the input from the attended portion of visual space, the client will be forced to attend to the contralesional visual space. It is important to remove the occlusion when the client is not engaged in therapy to ensure safety (Warren, 2006).

Positive effects of patching have been reported in the literature (e.g., Gillen et al., 2015), although the overall results of this treatment are mixed, including insufficient evidence to support the long-lasting impact of the intervention (Pierce & Buxbaum, 2002; Proto et al., 2009; Shinsha & Ishigami, 1999). Research has also reported that some clients do not tolerate patching well (Parton et al., 2004), and one review found that there was worsened function in some clients who received patching, especially when monocular patching was used (Barrett et al., 2006). As a result, patching should be used with caution, and clients with whom patching is used should be monitored carefully.

Limb Activation

Practitioners who use limb activation with clients encourage active use of the client's contralesional limb during activity. The hypothesis is that limb activation results in cortical stimulation in the damaged hemisphere, which can, in turn, lead to improvement in deficits, including hemi-inattention (Radomski & Giles, 2014; Figure 6-14). There is some evidence that indicates that this treatment can be effective in improving functioning for this population (Barrett et al., 2006; Pierce & Buxbaum, 2002; Proto et al., 2009; Radomski & Giles, 2014), especially for those with personal inattention and hemi-inattention in peripersonal space (Parton et al., 2004). One of the biggest limitations with this treatment is that it requires active use of the contralesional limb; passive movement does not show the same results. Because of the nature of ABI, it is likely that the person with hemi-inattention also has hemiparesis, which may limit their active use of the limb and make fewer people candidates for this intervention (Parton et al., 2004; Pierce & Buxbaum, 2002).

Some clients with active hemiparetic limb movement may also meet the criteria for constraint-induced movement therapy (CIMT), a treatment designed to improve functional use and decrease the likelihood of learned nonuse of the hemiparetic upper extremity. The qualifying criteria for CIMT are described in detail elsewhere, but typically include some degree of active finger and wrist extension, the ability to walk without assistive devices, and grossly intact cognition. Those who receive CIMT have their unaffected upper extremity constrained, such as by wearing a sling or a splint, for a prescribed number of hours per day and receive additional therapy, although the amount of time spent in sessions varies depending on the study. Research with this intervention has shown promising results with improving motor control of the hemiparetic limb

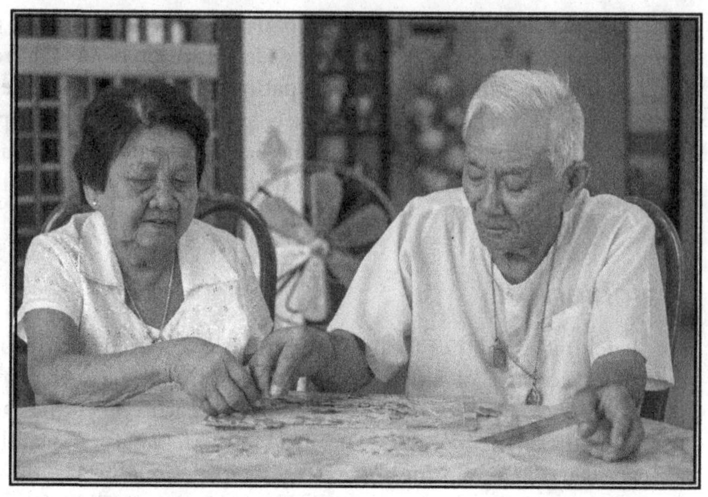

Figure 6-14. In limb activation therapy, clients are encouraged to use their hemiparetic limb actively in occupation. The theory is that active use of the limb increases neural activity in the damaged hemisphere and can increase attention contralesionally. (WitthayaP/shutterstock.com)

and decreasing the likelihood of learned nonuse for those with milder impairments (Rao, 2021). CIMT could also serve as a more intense form of limb activation for those with hemi-inattention.

In one study looking at the impact of CIMT on hemi-inattention, 27 people with a right-sided CVA and left hemi-inattention were randomized into one of three groups. The first group received CIMT, the second received CIMT and monocular eye patching on the right eye, and the third group received standard rehabilitation services. The researchers found that the participants in the CIMT group and the participants in the combined CIMT/eye patching group made significantly greater gains on the Catherine Bergego Scale than the control group. In addition, the CIMT group showed more frequent and longer visual fixations in the left visual field than either of the other two groups (Wu et al., 2013). For those with hemi-inattention and sufficient active use of the contralesional limb, CIMT and limb activation hold promise for improving function.

Alerts and Cueing

As stated previously, many clients with hemi-inattention also have deficits with arousal and other forms of attention, such as sustained attention. These clients may have better awareness and understanding of their general attentional issue than they have of hemi-inattention (Robertson et al., 1995). As a result, they may be more open to activities that work to improve sustained attention. Research has shown that interventions that work to treat sustained attention issues can also help lessen the impact of hemi-inattention (Robertson et al., 1995).

Increasing general attention can be accomplished in different ways, including using cues to remind the client to pay attention and to encourage the client to look to the unattended space. These cues can be verbal (e.g., "look left!"), auditory (e.g., with a bell or alarm), tactile (e.g., tapping the client on the arm), or kinesthetic (e.g., having the client reach into the unattended space; Barrett et al., 2006; Parton et al., 2004; Pierce & Buxbaum, 2002; Proto et al., 2009; Shinsha & Ishigami, 1999; Figure 6-15). Some forms of cueing may be more effective for some clients than others. For example, a client with aphasia may not benefit as much from a verbal cue as a tactile one. People can also be given cues in advance of an activity to increase their arousal and give them a warning that they will need to prepare themselves to attend to the activity. This preattentive cueing has been shown to increase the speed and accuracy of visual attention (Eimer, 1994; Robertson et al., 1998).

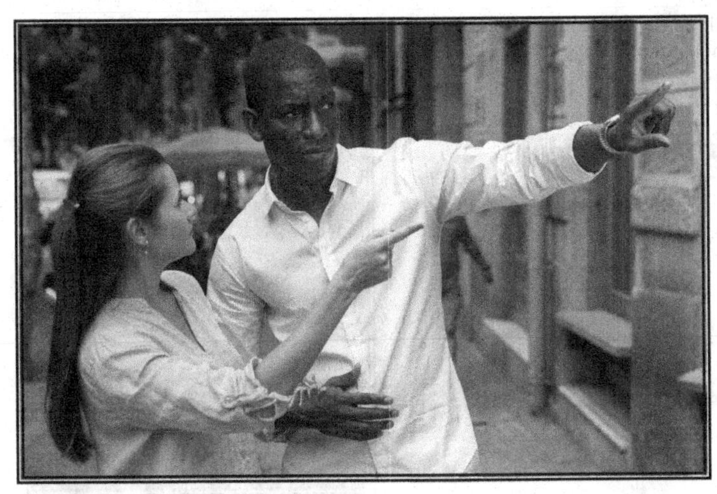

Figure 6-15. People with hemi-inattention often need cues to visually search the contralesional space. Cues can be external to the person, such as cues from another, or internal, when the person is able to cue themselves. (BearFotos/shutterstock.com)

At first, the cueing will be external, given to the client by occupational therapy practitioners and other team members, including family. These cues can at first be bewildering and frustrating for clients, especially if they are having difficulty understanding the nature of their condition. Researchers recommend that practitioners be aware of this and consider the way in which cues and feedback are provided to clients in the acute stage of recovery, including ensuring positive feedback when clients are successful (Klinke, Zahavi et al., 2015; Tham & Kielhofner, 2003). Over time, some clients can learn to cue themselves, such as by talking themselves through activities or by reminding themselves to look toward the contralesional side (Parton et al., 2004; Pierce & Buxbaum, 2002). However, being able to cue oneself requires insight, which not all clients will develop (Parton et al., 2004). In addition, cueing oneself to visually search and interact with contralesional space requires conscious effort, which can be exhausting and difficult for clients to maintain (Klinke, Zahavi et al., 2015). This type of cueing also slows down perceptual and cognitive processing, leading clients to need more time to accomplish tasks (Klinke, Zahavi et al., 2015). As a result, there will still likely be situations, such as in fast-moving and dynamic environments or while completing tasks that require more cognitive effort, when those with hemi-inattention with relatively complete recovery still do not attend to contralesional space even years postinjury (Tham & Kielhofner, 2003).

Transcutaneous Electrical Nerve Stimulation

Transcutaneous electrical nerve stimulation (TENS) has been widely used for treating people experiencing pain, but it has also been used to treat people with hemi-inattention after ABI (van Dijk et al., 2002). TENS units are small electrical units made up of one or more generators, a battery, and electrodes. They produce electrical currents and are programmable, with adjustments to amplitude, pulse width (the duration of the electrical input), and pulse rate (frequency) possible (Kaye, 2015). TENS is contraindicated with people with pacemakers and should be used with caution with those with somatosensory loss because of the possibility of burns (Kaye, 2015).

There is preliminary evidence for the use of TENS in the treatment of those with hemi-inattention either alone (Guariglia et al., 2000; Lafosse et al., 2003; van Dijk et al., 2002) or in conjunction with visual search training (Polanowska et al., 2009; Schröeder et al., 2008). TENS is thought to work by increasing the arousal of the person with hemi-inattention (van Dijk et al., 2002). However, the effect is not consistent, with some studies failing to find that TENS enhanced

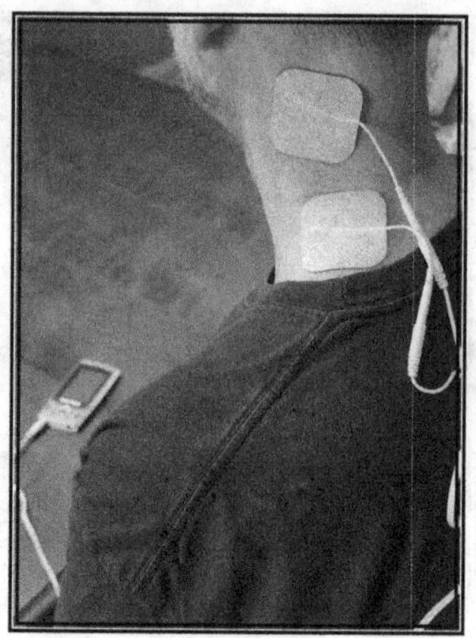

Figure 6-16. Using TENS to provide input to the contralesional side has shown promise as a treatment for hemi-inattention.

the impact of visual search training (Senіów et al., 2016). The long-term effects of TENS use are also unclear, with few studies examining lasting changes in hemi-inattention after treatment (van Dijk et al., 2002).

There is not universal agreement on the placement of electrodes or unit settings in this approach. Some studies have placed electrodes on the side of participants' necks (e.g., Guariglia et al., 2000; Figure 6-16), whereas others have placed electrodes on the dorsum of the participants' hands (e.g., Polanowska et al., 2009). Laterality does seem to be important, with electrode placement needing to be on the side of the hemi-inattention. Studies that have placed electrodes on the ipsilesional side have found no effect on hemi-inattention or a worsening of symptoms (van Dijk et al., 2002).

Although there is not agreement on the TENS unit settings, typically, the intensity is set in a range, from just above the threshold where participants are able to sense the input to a level where mild muscular twitches are observed. Frequency is usually set at 100 Hz. The duration of the treatment is also not agreed on, but TENS is usually applied for 10 to 20 minutes/session (van Dijk et al., 2002).

Mirror Therapy

When people participate in mirror therapy, they are seated with a mirror placed vertically at the midsagittal plane. They place their distal affected limb (upper or lower extremity) behind the mirror. Then, they move their nonaffected limb while watching the movement in the mirror (Ramachandran & Altschuler, 2009; Figure 6-17). Mirror therapy has been used in both the clinic and as a home program (Nilsen & DiRusso, 2014). The amount of time spent completing mirror therapy varies greatly in the literature. Individual session length varies from 15 to 60 minutes, sessions per week vary from 3 to 7, and program length varies from 2 to 8 weeks (Thieme et al., 2018).

Mirror therapy first emerged in the early 1990s as a treatment for people experiencing phantom limb pain after amputation (Ramachandran & Altschuler, 2009; Ramachandran & Rogers-Ramachandran, 1996). It has since been found useful in the treatment of other conditions, including complex regional pain syndrome (Ramachandran & Altschuler, 2009). There is also emerging evidence for the benefits of mirror therapy in the treatment of people with ABI. Mirror therapy appears to have benefit for the treatment of somatosensory loss (Doyle et al., 2010) and hemiparesis (Invernizzi et al., 2013; Nilsen & DiRusso, 2014; Park et al., 2015; Ramachandran &

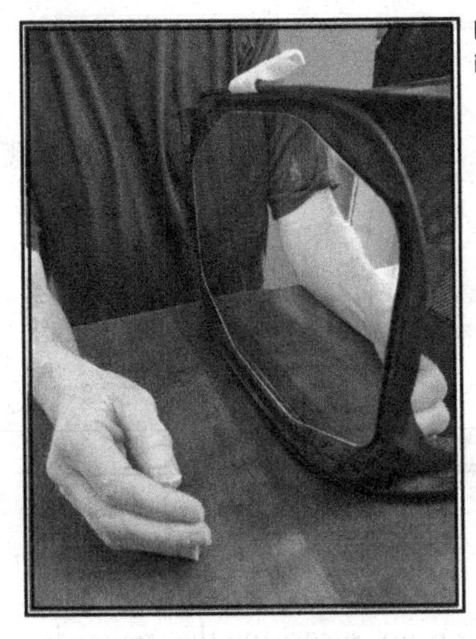

Figure 6-17. Mirror therapy shows promise as a treatment for hemi-inattention.

Altschuler, 2009; Samuelkamaleshkumar et al., 2014; Thieme et al., 2013, 2018). One advantage of mirror therapy is that it can be useful both for people with very severe hemiparesis as well as those with some voluntary motor control (Thieme et al., 2013).

In addition to its utility for people with motor and somatosensory loss after ABI, mirror therapy has been shown to have some benefit in the treatment of hemi-inattention. Several studies have been conducted using mirror therapy to treat people with hemi-inattention. These studies have found that those treated with mirror therapy have statistically significant improvements in their performance on hemi-inattention assessments, such as subtests of the BIT (Dohle et al., 2009; Klinke, Hafsteinsdottir et al., 2015; Pandian et al., 2014; Thieme et al., 2013). However, the effects of mirror therapy on functional performance are not well researched at this time. In addition, its long-term effects are not known, but some evidence indicates that there may be carryover for some clients (Pandian et al., 2014).

The underlying neural mechanism for mirror therapy is not fully understood, but research has been initiated to uncover it. Functional imaging studies have been completed with individuals without a brain injury. When these people move their limb while watching its reflection, there is cortical stimulation contralaterally, including in the sensorimotor cortex, the supplementary motor area, and the premotor cortex. This is expected because the contralateral hemisphere is controlling the movement of the limb. There is also ipsilateral stimulation, including to the sensorimotor cortex, cerebellum, and visual areas of the brain (Arya, 2016). For people with right-sided brain lesions, as is usually the case for those with hemi-inattention, moving the right hand while watching its reflection appears to stimulate multiple cortical regions in the right hemisphere. These include the occipital lobe, posterior parietal cortex (one of the areas implicated in hemi-inattention), intraparietal sulcus (which is important for visuomotor information processing), somatosensory cortex, motor cortex, and premotor cortex. Therefore, it seems that mirror therapy may lead to neural activation of the damaged hemisphere and may help to support and facilitate neuroplasticity after ABI (Arya, 2016).

Mirror therapy appears to be a viable treatment for people with hemi-inattention. It is noninvasive and has not been shown to have adverse side effects (Tyson et al., 2015). It is also a treatment that can be used at the clinic and at home (Nilsen & DiRusso, 2014) and can be self-directed by the client after training (Tyson et al., 2015). Mirror boxes are available commercially but are also simple and inexpensive to make with a cardboard box and a mirror tile.

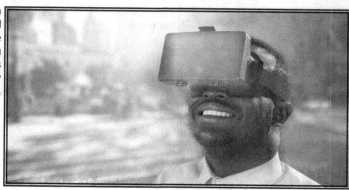

Figure 6-18. Virtual reality is an emerging therapy. It is being explored as a treatment modality for people with hemi-inattention, including as a way to practice with activities that are difficult to complete safely in real life, such as crossing streets. (vectorfusionart/shutterstock.com)

Emerging Treatments

Given the prevalence and complexity of hemi-inattention, it is not surprising that researchers are trialing new treatments on a regular basis. In addition, changes with technology allow opportunities for treatment that have not existed previously. Two examples of treatments for hemi-inattention that are gaining more attention are the use of virtual reality and the use of music.

Virtual reality may be used in different ways. One strategy uses virtual reality to allow clients to practice applying techniques in environments that would be unsafe or inaccessible to them during therapy. For example, clients can practice community navigation, including looking for traffic and crossing streets, in a virtual environment more easily and safely than they can in a real-life environment, especially if the practitioner wants to allow the client to make and learn from mistakes (Katz et al., 2005; Navarro et al., 2013; Figure 6-18). Virtual reality can also allow clients to explore space safely to allow for the formation of new spatial maps and get feedback as they interact with contralesional space (Castiello et al., 2004; Kim et al., 2011; Mainetti et al., 2013). One study using virtual reality in this way found that clients who used the system had an improved ability to locate objects on their left, although the researchers did not examine the long-lasting impact, so the sustainability of the gains were not known (Castiello et al., 2004). Virtual reality holds promise for treating this population, especially because some of the studies have demonstrated moderate to large effect sizes (Lisa et al., 2013).

Another emerging treatment strategy is the use of music. This treatment technique is primarily focused on improving alertness and general sustained attention (Shinsha & Ishigami, 1999). One study with 16 people with hemi-inattention found that listening to classical music improved performance on conventional tests of hemi-inattention more than listening to white noise or silence (Tsai et al., 2013). Active engagement with music may also help. A small study with two participants with a right CVA and hemi-inattention was conducted looking at the impact of instrument playing on conventional tests of hemi-inattention. In this study, participants were asked to play scales on a keyboard that was set up in such a way that the participants needed to move from their right to the left, unattended space. The researchers found that both participants improved with performance on some of the conventional tests of hemi-inattention, with one participant's improvement lasting for at least 1 week post-treatment (Bodak et al., 2014).

Tips for Improving the Likelihood of Generalization

As described previously, one of the biggest challenges with treating people with hemi-inattention is that gains observed in treatment sessions often do not generalize well. As a result, although clients and study participants may show improvement in certain situations that are identical or very similar to those in which they were trained, they do not often use compensatory strategies in new circumstances. This can lead to continued dependence on others (Barrett et al., 2006; Longley et al., 2021; Proto et al., 2009). Therefore, it is essential that treating practitioners take steps to assist clients in generalizing the use of compensatory strategies. There are several techniques that may be able to help with this goal.

One essential technique is the provision of opportunities to practice using the compensatory strategy being taught in multiple environments. It can be difficult to help clients transfer the use of compensatory strategies from one situation to another. One model of treatment that may be helpful in systematically assisting clients to use techniques in different environments is the multicontext approach. This model describes how to train clients to use compensatory strategies in increasingly different situations and is relevant for use with people with hemi-inattention (Toglia, 2018). For more details about the multicontext approach, see Chapter 10. In addition to practicing the compensatory strategy in different situations, the practitioner can also consider the intensity of instruction and the consistency of cues. To encourage generalization, it is essential that all members of the rehabilitation team, including the client and family members, are aware of the strategies that are being taught and encourage their use in a variety of situations. The team also needs to cue the client in consistent ways, using the approach that has been found to be most useful for that client (e.g., a specific verbal or visual cue; Cicerone et al., 2000; Kaldenberg, 2014; Proto et al., 2009).

An example of the successful use of these strategies (i.e., intensity, consistency, practice, and multiple settings) was described in a case study by Niemeier (2002). In this case study, a woman with a right CVA and hemi-inattention was taught to use the lighthouse strategy (described previously) to assist with conducting a complete and systematic visual search. The practitioner worked with the client, the client's husband, and the inpatient team to consistently cue the woman to use the lighthouse strategy during a wide variety of activities. In addition, pictures of a lighthouse were posted in highly visible locations to remind the client about the strategy. Over the course of a 4-week rehabilitation period, the client had numerous opportunities to practice the technique throughout the day. At the time of discharge, she and her husband were reminded to continue use of the lighthouse strategy at home. At a 1-month follow-up visit, the client was continuing to use the strategy independently (Niemeier, 2002). It is unwise to assume that these results would be found for all people with hemi-inattention after ABI, but there are several interesting findings in this case study, including the impact for this participant of repetition, consistency, and opportunities for practicing the strategy with a wide variety of activities.

In addition to these techniques, additional methods that can assist clients in the use of compensatory strategies are making training activities meaningful and relevant to the client and allowing time for mistakes and exploration. This was illustrated in a qualitative study that was conducted with four women with right CVA and hemi-inattention (Tham et al., 1999; Tham & Kielhofner, 2003). These women were interviewed at numerous times during their inpatient rehabilitation about their adjustment to life with hemi-inattention and the treatment methods that they found most helpful. The women explained that they felt that people around them assisted too quickly and that they wanted and needed more time to experiment and explore in order to problem solve for themselves. They also expressed a desire for more time for reflection about what was happening and what helped them function better, which is consistent with recommendations to have people predict and then reflect on performance in order to encourage improved insight into deficits (Ronchi et al., 2014; Warren, 2006). In addition, the women emphasized the importance of activities that were meaningful, with one woman stating, "I can see things if I am interested in seeing them" (Tham et al., 1999, p. 403). As a result of these findings, the authors recommended that clinicians allow clients to have time for processing and reflection to develop insight into their deficits and that meaningful activities be used to encourage clients to learn compensatory strategies (Tham et al., 1999; Tham & Kielhofner, 2003).

Conclusion

Hemi-inattention is a complex and heterogenous disorder that impacts many people after ABI, especially those with damage to the right cerebral hemisphere. It can manifest in a variety of ways, most commonly observed when clients visually search their environments. Hemi-inattention can have a sizable impact on functioning, leading to longer hospital stays and decreased independence. The evaluation of this population should be conducted with a battery of tests to consider hemi-inattention in personal, peripersonal, and extrapersonal space and in both static and dynamic environments. Treatment may make use of a variety of techniques as well, including environmental modification, instruction in strategies to use an organized and systematic search pattern, prisms, limb activation, and so forth. It is also important for clinicians to consider the impact of anosognosia and work to improve clients' insight into their deficits to enable them to make better use of treatment techniques and generalize their use.

References

Aloiso, L. (2004). Visual dysfunction. In G. Gillen & A. Burkhardt (Eds.), *Stroke rehabilitation: A function-based approach* (2nd ed., pp. 338-357). Mosby Inc.

Anderson, A. J., Shuey, N. H., & Wall, M. (2009). Rapid confrontation screening for peripheral visual field defects and extinction. *Clinical and Experimental Optometry, 92*, 45-48. https://doi.org/10.1111/j.1444-0938.2008.00280.x

Árnadóttir, G. (1990). *The brain and behavior: Assessing cortical dysfunction through activities of daily living.* C. V. Mosby Company.

Árnadóttir, G. (2021). *Impact of neurobehavioral deficits on activities of daily living. In G. Gillen & D. M. Nilsen (Eds.). Stroke rehabilitation: A function-based approach* (5th ed., pp. 556-592). Elsevier.

Arya, K. N. (2016). Underlying neural mechanisms of mirror therapy: Implications for motor rehabilitation in stroke. *Neurology India, 64*, 38-44. https://doi.org/10.4103/0028-3886.173622

Azouvi, P., Marchal, F., Samuel, C., Morin, L., Renard, C., Louis-Dreyfus, A., Jokie, C., Wiart, L., Pradat-Diehl, P., Deloche, G., & Bergego, C. (1996). Functional consequences and awareness of unilateral neglect: Study of an evaluation scale. *Neuropsychological Rehabilitation, 6*, 133-150. https://doi.org/10.1080/713755501

Azouvi, P., Olivier, S., de Montety, G., Samuel, C., Louis-Dreyfus, A., & Tesio, L. (2003). Behavioral assessment of unilateral neglect: Study of the psychometric properties of the Catherine Bergego Scale. *Archives of Physical Medicine and Rehabilitation, 84*, 51-57. https://doi.org/10.1053/apmr.2003.50062

Azouvi, P., Samuel, C., Louis-Dreyfus, A., Bernati, T., Bartolomeo, P., Beis, J.-M., Chokron, S., Leclercq, M., Marchal, F., Martin, Y., de Montety, G., Olivier, S., Perennou, D., Pradat-Diehl, P., Prairial, C., Rode, G., Siéroff, E., Wiart, L., & Rousseaux. M. (2002). Sensitivity of clinical and behavioural tests of spatial neglect after right hemisphere stroke. *Journal of Neurology, Neurosurgery and Psychiatry, 73*, 160-166. https://doi.org/10.1136/jnnp.73.2.160

Bailey, M. J., Riddoch, M. J., & Crome, P. (2000). Evaluation of a test battery for hemineglect in elderly stroke patients for use by therapists in clinical practice. *NeuroRehabilitation, 14*, 139-150. https://doi.org/10.3233/NRE-2000-14303

Bailey, M. J., Riddoch, M. J., & Crome, P. (2004). Test-retest stability of three tests for unilateral visual neglect in patients with stroke: Star cancellation, line bisection, and the Baking Tray Task. *Neuropsychological Rehabilitation, 14*, 403-419. https://doi.org/10.1080/09602010343000282

Barrett, A. M., Buxbaum, L. J., Coslett, H. B., Edwards, E., Heilman, K. M., Hillis, A. E., Milberg, W. P., & Robertson, I. H. (2006). Cognitive rehabilitation interventions for neglect and related disorders: Moving from bench to bedside in stroke patients. *Journal of Cognitive Neuroscience, 18*, 1223-1236. https://doi.org/10.1162/jocn.2006.18.7.1223

Bisiach, E., & Luzzatti, C. (1978). Unilateral neglect of representational space. *Cortex, 14*, 129-133. https://doi.org/10.1016/S0010-9452(78)80016-1

Bodak, R., Malhotra, P., Bernardi, N., Cocchini, G., & Stewart, L. (2014). Reducing chronic visuo-spatial neglect following right hemisphere stroke through instrument playing. *Frontiers in Human Neuroscience, 8*, 1-8. https://doi.org/10.3389/fnhum.2014.00413

Castiello, U., Lusher, D., Burton, C., Glover, S., & Disler, P. (2004). Improving left hemispatial neglect using virtual reality. *Neurology, 62*, 1958-1962. https://doi.org/10.1212/01.WNL.0000128183.63917.02

Chan, D. Y. W., & Man, D. W. K. (2013). Unilateral neglect in stroke. *Topics in Geriatric Rehabilitation, 29*, 126-134. https://doi.org/10.1097/TGR.0b013e31827ea7c9

Chen, P., Chen, C. C., Hreha, K., Goedert, K. M., & Barrett, A. M. (2015). Kessler Foundation Neglect Assessment Process uniquely measures spatial neglect during activities of daily living. *Archives of Physical Medicine and Rehabilitation, 96*, 869-876. https://doi.org/10.1016/j.apmr.2014.10.023

Chen, P., & Hreha, K. (2015). *Kessler Foundation Neglect Assessment Process 2015 manual.* Kessler Foundation.

Chen, P., Hreha, K., Fortis, P., Goedert, K. M., & Barrett, A. M. (2012). Functional assessment of spatial neglect: A review of the Catherine Bergego Scale and an introduction of the Kessler Foundation Neglect Assessment Process. *Topics in Stroke Rehabilitation, 19*, 423-435. https://doi.org/10.1310/tsr1905-423

Chen-Sea, M.-J. (2000). Validating the Draw-A-Man test as a personal neglect test. *American Journal of Occupational Therapy, 54*(4), 391-397. https://doi.org/10.5014/ajot.54.4.391

Chen Sea, M. J., Henderson, A., & Cermak, S. (1993). Patterns of visual spatial inattention and their functional significance in stroke patients. *Archives of Physical Medicine and Rehabilitation, 74*, 355-360.

Chen Sea, M. J., & Henderson, A. (1994). The reliability and validity of visuospatial inattention tests with stroke patients. *Occupational Therapy International, 1*, 36-48. https://doi.org/10.1002/oti.6150010106

Christy, K., & Huffine, N. (2021). Visual perceptual assessment and intervention. In D. P. Dirette & S. A. Gutman (Eds.) *Occupational therapy for physical dysfunction* (8th ed., pp. 117-142). Lippincott Williams & Wilkins.

Cicek, M., Gitelman, D., Hurley, R. S. E., Nobre, A., & Mesulam, M. (2007). Anatomical physiology of spatial extinction. *Cerebral Cortex, 17*, 2892-2898. https://doi.org/10.1093/cercor/bhm014

Cicerone, K. D., Dahlberg, C., Kalmar, K., Langenbahn, D. M., Malec, J. F., Bergquist, T. F., Felicetti, T., Giacino, J. T., Harley, J. P., Harrington D. E., Herzog, J., Kneipp, S., Laatsch, L., & Morse, P. A. (2000). Evidence-based cognitive rehabilitation: Recommendations for clinical practice. *Archives of Physical Medicine and Rehabilitation, 81*, 1596-1615. https://doi.org/10.1053/apmr.2000.19240

DiPelligrino, G., Basso, G., & Frassinetti, F. (1997). Spatial extinction on double asynchronous stimulation. *Neuropsychologia, 35*, 1215-1223. https://doi.org/10.1016/S0028-3932(97)00044-4

Dohle, C., Pullen, J., Nakaten, A., Kust, J., Rietz, C., & Karbe, H. (2009). Mirror therapy promotes recovery from severe hemiparesis: A randomized controlled trial. *Neurorehabilitation and Neural Repair, 23*, 209-217. https://doi.org/10.1177/1545968308324786

Donoso-Brown, E. V., & Powell, J. M. (2017). Assessment of unilateral neglect in stroke: Simplification and structuring of test items. *British Journal of Occupational Therapy, 80*, 448-452. https://doi.org/10.1177/0308022616685582

Doyle, S., Bennett, S., Fasoli, S. E., & McKenna, K. T. (2010). Interventions for sensory impairment in the upper limb after stroke. *Cochrane Database of Systematic Reviews, 2010*(6). https://doi.org/10.1002/14651858.CD006331.pub2

Eimer, M. (1994). An ERP study on visual spatial priming with peripheral onsets. *Psychophysiology, 31*, 154-163. https://doi.org/10.1111/j.1469-8986.1994.tb01035.x

Ellis, A. W., Jordan, J. L., & Sullivan, C.-A. (2006). Unilateral neglect is not unilateral: Evidence for additional neglect of extreme right space. *Cortex, 42*, 861-868. https://doi.org/10.1016/S0010-9452(08)70429-5

Ferber, S., & Karnath, H. O. (2001). How to assess spatial neglect—Line bisection or cancellation tests? *Journal of Clinical and Experimental Neuropsychology, 23*, 599-607. https://doi.org/10.1076/jcen.23.5.599.1243

Frassinetti, F., Angeli, V., Meneghello, F., Avanzi, S., & Ladavas, E. (2002). Long-lasting amelioration of visuospatial neglect by prism adaptation. *Brain, 125*, 608-623. https://doi.org/10.1093/brain/awf056

Gardarsdóttir, S., & Kaplan, S. (2002). Validity of the Árnadóttir OT-ADL Neurobehavioral Evaluation (A-ONE): Performance in activities of daily living and neurobehavioral impairments of persons with left and right hemisphere damage. *American Journal of Occupational Therapy, 56*, 499-508. https://doi.org/10.5014/ajot.56.5.499

Gauthier, L., Dehaut, F., & Joanette, Y. (1989). The Bells Test: A quantitative and qualitative test for visual neglect. *International Journal of Clinical Neuropsychology, 11*, 49-54. https://doi.org/10.1037/t28075-000

Gillen, G., Nilsen, D., Attridge, J., Banakos, E., Morgan, M., Winterbottom, L., & York, W. (2015). Effectiveness of interventions to improve occupational performance of people with cognitive impairments after stroke: An evidence-based review. *American Journal of Occupational Therapy, 69*, 1-9. https://doi.org/10.5014/ajot.2015.012138

Goedert, K., Chen, P., Boston, R., Foundas, A., & Barrett, A. M. (2013). Presence of motor-intentional aiming deficit predicts functional improvement of spatial neglect with prism adaptation. *Neurorehabilitation and Neural Repair, 28*, 483-493. https://doi.org/10.1177/1545968313516872

Gordon, W. A., Hibbard, M. R., Egelko, S., Diller, L., Shaver, M. S., Lieberman, A., & Ragnarsson, K. (1985). Perceptual remediation in patients with right brain damage: A comprehensive program. *Archives of Physical Medicine and Rehabilitation, 66*, 353-359.

Grabowska, A., Marchewka, A., Seniów, J., Polanowska, K., Jednoróg, K., Królicki, L., Kossut, M. & Czlonkowska, A. (2011). Emotionally negative stimuli can overcome attentional deficits in patients with visuo-spatial hemineglect. *Neuropsychologia, 49*, 3327-3337. https://doi.org/10.1016/j.neuropsychologia.2011.08.006

Guariglia, C., Coriale, G., Cosentino, T., & Pizzamiglio, L. (2000). TENS modulates spatial reorientation in neglect patients. *Neuroreport, 11*, 1945-1948. https://doi.org/10.1097/00001756-200006260-00027

Halligan, P. W., & Marshall, J. C. (1991). Left neglect for near but not far space in man. *Nature, 350*, 498-500. https://doi.org/10.1038/350498a0

Hannaford, S., Gower, G., Potter, J. M., Guest, R. M., & Fairhurst, M. C. (2003). Assessing visual inattention: Study of inter-rater reliability. *British Journal of Therapy and Rehabilitation, 10*(2), 72-75. https://doi.org/10.12968/bjtr.2003.10.2.13574

Hartman-Maeir, A., & Katz, N. (1995). Validity of the Behavioural Inattention Test (BIT): Relationships with functional tasks. *American Journal of Occupational Therapy, 49*, 507-516. https://doi.org/10.5014/ajot.49.6.507

Heilman, K. M., Valenstein, E., & Watson, R. T. (2000). Neglect and related disorders. *Seminars in Neurology, 20*, 463-470. https://doi.org/10.1055/s-2000-13179

Invernizzi, M., Negrini, S., Carda, S., Lanzotti, L., Cisari, C., & Baricich, A. (2013). The value of adding mirror therapy for upper limb motor recovery of subacute stroke patients: A randomized controlled trial. *European Journal of Physical and Rehabilitation Medicine, 49*, 311-317.

Kaldenberg, J. (2014). Optimizing vision and visual processing. In M. V. Radomski & C. A. Trombly Latham (Eds.), *Occupational therapy for physical dysfunction* (7th ed., pp 699-724). Lippincott Williams & Wilkins.

Katz, N., Ring, H., Naveh, Y., Kizony, R., Feintuch, U., & Weiss, P. L. (2005). Interactive virtual environment training for safe street crossing of right hemisphere stroke patients with unilateral spatial neglect. *Disability and Rehabilitation, 27*, 1235-1243. https://doi.org/10.1080/09638280500076079

Kaye, V. (2015). Transcutaneous electrical nerve stimulation. Medscape. http://emedicine.medscape.com/article/325107-overview#a1

Kelly, J. P. (1985). Anatomy of the central visual pathways. In E. R. Kandel & J. H. Schwartz (Eds.), *Principles of neural science* (2nd ed., pp. 356-365). Elsevier Science.

Kessels, R. P. C., & de Haan, E. H. F. (2003). Implicit learning in memory rehabilitation: A meta-analysis on errorless learning and vanishing cues methods. *Journal of Clinical and Experimental Neuropsychology, 25*, 805-814. https://doi.org/10.1076/jcen.25.6.805.16474

Kim, Y. M., Chun, M. H., Yun, G. J., Song, Y. J., & Young, H. E. (2011). The effect of virtual reality training on unilateral spatial neglect in stroke patients. *Annals of Rehabilitation Medicine, 35*, 309-315. https://doi.org/10.5535/arm.2011.35.3.309

Kinsella, G., Packer, S., Ng, K., Olver, J., & Stark, R. (1995). Continuing issues in the assessment of neglect. *Neuropsychological Rehabilitation, 5*, 239-258. https://doi.org/10.1080/09602019508401469

Klinke, M. E., Hafsteinsdottir, T. B., Hjaltason, H., & Jonsdottir, H. (2015). Ward-based interventions for patients with hemispatial neglect in stroke rehabilitation: A systematic literature review. *International Journal of Nursing Studies, 52*, 1375-1403. https://doi.org/10.1016/j.ijnurstu.2015.04.004

Klinke, M. E., Zahavi, D., Hjaltason, H., Thorsteinsson, B., & Jonsdottir, H. (2015). "Getting the left right": The experience of hemispatial neglect after stroke. *Qualitative Health Research, 12*, 1623-1636. https://doi.org/10.1177/1049732314566328

Lafosse, C. K., Kerckhofs, E., Troch, M., Vandenbussche, E. (2003). Upper limb exteroceptive somatosensory and proprioceptive sensory afferent modulation of hemispatial neglect. *Journal of Clinical & Experimental Neuropsychology, 25*, 308-323. https://doi.org/10.1076/jcen.25.3.308.13807

Lisa, L. P., Jughters, A., & Kerckhofs, E. (2013). The effectiveness of different treatment modalities for the rehabilitation of unilateral neglect in stroke patients: A systematic review. *NeuroRehabilitation, 33*, 611-620. https://doi.org/10.3233/NRE-130986

Longley, V., Hazelton, C., Heal, C., Pollock, A., Woodward-Nutt, K., Mitchell, C., Pobric, G., Vail, A., & Brown, A. (2021). Non-pharmacological interventions for spatial neglect or inattention following stroke and other non-progressive brain injury. *Cochrane Database of Systematic Reviews, 2021*(7). https://doi.org/10.1002/14651858.CD003586.pub4

Luauté , J., Halligan, P., Rode, G., Jacquin-Courtois, S., & Boisson, D. (2006). Prism adaptation first among equals in alleviating left neglect: A review. *Restorative Neurology and Neuroscience, 24*(4-6), 409-418.

Lucas, N., & Vuilleumier, P. (2008). Effects of emotional and non-emotional cues on visual search in neglect patients: Evidence for distinct sources of attentional guidance. *Neuropsychologia, 46*, 1401-1414. https://doi.org/10.1016/j.neuropsychologia.2007.12.027

Lundy-Ekman, L. (2018). *Neuroscience: Fundamentals for rehabilitation* (5th ed.). Elsevier.

MacDonald, J. (1960). An investigation of body scheme in adults with cerebral vascular accident. *American Journal of Occupational Therapy, 14*, 72-79.

Maeshima, S. O., Truman, G., Smith, D. S., Dohi, N., Shigeno, K., Itakura, T., & Komai, N. (2001). Factor analysis of the components of 12 standard test batteries, for unilateral spatial neglect, reveals that they contain a number of discrete and important clinical variables. *Brain Injury, 15*, 125-137. https://doi.org/10.1080/026990501458362

Mainetti, R., Sedda, A., Ronchetti, M., Bottini, G., & Borghese, N. A. (2013). Duckneglect: Video-games based neglect rehabilitation. *Technology and Health Care, 21*, 97-111. https://doi.org/10.3233/THC-120712

Maloney, M. P., & Payne L. (1969). Validity of the Draw-a-Person test as a measure of body image. *Perceptual and Motor Skills, 29*, 119-122. https://doi.org/10.2466/pms.1969.29.1.119

Mapstone, M., Weintraub, S., Nowinski, C., Kaptanoglu, G., Gitelman, D. R., & Mesulam, M.-M. (2003). Cerebral hemispheric specialization for spatial attention: Spatial distribution of search-related eye fixations in the absence of neglect. *Neuropsychologia, 41*, 1396-1409. https://doi.org/10.1016/S0028-3932(03)00043-5

Marsh, E. B., & Hillis, A. E. (2008). Dissociation between egocentric and allocentric visuospatial and tactile neglect in acute stroke. *Cortex, 44*, 1215-1220. https://doi.org/10.1016/j.cortex.2006.02.002

Marsh, N. V., & Kersel, D. A. (1993). Screening tests for visual neglect following stroke. *Neuropsychological Rehabilitation, 3*, 245-257. https://doi.org/10.1080/09602019308401439

Mattingley, J. B., Driver, J., Beschin, N., & Robertson, I. H. (1997). Attention competition between modalities: Extinction between touch and vision after right hemisphere damage. *Neuropsychologia, 35*, 867-880. https://doi.org/10.1016/S0028-3932(97)00008-0

Mesulam, M.-M. (1981). A cortical network for directed attention and unilateral neglect. *Annals of Neurology, 10*, 309-325. https://doi.org/10.1002/ana.410100402

Mesulam, M.-M. (1990). Large-scale neurocognitive networks and distributed processing for attention, language, and memory. *Annals of Neurology, 28*, 597-613. https://doi.org/10.1002/ana.410280502

Mesulam, M.-M. (1994). The multiplicity of neglect phenomena. *Neuropsychological Rehabilitation, 4*, 173-176. https://doi.org/10.1080/09602019408402278

Mesulam, M.-M. (1999). Spatial attention and neglect: Parietal, frontal and cingulate contributions to the mental representation and attentional targeting of salient extrapersonal events. *Philosophical Transactions of the Royal Society of London, 354*, 1325-1346. https://doi.org/10.1098/rstb.1999.0482

Navarro, M.-D., Llorens, R., Noe, E., Ferri, J., & Alcaniz, M. (2013). Validation of a low-cost virtual reality system training street-crossing. A comparative study in healthy, neglected and non-neglected stroke individuals. *Neuropsychological Rehabilitation, 23*, 597-618. https://doi.org/10.1080/09602011.2013.806269

Niemeier, J. P. (1998). The lighthouse strategy: Use of a visual imagery technique to treat visual inattention in stroke patients. *Brain Injury, 12*, 399-406. https://doi.org/10.1080/026990598122511

Niemeier, J. P. (2002). Visual imagery training for patients with visual perceptual deficits following right hemisphere cerebrovascular accidents: A case study presenting the lighthouse strategy. *Rehabilitation Psychology, 47*, 426-437. https://doi.org/10.1037/0090-5550.47.4.426

Niemeier, J. P., Cifu, D. X., & Kishore, R. (2001). The lighthouse strategy: Improving the functional status of patients with unilateral neglect after stroke and brain injury using a visual imagery intervention. *Topics in Stroke Rehabilitation, 8*, 10-18. https://doi.org/10.1310/7UKK-HJ0F-GDWF-HHM8

Nilsen, D. M., & DiRusso, T. (2014). Using mirror therapy in the home environment: A case report. *American Journal of Occupational Therapy, 68*, e84-e89. https://doi.org/10.5014/ajot.2014.010389

Pandian, J. D., Arora, R., Kaur, P., Sharma, D., Vishwambaran, D. K., & Arima, H. (2014). Mirror therapy in unilateral neglect after stroke (MUST trial): A randomized controlled trial. *Neurology, 83*, 1012-1017. https://doi.org/10.1212/WNL.0000000000000773

Park, Y., Chang, M., Kim, K.-M., & An, D.-H. (2015). The effects of mirror therapy with tasks on upper extremity function and self-care in stroke patients. *Journal of Physical Therapy Science, 27*, 1499-1501. https://doi.org/10.1589/jpts.27.1499

Parton, A., Malhotra, P., & Husain, M. (2004). Hemispatial neglect. *Journal of Neurology, Neurosurgery and Psychiatry, 75*, 13-21.

Pierce, S. R., & Buxbaum, L. J. (2002). Treatments of unilateral neglect: A review. *Archives of Physical Medicine and Rehabilitation, 83*, 256-268. https://doi.org/10.1053/apmr.2002.27333

Plummer, P., Morris, M. E., & Dunai, J. (2003). Assessment of unilateral neglect. *Physical Therapy, 83*, 732-740. https://doi.org/10.1093/ptj/83.8.732

Polanowska, K., Seniów, J., Paprot, E., Lesniak, M., & Czlonkowska, A. (2009). Left-hand somatosensory stimulation combined with visual scanning training in rehabilitation for post-stroke hemineglect: A randomised, double-blind study. *Neuropsychological Rehabilitation, 19*, 364-382. https://doi.org/10.1080/09602010802268856

Proto, D., Pella, R. D., Hill, B. D., & Gouvier, W. D. (2009). Assessment and rehabilitation of acquired visuospatial and proprioceptive deficits associated with visuospatial neglect. *NeuroRehabilitation, 24*, 145-157. https://doi.org/10.3233/NRE-2009-0463

Radomski, M. V., & Giles, G. M. (2014). Optimizing cognitive performance. In M. V. Radomski & C. A. Trombly Latham (Eds.), *Occupational therapy for physical dysfunction* (7th ed., pp. 725-752). Lippincott Williams & Wilkins.

Ramachandran, V. S., & Altschuler, E. L. (2009). The use of visual feedback, in particular mirror visual feedback, in restoring brain function. *Brain, 132*, 1693-1710. https://doi.org/10.1093/brain/awp135

Ramachandran, V. S., & Rogers-Ramachandran, D. (1996). Synaesthesia in phantom limbs induced with mirrors. *Proceedings of the Royal Society B: Biological Sciences, 263*, 377-386. https://doi.org/10.1098/rspb.1996.0058

Rao, A. K. (2021). Approaches to motor control dysfunction: An evidence-based review. In G. Gillen & D. M. Nilsen (Eds.), *Stroke rehabilitation: A function-based approach* (5th ed., pp. 332-348). Elsevier.

Rich, T. J. (2020). *The contributions of spatial processing and selection attention to the deficits of patients with spatial neglect and neglect dyslexia* [Unpublished doctoral dissertation]. University of Washington.

Robertson, I. H., Mattingley, J. B., Rorden, C., & Driver, J. (1998). Phasic alerting of neglect patients overcomes their spatial deficit in visual awareness. *Nature, 395*, 169-172. https://doi.org/10.1038/25993

Robertson, I. H., Tegner, R, Tham, K., Lo, A., & Nimmo-Smith, I. (1995). Sustained attention training for unilateral neglect: Theoretical and rehabilitation implications. *Journal of Clinical and Experimental Neuropsychology, 17*, 416-430. https://doi.org/10.1080/01688639508405133

Ronchi, R., Bolognini, N., Gallucci, M., Chiapella, L., Algeri, L., Spada, M. S., & Vallar, G. (2014). (Un)awareness of unilateral spatial neglect: A quantitative evaluation of performance in visuo-spatial tasks. *Cortex, 61*, 167-182. https://doi.org/10.1016/j.cortex.2014.10.004

Saj, A., Honore, J., Braem, B., Bernati, T., & Rousseaux, M. (2012). Time since stroke influences the impact of hemianopia and spatial neglect on visual-spatial tasks. *Neuropsychology, 26*, 37-44. https://doi.org/10.1037/a0025733

Samuelkamaleshkumar, S., Reethajanetsureka, S., Pauljebaraj, P., Benshamir, B., Padankatti, S. M., & David, J. A. (2014). Mirror therapy enhances motor performance in the paretic upper limb after stroke: A pilot randomized controlled trial. *Archives of Physical Medicine and Rehabilitation, 95*, 2000-2005. https://doi.org/10.1016/j.apmr.2014.06.020

Schenkenberg, T., Bradford, D. C., & Ajax, E. T. (1980). Line bisection and unilateral visual neglect in patients with neurological impairment. *Neurology, 30*, 509-517. https://doi.org/10.1212/WNL.30.5.509

Schröder, A., Wist, E., & Hömberg, V. (2008). TENS and optokinetic stimulation in neglect therapy after cerebrovascular accident: A randomized controlled study. *European Journal of Neurology, 15*, 922-927. https://doi.org/10.1111/j.1468-1331.2008.02229.x

Seniów, J., Polanowska, K., Lesniak, M., & Czlonkowska, A. (2016). Adding transcutaneous electrical nerve stimulation to visual scanning training does not enhance treatment effect on hemispatial neglect: A randomized, controlled, double-blind study. *Topics in Stroke Rehabilitation, 23*, 377-383. https://doi.org/10.1179/1074935715Z.00000000058

Shinsha, N., & Ishigami, S. (1999). Rehabilitation approach to patients with unilateral spatial neglect. *Topics in Stroke Rehabilitation, 6*, 1-14. https://doi.org/10.1310/P4PC-KWCA-DVYU-H4FP

Stein, M. S., Maskill, D., & Marston, L. (2009). Impact of visual-spatial neglect on stroke functional outcomes, discharge destination and maintenance of improvement post-discharge. *British Journal of Occupational Therapy, 72*, 219-225. https://doi.org/10.1177/030802260907200508

Suter, P. S. (2018). Rehabilitation and management of visual dysfunction following traumatic brain injury. In M. J. Ashley & D. A. Hovda (Eds.), *Traumatic brain injury: Rehabilitation, treatment and case management* (4th ed., pp. 451-486). CRC Press.

Tham, K., Borell, L., & Gustavsson, A. (1999). The discovery of disability: A phenomenological study of unilateral neglect. *American Journal of Occupational Therapy, 54*, 398-406. https://doi.org/10.5014/ajot.54.4.398

Tham, K., Ginsberg, E., Fisher, A. G., & Tegner, R. (2001). Training to improve awareness of disabilities in clients with unilateral neglect. *American Journal of Occupational Therapy, 55*, 46-53. https://doi.org/10.5014/ajot.55.1.46

Tham, K., & Kielhofner, G. (2003). Impact of the social environment on occupational experience and performance among persons with unilateral neglect. *American Journal of Occupational Therapy, 57*, 403-412. https://doi.org/10.5014/ajot.57.4.403

Tham, K., & Tegner, R. (1996). The baking tray task: A test of spatial neglect. *Neuropsychological Rehabilitation, 6*, 19-25. https://doi.org/10.1080/713755496

Thieme, H., Bayn, M., Wurg, M., Zange, C., Pohl, M., & Behrens, J. (2013). Mirror therapy for patients with severe arm paresis after stroke—A randomized controlled trial. *Clinical Rehabilitation, 27*, 314-324. https://doi.org/10.1177/0269215512455651

Thieme, H., Morkisch, N., Mehrholz, J., Pohl, M., Behrens, J., Borgetto, B., & Dohle, C. (2018). Mirror therapy for improving motor function after stroke. *Cochrane Database of Systematic Reviews, 2018*(7). https://doi.org/10.1002/14651858.CD008449.pub3

Toglia, J. (2018). The dynamic interactional model and the multicontext approach. In N. Katz & J. Toglia (Eds.), *Cognition, occupation, and participation across the life span: Neuroscience, neurorehabilitation, and models of intervention in occupational therapy* (4th ed., pp. 355-386). AOTA Press.

Toglia, J., & Cermak, S. A. (2009). Dynamic assessment and prediction of learning potential in clients with unilateral neglect. *American Journal of Occupational Therapy, 64*, 569-579. https://doi.org/10.5014/ajot.63.5.569

Tsai, P., Chen, M., Huang, Y., Lin, K., Chen, K., & Hsu, Y. (2013). Listening to classical music ameliorates unilateral neglect after stroke. *American Journal of Occupational Therapy, 67*, 328-335. https://doi.org/10.5014/ajot.2013.006312

Tyson, S., Wilkinson, J., Thomas, N., Selles, R., McCabe, C., Tyrrell, P., & Vail, A. (2015). Phase II pragmatic randomized controlled trial of patient led mirror therapy and lower limb exercises in acute stroke. *Neurorehabiltation and Neural Repair, 29*, 818-26. https://doi.org/10.1177/1545968314565513

van Dijk, K. R. A., Scherder, E. J. A., Scheltens, P., & Sergeant, J. A. (2002). Effects of transcutaneous electrical nerve stimulation (TENS) on non-pain related cognitive and behavioural functioning. *Reviews in the Neurosciences, 13*, 257-270. https://doi.org/10.1515/REVNEURO.2002.13.3.257

Warren, M. L. (1990). Identification of visual scanning deficits in adults after cerebrovascular accident. *American Journal of Occupational Therapy, 44*(5), 391-399. https://doi.org/10.5014/ajot.44.5.391

Warren, M. (1998). *Brain Injury Visual Assessment Battery for Adults: Test manual.* VisAbilities Rehab Services Inc.

Warren, M. (2006). Evaluation and treatment of visual deficits following brain injury. In H. M. Pendleton & W. Schultz-Krohn (Eds.), *Pedretti's occupational therapy: Practice skills for physical dysfunction* (6th ed., pp. 532-572). Mosby Elsevier.

Warren, M. (2018). Evaluation and treatment of visual deficits after brain injury. In H. M. Pendleton & W. Shultz-Krohn (Eds.), *Pedretti's occupational therapy: Practice skills for physical dysfunction* (8th ed., pp. 594-630). Mosby Elsevier.

Weisser-Pike, O. (2014). Assessing abilities and capacities: Vision and visual processing. In M. V. Radomski & C. A. Trombly Latham (Eds.), *Occupational therapy for physical dysfunction* (7th ed., pp. 103-120). Lippincott Williams & Wilkins.

Wiart, L., Bon Saint Come, A., Debelleix, X., Petit, H., Joseph, P. A., Mazaux, J. M., & Barat, M. (1997). Unilateral neglect syndrome rehabilitation by trunk rotation and scanning training. *Archives of Physical Medicine and Rehabilitation, 78*, 424-429. https://doi.org/10.1016/S0003-9993(97)90236-7

Wilson, B., Cockburn, J., & Halligan, P. (1987). *Behavioural Inattention Test.* Thames Valley Test Co.

Wong, C. E. I., Branco, L. D., Cotrena, C., Joanette, Y., & Fonseca, R. P. (2018). [Reliability and construct validity of the Bells.] *Avaliação Psicológica, 17*(1), 28-36. https://doi.org/10.15689/ap.2017.1701.04.13128

Wu, C.-Y., Wang, T.-N., Chen, Y.-T., Lin, K.-C., Chen, Y.-A., Li, H.-T., & Tsai, P.-L. (2013). Effects of constraint-induced therapy combined with eye patching on functional outcomes and movement kinematics in poststroke neglect. *American Journal of Occupational Therapy, 67*, 236-245. https://doi.org/10.5014/ajot.2013.006486

Yoon, T. H., Yi, T. I., & Park, S. G. (2012). The effect of video feedback on unilateral spatial neglect in stroke patients. *Journal of Rehabilitation Medicine, 52*(Suppl.), 87.

Zoltan, B., Jabri, J., Panikoff, L., & Rychman, D. (1983). *Perceptual motor evaluation for head injured and other neurologically impaired adults.* Santa Clara Valley Medical Center.

CHAPTER 7

Aspects of Cognition

Cognition is complex and multifaceted with a wide variety of cognitive skills necessary for independent living and maximal occupational performance. These cognitive skills are highly interconnected, with each influencing the functioning of the others. As a result of this interconnection, it is rare to have only one type of cognitive functioning impacted after acquired brain injury (ABI). This chapter focuses on the cognition skills of attention, memory, and executive functioning, including the neurological structures that underlie these cognitive abilities. We also discuss apraxia, a cognitive skill that is essential for motor planning and execution. The evaluation and treatment approaches for clients with cognitive deficits are considered in Chapters 8, 9, and 10.

Attention

Attention is an active process that helps individuals focus on sensations and experiences that are relevant to them. As sensory stimuli are received, the nervous system begins to process them and determine which are important to an individual's needs or goals. Those stimuli will be prioritized so that the individual can focus on them, a process called *selectivity* (Heilman et al., 2000). Selectivity enables a target stimulus to receive priority in focus over a nontarget stimulus, allowing an individual to respond to a specific event and ignore other events that are happening simultaneously (Lundy-Ekman, 2018; Mateer, 2000; Parenté & Herrmann, 2010). Attention encompasses several skills, including the ability to narrow focus to a single target, the ability to sustain focus on a target, and the ability to shift focus from one target to another (Lundy-Ekman, 2018; Maeir & Rotenberg-Shpigelman, 2015). Attention requires effort and is flexible in how it is used (Lundy-Ekman, 2018). It can be used broadly, such as when a person attends to an auditorium full of people, or focused, such as when attending to an individual speaker in a crowd. Attention can be directed to extrapersonal space, such as the physical environment, or intrapersonal space, such as bodily sensations (Parker, 2012).

Kaminsky, T. A., & Powell, J. M.
Zoltan's Vision, Perception, and Cognition: Evaluation and Treatment of the Adult With Acquired Brain Injury, Fifth Edition (pp. 177-201).

Attention is an essential precursor for other cognitive functions and types of learning (Ashley et al., 2018; Devinsky & D'Esposito, 2004). For example, attending to a stimulus is the first step in committing that stimulus to memory; not noticing something will not enable a person to remember it (Ashley et al., 2018; Gillen, 2018; Lundy-Ekman, 2018; Parenté & Herrmann, 2010). Just as attention influences other types of cognition, it, in turn, is affected by other aspects of a person's functioning. Consciousness, awareness, and arousal are necessary for a person to be alert enough to attend to stimuli. In addition, attention is impacted by affect and motivation (Devinsky & D'Esposito, 2004; Lundy-Ekman, 2018). For example, imagine that you are attending class in the morning after getting only a few hours of sleep. The classroom is warm, the lights are dim, and the professor is lecturing on a topic in which you have little interest. It is likely that these factors will decrease your arousal level, making it difficult for you to attend to what the professor is saying. Imagine, instead, that you are in your favorite class after a full night's sleep and that the professor is leading a discussion on a topic that you feel passionately about. These factors are more likely to increase your arousal level and better enable you to focus your attention on the class activities (Lundy-Ekman, 2018).

In addition to being affected by arousal level, attention is heavily influenced by the circumstances that surround the person. Toglia (1993) suggested that occupational therapy practitioners consider attentional function/dysfunction as an interaction among task characteristics, environment, and the individual's capabilities. The complexity or familiarity of a given task will determine the extent to which attention is required, with more focused and selective attention needed for novel tasks (Lundy-Ekman, 2018; Toglia, 1993). In this way, more conscious processing is used when new information is being considered. On the other hand, automatic processing occurs at a subcortical level. Once a task becomes more automatic, significant conscious attentional resources are no longer required, and attention can be directed to other more novel aspects of a particular task (Lundy-Ekman, 2018). As a result, the demands placed on attention can differ depending on the situation. You can likely relate to this with a variety of tasks in which you are engaged each day. For example, think back to when you were first learning to drive. You focused a lot of conscious attention on the task of driving, thinking carefully about the different steps of starting the car, steering, braking, changing lanes, and so forth while also being highly focused on your environment. As you gained skills and experience, you were able to expend less conscious effort on attending to driving and started to be able to listen to music or carry on conversations with passengers in the car as you drove (Lundy-Ekman, 2018).

Often, the term *attention* is used interchangeably with other terms such as *alertness*, *vigilance*, or *effort*. This can create confusion and make it more difficult for the clinician to identify deficits and design treatment programs. Therefore, these and other related terms are described in an effort to clarify the related concepts.

- Alerting: Alerting is a subconscious skill that prepares the individual to mobilize attention. It is heavily modulated by the reticular activating system in the brainstem, which helps to control sleep–wake cycles (Garcia-Rill, 2009).
- Attention: Attention provides the means by which individuals can focus on objects or events in order to receive incoming information (Dirette & McCormack, 2021; Parenté & Herrmann, 2010). There are several subcategories of attention (Dirette & McCormack, 2021; Sohlberg & Mateer, 2001):
    - Focused attention: Focused attention directs and orients the individual toward the stimulus of interest (Radomski & Morrison, 2014; Sohlberg & Mateer, 2001). It has both physical and mental components, allowing the person to physically position the body and mentally orient in such a way that the individual is able to receive sensory information and take motor action (Parker, 2012). With focused attention, the mind is free of extraneous thoughts, and an effort is made to keep sensory channels open to incoming information

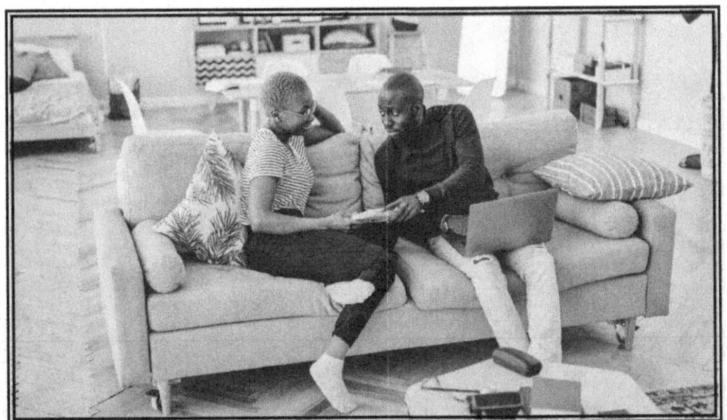

Figure 7-1. Focused attention in a conversation. To attend more carefully to what the woman is saying, this man has oriented his body toward her and away from his computer so that he can better focus on the conversation. (GaudiLab/shutterstock.com)

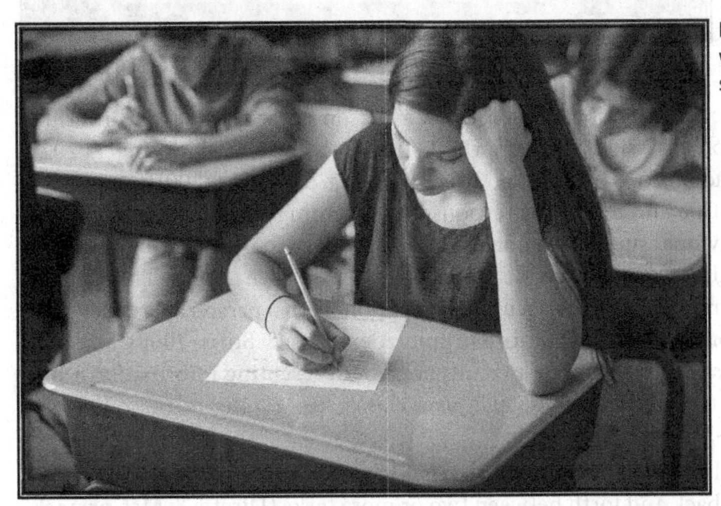

Figure 7-2. Sustained attention while taking a test. (antoniodiaz/shutterstock.com)

(Parker, 2012; Sohlberg & Mateer, 2001). For example, imagine having an important conversation with another person. To best focus attention on your conversation partner, you turn toward them and look at them. You may also remove distractions, such as shutting off a television that is on or silencing your phone so that you are not interrupted (Figure 7-1).

- Sustained attention: Sustained attention allows an individual to attend to stimuli for an extended period of time (Dirette & McCormack, 2021). This term describes the ability of an individual to consciously process stimuli with repetitive, nonarousing qualities that would otherwise cause habituation and distraction to other stimuli (Manly et al., 2002; Sohlberg & Mateer, 2001). The ability to sustain attention over a period of time is also sometimes called *vigilance* (Parenté & Herrmann, 2010; Radomski & Morrison, 2014). It is this aspect of attention that appears particularly vulnerable to brain damage (Stuss & Alexander, 2000). For example, imagine taking a test in a course. While the test is administered, you need to keep your attention on the test questions rather than on other things, such as what you need to get at the grocery store or the story line of your favorite television program. It is your sustained attention that allows you to accomplish this task (Figure 7-2).

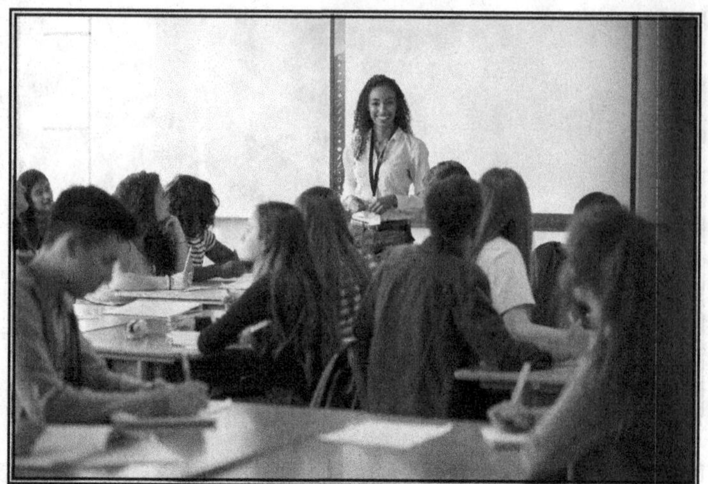

Figure 7-3. Students in a classroom use selective attention when listening to the instructor and ignoring other students. (Monkey Business Images/shutterstock.com)

- Selective attention: Selective attention is used when a person ignores irrelevant information and focuses attention exclusively on important stimuli (Dirette & McCormack, 2021; Lundy-Ekman, 2018; Radomski & Morrison, 2014; Sohlberg & Mateer, 2001). Achieving this requires both activating and inhibiting responses to incoming stimuli. Selective attention ensures that an individual suppresses nonattended stimuli such that only one stimulus is processed at a given time in higher cortical areas (Nieber & Koch, 2000). This enables goal-directed behavior and is critical for accurate perception, with a person able to separate relevant information from that which is unimportant (Alexander & Stuss, 2000). Selective attention is what enables you to attend to a faculty member presenting information while ignoring other stimuli in your classroom, such as a classmate's typing or the noise of a projector's fan (Figure 7-3).
- Alternating attention (also called *attentional flexibility*): Alternating attention allows an individual to shift focus back and forth between two or more tasks (Dirette & McCormack, 2021; Radomski & Morrison, 2014; Sohlberg & Mateer, 2001). For example, in a meal preparation activity, a person would use alternating attention to chop vegetables while periodically checking food on the stove. In this case, alternating attention allows the person to pause in chopping vegetables to attend to the food on the stove and then return to chopping vegetables, smoothly resuming the prior activity (Figure 7-4).
- Divided attention (also called *multitasking*): Divided attention allows people to do two or more things at once (Dirette & McCormack, 2021; Lundy-Ekman, 2018; Radomski & Morrison, 2014; Sohlberg & Mateer, 2001), such as making a meal while carrying on a conversation on the telephone. Driving is another task that requires good divided attention so that the driver is able to attend to multiple factors simultaneously (Lundy-Ekman, 2018). Divided attention requires the ability to allocate attentional resources, rapidly switching attention between tasks. It is best achieved when one or both of the tasks is routine and do not use the same skills (Ashley et al., 2018; Mateer, 2000; Sohlberg & Mateer, 2001). For example, let us return to the meal-making example provided previously. You are likely able to have a conversation and cook, especially if you are familiar with the dish you are making (Figure 7-5). It is much more difficult to have a conversation and read a recipe. In this case, talking and reading both rely on language skills. When faced with this situation, you probably ask your conversation partner to give you a moment while you consult the recipe. After getting the information you need, you are then able to return to both the conversation and the cooking itself. This example also shows the interplay among different types

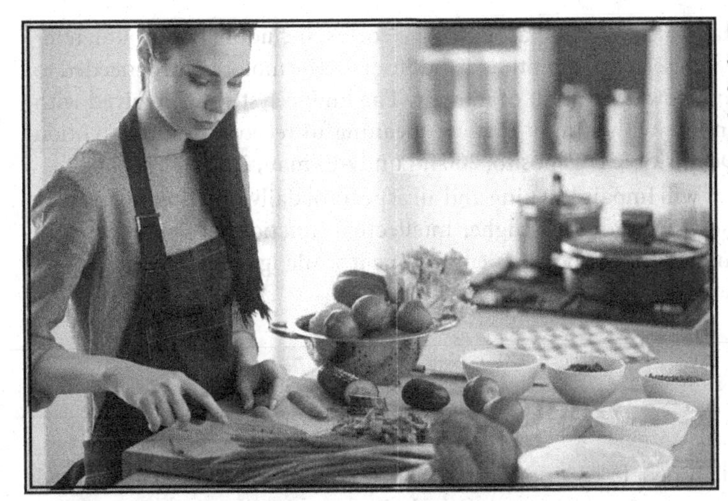

Figure 7-4. Using alternating attention during meal preparation allows this woman to work on making a salad, pause to check pasta cooking on the stove, and then return to salad making. (lenetstan/shutterstock.com)

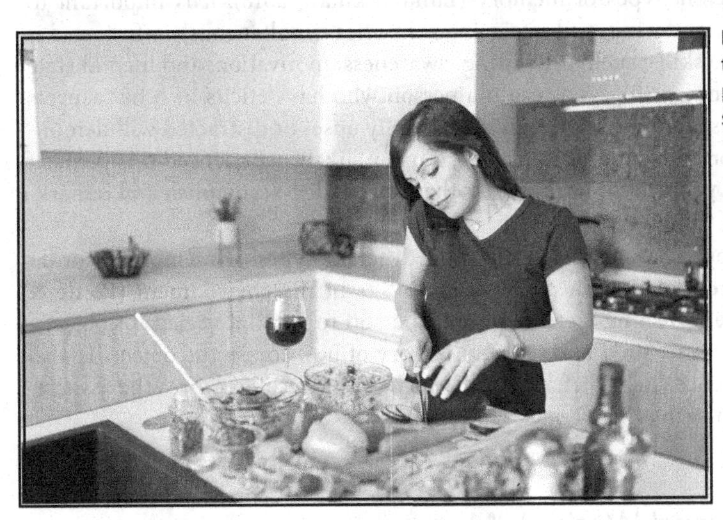

Figure 7-5. Using divided attention to prepare a meal and talk on the phone simultaneously. (antoniodiaz/shutterstock.com)

of attention. While cooking and talking, you are making use of divided attention. Pausing both cooking and talking while reading the recipe and then returning to the original tasks makes use of alternating attention.

Attention deficits are common after ABI (Ashley et al., 2018; Chan, 2000; Cicerone, 2002; Devinsky & D'Esposito, 2004; Manly et al., 2002). Deficits can vary and can result in difficulty focusing, distractibility, and difficulty with attentional flexibility (Mateer, 2000). Clients may display poor performance in noisy or busy environments because of distractibility, have difficulty maintaining attention on a task through completion, or have challenges with shifting focus or with multitasking (Ashley et al., 2018). Other signs of impairment in attention can be observed with clients who exhibit slow processing, fatigue, irritability, complaints of headache when concentrating on tasks, or difficulty staying on task (Constantinidou & Thomas, 2018; Mateer, 2000).

Attention is accomplished by a network of highly interconnected anatomical areas (Ashley et al., 2018). As a result, attentional deficits can arise from damage to multiple portions of the brain including the frontal and temporal lobes; the limbic system; and subcortical structures, such as the reticular activating system, superior colliculi, and the basal ganglia (Ashley et al., 2018; Chan, 2000; Devinsky & D'Esposito, 2004; Gazzaniga et al., 2019; Lundy-Ekman, 2018). Each of these areas is responsible for a different aspect of attention, and all communicate with each other. The reticular activating system mediates alertness and arousal. The cortex, including the frontal, temporal, and parietal lobes, assists with selective attention, in addition to the motor control needed to physically direct the eyes and body toward stimuli of interest. The limbic system is involved with the motivational aspects of attention, with stimuli that are meaningful receiving more attention than those that are irrelevant (Devinsky & D'Esposito, 2004; Lundy-Ekman, 2018).

Any type of attentional deficit will impair learning and all aspects of daily functioning (Ashley et al., 2018). Memory, problem solving, and other higher intellectual functions are all dependent on the ability to focus on relevant information in the environment while ignoring or paying less attention to irrelevant information.

Memory

Memory is a process by which people encode, store, and retrieve information. It is a broad term that includes several different types of memory (Lundy-Ekman, 2018). It is important to realize that the process of creating, storing, and retrieving memories simultaneously affects and is affected by a variety of cognitive skills, such as learning, awareness, motivation, and mental state (Levy, 2018; Parenté & Herrmann, 2010). As a result, a person who has deficits in other aspects of cognitive functioning, such as attention, or who is emotionally upset or distracted will demonstrate difficulty with memory formation and/or retrieval. You have likely experienced this yourself when in times of stress you find yourself forgetting tasks that you need to accomplish and remarking that you are "losing track of things."

The completion of many everyday tasks is reliant on different types of memory in order for individuals to interact appropriately with people and objects in the environment (Forde & Humphries, 2000). For example, brushing teeth requires a person to recall a variety of objects, including the toothbrush, toothpaste, sink, and faucet. Memory of how to use the objects is also essential, which relies on experience (Ashley et al., 2018). Much of this recall requires the association of objects or situations with each other (Lou & Lane, 2005).

Sensory, Perceptual, and Working Memory

The memory process begins with the input of sensations. Individuals selectively attend to the environment depending on their interests at the time. This input creates sensory memory, which is the first phase of an individual's information processing. Sensory memory allows individuals to process enormous amounts of information in a short period of time (Gazzaniga et al., 2019; Parenté & Herrmann, 2010; Radomski & Morrison, 2014). Sensory memory is very short in duration (several seconds at most), is modality specific, and either transfers for further analysis or degenerates rapidly (Lou & Lane, 2005). Fuster (1998) placed sensory memory at the base of a hierarchy of perceptual memory. The top of the hierarchy is composed of abstract concepts that, although originally acquired by sensory experience, have become independent from these experiences through processing (Fuster, 1998). It is important to remember that if information is distorted at the stage of sensory memory, then the encoding process in all other areas of memory will be adversely affected (Parenté & Herrmann, 2010).

The creation of memory continues from sensory memory to working memory (Fuster, 1998), which may be considered a form of short-term memory (Radomski & Morrison, 2014). Information that is in our conscious thoughts is stored in working memory. Working memory allows short-term storage of information without concurrent sensory input and also enables information to be available for use, including for mental manipulation (Devinsky & D'Esposito, 2004;

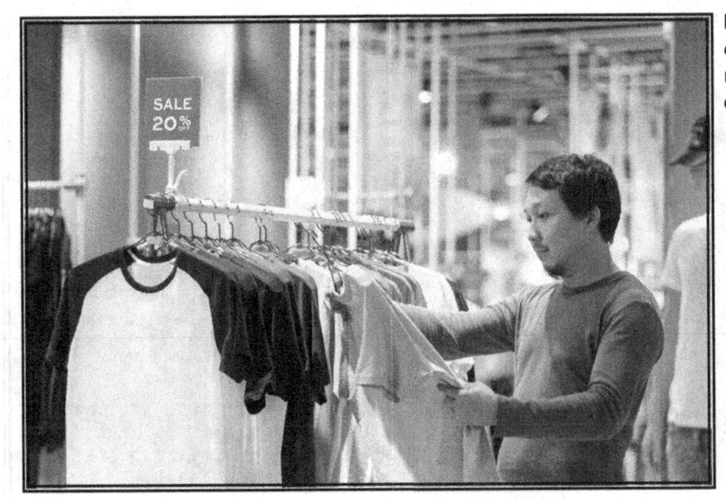

Figure 7-6. Calculating a sale price on a piece of clothing uses working memory. (TZIDO SUN/shutterstock.com)

Eriksson et al., 2015; Gazzaniga et al., 2019; Lundy-Ekman, 2018; Radomski & Morrison, 2014). Fletcher and Henson (2001) described working memory as a mental workspace that allows information to be manipulated for complex problem solving. This can include bringing in information from long-term memory. It is involved in the processing of information while performing a wide variety of daily tasks (Lundy-Ekman, 2018). For example, a person who is calculating the sale price on a piece of clothing is using working memory to manipulate the numbers (Figure 7-6). Working memory makes use of a wide cortical network, including the prefrontal cortex, parietal cortex, medial temporal lobe, and basal ganglia, especially the striatum (Eriksson et al., 2015). Although information in working memory has a longer storage time than in sensory memory, it is still quite brief (approximately 10 to 15 seconds). In order to keep information active in working memory, it must be repeated or otherwise processed in some way (Eriksson et al., 2015). Neuroimaging studies have found that the specific cortical areas that are active during working memory tasks depend on the features of the information being processed (Eriksson et al., 2015). For example, areas on the left side of the prefrontal cortex are more likely to be active if verbal memory is being processed, and areas on the right side of the prefrontal cortex are more likely to be active if the information is spatial in nature. Similarly, the medial temporal lobe is more likely to be active if working memory is manipulating information rather than maintaining it (Eriksson et al., 2015).

From working memory, items are consolidated into long-term memory, which allows the new memories to be integrated with the existing ones (Parenté & Herrmann, 2010). This process is called *encoding* and is what allows information to be stored efficiently in long-term memory (Gazzaniga et al., 2019; Parenté & Herrmann, 2010). The consolidation process can take minutes or hours and results in a permanent change to the cell structure in the brain (Lundy-Ekman, 2018). Items can be stored in long-term memory for extended periods of time (in some cases, for life). The storage of long-term memories does not occur at a single place in the brain. Information is stored differently depending on its type and age (Lundy-Ekman, 2018).

A variety of factors influence encoding. For example, the type of rehearsal that occurs during working memory determines the success of the encoding process. Craik and Kester (2000) described two types of rehearsal: (a) maintenance rehearsal, when information is kept passively in mind (i.e., rote repetition), and (b) elaborative rehearsal, when information is meaningfully related to other information presented either previously or currently.

Encoding and storing information in long-term memory are only two of the steps necessary to use long-term memories effectively. It is also essential that a person be able to subsequently retrieve memories. Retrieval is the final aspect of the memory process and results in recovering previously saved information and then converting it into conscious experience (Craik & Kester,

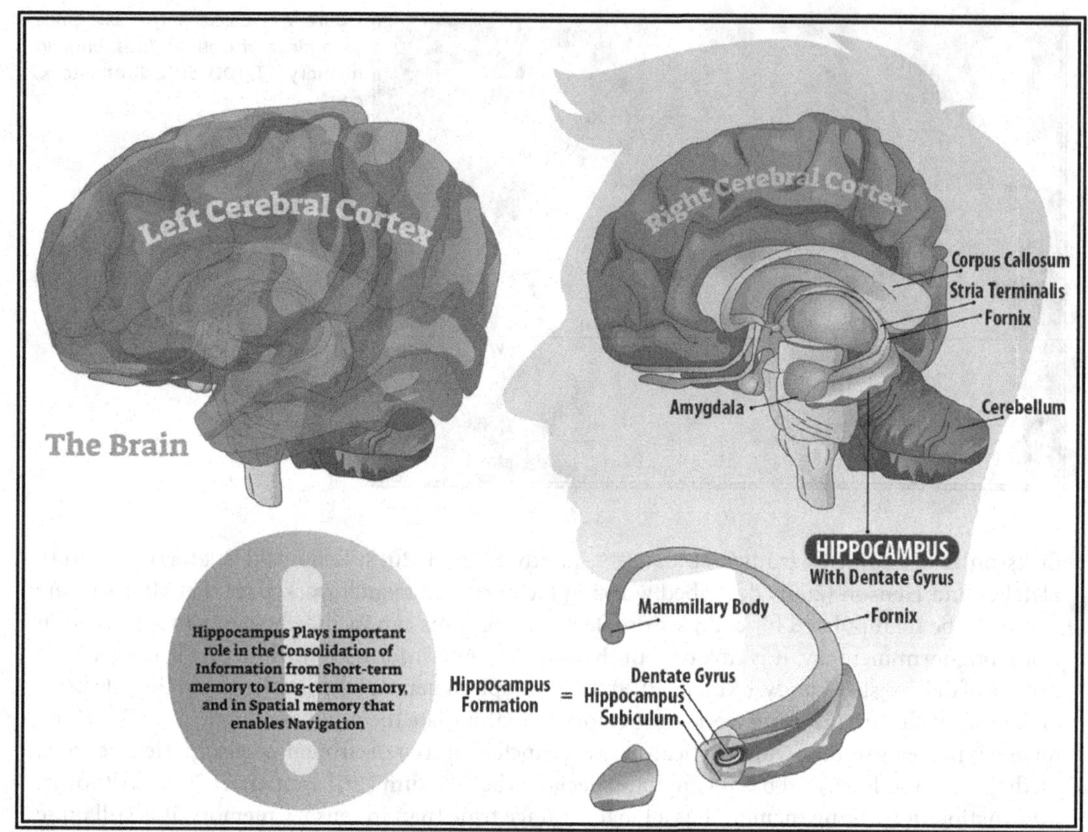

Figure 7-7. The hippocampus and medial temporal lobe are important for consolidating and encoding long-term memories. (VectorMine/shutterstock.com)

2000; Gazzaniga et al., 2019). Elaborative rehearsal typically results in better recall because more connections are made that then can be used later to bring the memory back to conscious thought (Craik & Kester, 2000).

There are several types of memories, all of which play an important role in an individual's ability to function and communicate successfully. These categories of memory include declarative/explicit memory (with the two subtypes of semantic and episodic), nondeclarative/implicit/procedural memory, and prospective memory. The client with ABI may have any aspect or type of memory impaired, and the type of memory that is impacted can influence performance (Dirette & McCormack, 2021). Therefore, the clinician should have an understanding of the types of memory that exist.

Explicit/Declarative and Implicit/Procedural Memory

Explicit memory, also referred to as *declarative memory*, consists of information that can be consciously stated or "declared" to have been learned or experienced, meaning that people must be able to access the information in a conscious way and demonstrate awareness of their previous interactions with those memories (Ashley et al., 2018; Lundy-Ekman, 2018). There are two types of declarative memory: semantic (facts) and episodic (events; Ashley et al., 2018; Devinsky & D'Esposito, 2004; Lundy-Ekman, 2018). Neurologically, both types of declarative memory depend on the medial temporal lobe, including the hippocampus, and the limbic system for encoding and consolidating information (Ashley et al., 2018; Gazzaniga et al., 2019; Markowitsch et al.,

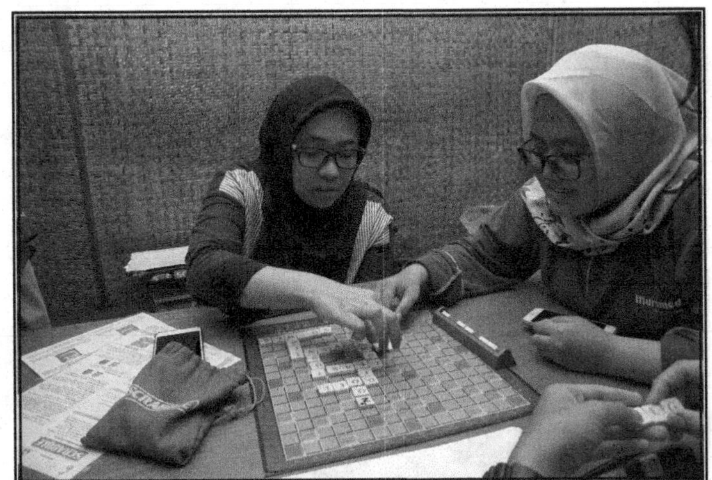

Figure 7-8. Playing a board game that involves spelling is dependent on semantic declarative memory, which enables people to remember facts. (Learnmoreandmore/shutterstock.com)

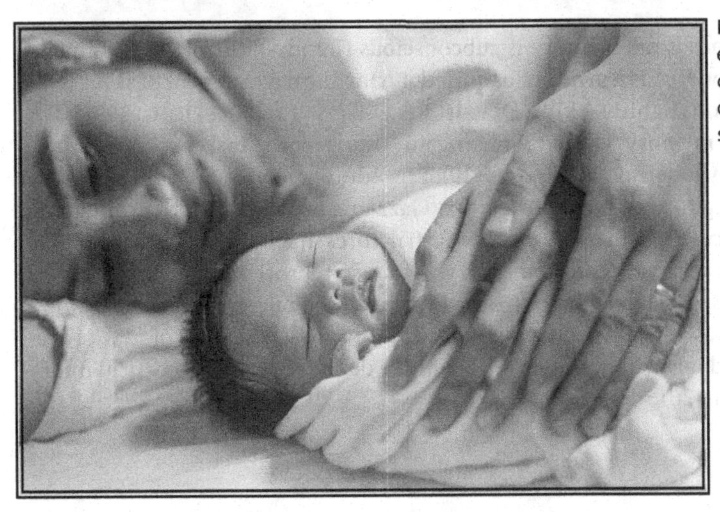

Figure 7-9. Recalling the details of an event in one's life, such as the birth of a child, is an example of episodic declarative memory. (paulaphoto/shutterstock.com)

1999; Figure 7-7). The frontal and temporal lobes are important for declarative memory retrieval (Markowitsch et al., 1999).

The first type of declarative memory, semantic, involves general facts or knowledge about the self or the world (Ashley et al., 2018). The range of personal semantic memory can include basic autobiographical knowledge expressed in a verbal form (e.g., by stating one's name, age, family, schooling) or a nonverbal form (e.g., the ability to recognize family members as familiar; Kapur, 1999). Semantic memory is not related to the person themselves and can include such things as remembering the names of the cranial nerves or dates of historical events or how to spell words (Figure 7-8).

The other type of declarative memory, episodic, consists of knowledge of a previous personally experienced event along with the awareness or understanding that the event occurred in a person's past (Ashley et al., 2018; Devinsky & D'Esposito, 2004; Klein et al., 2002). Episodic memory includes remembering the context in which the item was studied or an event occurred (Cansino et al., 2002). Episodic memory allows an individual to mentally travel back in time and re-experience events that occurred minutes ago or decades ago (Klein et al., 2002). Examples of episodic memory include remembering momentous occasions, such as the first day of college or the birth of a child, or more everyday events, such as what you ate for dinner last night (Figure 7-9).

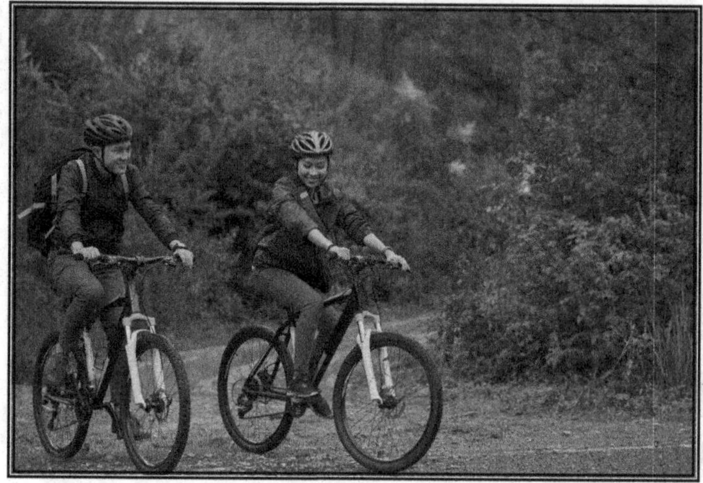

Figure 7-10. Procedural memory results in the ability to complete activities without conscious thought, such as when a person is skilled with riding a bicycle. (Dragon Images/shutterstock.com)

In contrast, implicit, or procedural, memory is subconscious (Lundy-Ekman, 2018). Implicit memory refers to the information that is learned or acquired during the development of skills (e.g., motor skills, perceptual skills, and cognitive skills; Devinsky & D'Esposito, 2004; Fuster, 1998). For example, a person uses implicit memory when completing an "overlearned" task, such as riding a bike, walking, or keyboarding by touch alone (Figure 7-10). Procedural memory appears to involve structures such as the basal ganglia and the motor cortex (Gazzaniga et al., 2019). Neuroimaging studies have identified that the cerebellum and subcortical structures, including the basal ganglia, are some of the areas associated with procedural memory. As a result, procedural memory can be spared in cases of cortically based memory impairment (Maeir & Rotenberg-Shpigelman, 2015). This is important for allowing task-specific training to occur through the creation of new procedural memory even with individuals with more severe cognitive deficits because of cortical injury (Maeir & Rotenberg-Shpigelman, 2015).

Prospective Memory

Prospective memory is remembering to complete an activity or carry out a task at some point in the future (Gillen, 2018; Krellman et al., 2018; Toglia et al., 2019). It involves committing to memory what one intends to do as well as remembering to actually complete that activity at the appropriate time and in the appropriate way (Krellman et al., 2018). Prospective memory allows an individual to carry out an intended action in the future without performing continuous rehearsal of the intention until the appropriate time has occurred (Krellman et al., 2018). McDaniel et al. (1999) identified two types of prospective memory: (a) event-based prospective memory, when some environmental event signals that it is time to complete the intended action (e.g., running to first base after hitting a baseball), and (b) time-based prospective memory, when a particular time or a particular amount of elapsed time signals that it is time to complete the intended action (e.g., attending a doctor's appointment at 3:00 p.m. on Tuesday). Other examples of prospective memory include activities such as remembering to buy bread when passing the store on the way home, remembering to take medications in the morning, or remembering to make a phone call (McDaniel et al., 1999; Figure 7-11).

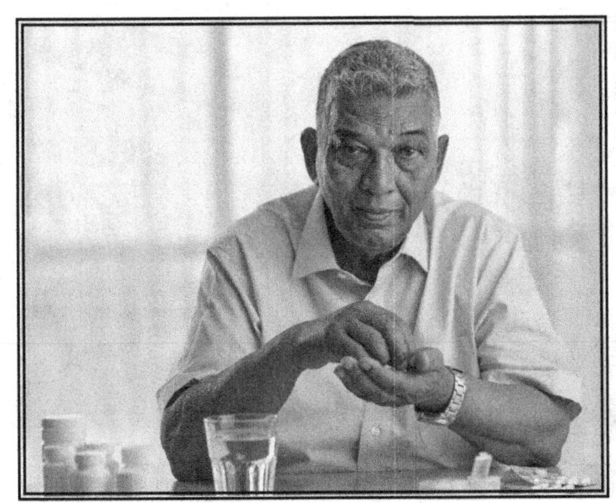

Figure 7-11. Remembering to take prescription medication at the appropriate time and in the appropriate way (e.g., with food) requires the use of prospective memory. (Dragon Images/shutterstock.com)

Memory Deficits After Acquired Brain Injury

Memory loss has been well documented as one of the most common consequences of ABI (Gillen, 2018; Makatura et al., 1999). Even those classified as having a mild traumatic brain injury are often shown to have impaired working memory processes (McAllister et al., 1999). These deficits may be long lasting as well. Research has shown that memory deficits persist for numerous clients 6 months or more after a stroke, although the incidence is often lower than during the more acute stage (Mellon et al., 2015). The client with ABI can have impairment in one or more types of memory, and different types of memory can be affected differently in individuals (Gillen, 2018; Parenté & Herrmann, 2010).

The nature of the deficit depends on the extent and location of cortical and/or subcortical damage (Devinsky & D'Esposito, 2004). Memory loss associated with ABI can significantly affect occupational performance. Deficits in memory processing, storage, and retrieval affect client insight, awareness, and motivation (Lou & Lane, 2005). These deficits can also affect the client's ability to follow a conversation; plan activities; travel independently; recall and initiate the use of compensatory strategies; perform activities of daily living (ADLs); and, ultimately, live an independent life (Makatura et al., 1999).

Orientation

Orientation refers to knowledge about different aspects of self and the environment (mostly temporal and physical) surrounding the self (Dirette & McCormack, 2021). When considering orientation, the areas that are typically assessed include person, place, time, and circumstances. Those who are oriented to person are knowledgeable regarding facts about themselves, such as their name, age, and gender identity (Radomski & Morrison, 2014). Orientation to time includes knowledge of the year, season, month, day of the week, date, and time of day (Figure 7-12). Orientation to place allows people to know where they are, including the country, state, city, and specific location, such as the name of the facility in which they are being treated (Glogoski et al., 2006). Finally, orientation to circumstances enables people to know what has happened to them, such as why they are hospitalized (Radomski & Morrison, 2014).

Individuals who are fully oriented are able to identify and understand aspects of themselves and to situate themselves in relation to time and place within their personal environment (Toglia et al., 2019). This ability depends on the integration of several cognitive abilities that are

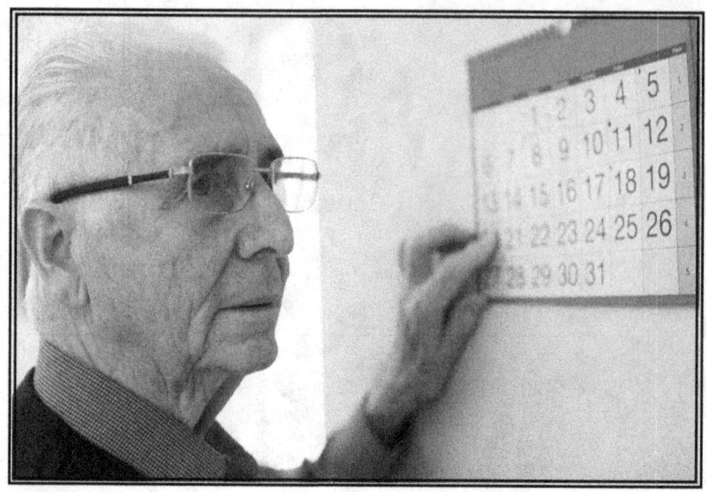

Figure 7-12. Orientation to person, place, time, and circumstances can be disrupted in people with ABI. Orientation to time (e.g., day of the week, date) is often the most significantly disrupted. (Daisy Daisy/shutterstock.com)

represented in different areas of the brain (Toglia et al., 2019). As a result, disorientation is very common after a brain injury (Deitz et al., 1992) and may be caused by different deficits, such as retrograde memory loss or problems with new learning (Sohlberg et al., 2000). For example, disorientation to person results from retrograde memory loss of autobiographical information (Deitz et al., 1992). On the other hand, orientation to date, place, and present circumstances requires the ability to take in, store, and later recall new information (Radomski & Morrison, 2014).

Different aspects of orientation are affected by a brain injury differently. Orientation to time appears to be the most vulnerable to being lost after a brain injury, with orientation to person most resistant to breakdown (Deitz et al., 1992; Radomski & Morrison, 2014). Similarly, the recovery of different aspects of orientation varies. The most common sequence of recovery of orientation after a brain injury is person followed by place and circumstances, with time recovered last (Deitz et al., 1992). Clients with ABI who are disoriented are unsure of time, person, and/or place, which can lead to confusion and agitation. In fact, disorientation has been found to be a key factor in the behavior problems sometimes present in the adult client with ABI (Persel & Persel, 2018). Disorientation can be temporary or long lasting with long-lasting disorientation being a negative prognostic indicator for recovery because it is a barrier to independent living (Deitz et al., 1992).

Executive Function

The term *executive function* refers to a variety of skills that coordinate and control other aspects of cognition, allowing us to complete a number of tasks, including setting and accomplishing goals (Constantinidou & Thomas, 2018; Dirette & McCormack, 2021; Gillen, 2018; Lundy-Ekman, 2018). These skills come into play primarily during nonroutine and/or complex activity. As a result, disorders of executive function are most apparent in novel, complex, and/or unstructured situations (Toglia & Katz, 2018; Toglia et al., 2019). Impairments are sometimes called *dysexecutive syndrome* and are common after ABI (Dorsey et al., 2019; Gillen 2018).

Executive function is conceptualized as a supervisory control system responsible for planning, correcting errors, directing attention, processing information, and inhibiting habitual responses (Gillen, 2021; Toglia et al., 2019). Ylvisaker and Szekeres (1989) described two categories of executive function. The first category is the knowledge base, which is an organized system consisting of general information, learned skills or routines, rules, and procedures. Without this knowledge base, new information is difficult to interpret, organize, and remember. The second category is

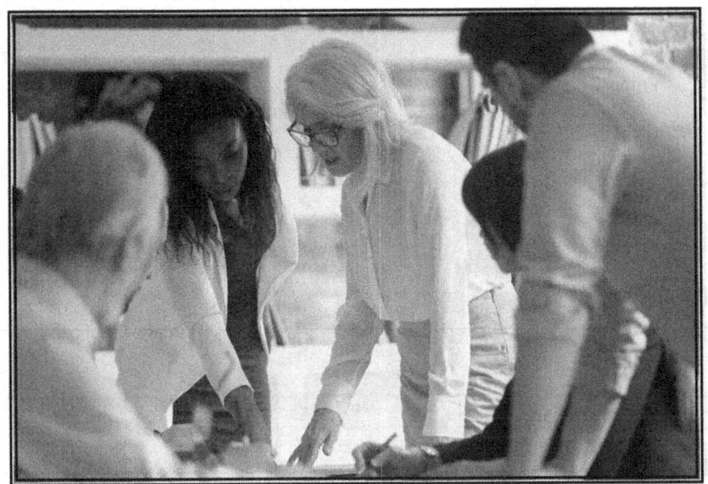

Figure 7-13. Executive function is especially important for novel, dynamic, and complex tasks, including work and IADLs. (fizkes/shutterstock.com)

the executive system, which deals with the mental functions related to setting and achieving goals, creating plans, monitoring the implementation of those plans, making corrections, and problem solving (Ylvisaker & Szekeres, 1989).

Executive function also encompasses metacognition (i.e., people's understanding and manipulation of their own cognitive and perceptual processes; Toglia & Maeir, 2018). The ability to evaluate a task's level of difficulty in relation to one's strengths or weaknesses and predict success is one way that metacognition is demonstrated (Toglia & Maeir, 2018). These self-regulating processes are thought to begin developing during early childhood and are believed to be dependent on the maturation and integrity of the prefrontal cortex. This theory is supported by studies that have examined cognitive changes undergone by adolescents, including during puberty, when the prefrontal cortex undergoes significant changes, into young adulthood with resultant maturation of executive functions and metacognition (Chaku & Hoyt, 2019). In addition to their importance for realistic evaluation of one's own skills and performance, metacognitive abilities have also been viewed as critical components for generalization. People who generalize are able to use the skills and strategies they have learned in numerous contexts rather than solely in the training situation (Josman & Jarus, 2001; Toglia, 2018).

Adequate executive function allows for effective adaptation and accommodation to changing environmental demands. These skills are essential for the successful completion of complex or novel tasks and for those completed in dynamic, changing environments. Examples of instrumental activities of daily living (IADLs) that rely on executive function skills are driving, making a multicourse meal, and organizing a weekly schedule for a busy family of four (Toglia & Katz, 2018; Toglia et al., 2019). In addition to its role in IADLs, executive function is essential for other types of occupation, including social participation and work (Dorsey et al., 2019; Goverover & Hinojosa, 2002; Figure 7-13).

Impaired executive function has mostly been associated with frontal lobe damage, although subcortical structures, including the basal ganglia, are implicated (Constantinidou & Thomas, 2018; Figure 7-14). Neuroimaging studies have shown that the neurological structures that contribute to executive functions are widely distributed rather than in discrete locations in the brain (Ashley et al., 2018). For example, it is believed that different regions within the prefrontal cortex are associated with different aspects of executive functioning (Dirette & McCormack, 2021; Gillen, 2018). This results in different clinical presentation depending on which area of the frontal lobe is damaged. When damage occurs to the dorsolateral prefrontal cortex, people usually present with flat emotion and slowed cognitive and motor processing. In contrast, when damage

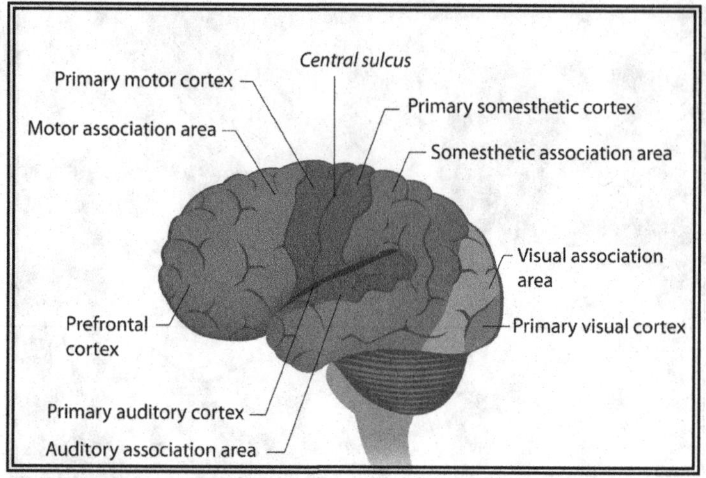

Figure 7-14. Many areas of the brain contribute to executive function, but the prefrontal cortex is especially important. (Alila Medical Media/shutterstock.com)

occurs to the orbitofrontal cortex, individuals usually present with disinhibition, poor judgment, and emotional lability (Schenkman et al., 2013).

It is important to remember that executive dysfunction is a common deficit after ABI even with mild infarcts and that these deficits are often the most persistent of the cognitive impairments that can be observed after ABI (McDonald et al., 2000). Executive dysfunction is also a prognostic indicator for the amount of functional recovery a person may be able to achieve. In a study of 90 people with traumatic brain injury, executive functioning along with memory and premorbid intelligence were predictors of functional dependence after discharge (Hanks et al., 1999). In a sizable study of 7740 people with a cerebrovascular accident, almost half (49.3%) were found to have had a mild stroke. These people were discharged from the hospital with little to no rehabilitation services, but many had executive dysfunction that limited their ability to successfully return to complex activities, such as paid employment. Of those who did return to work, approximately half reported difficulties, such as deficits with organization or inefficiency, which are symptoms of executive dysfunction (Wolf et al., 2009).

Impairment in executive function leads to deficits in initiation, planning and organization, problem solving, mental flexibility, concept formation or abstraction, categorization, decision making, self-error correction, and self-monitoring (Constantinidou & Thomas, 2018; Dirette & McCormack, 2021; Gillen, 2018; Toglia & Katz, 2018, Toglia et al., 2019). Executive dysfunction also often manifests in difficulties with behavioral regulation (Constantinidou & Thomas, 2018). Clients with poor executive function are often impulsive, have tangential conversations, make perseverative comments, and are socially inappropriate. They may not be able to adequately monitor social situations or their relations with others. These clients will often judge their own performance in general or global terms rather than looking specifically and objectively at what they have done. When trying to solve a problem, they will also only consider one possible solution and will fail to consider relevant information in choosing the best solutions. Activities that previously required little or no effort may instead require deliberate control and effort, which results in decreased efficiency (Constantinidou & Thomas, 2018).

Apraxia

Praxis is a complex system that enables people to plan and then perform tasks involving motor actions in a coordinated and effective manner. The motor planning that occurs with praxis allows people to accomplish everyday, simple tasks, such as hair combing, in addition to more complex or extended tasks and routines, such as grooming or dressing (Giovannetti et al., 2002). In order to physically perform tasks such as these, people need to be able to complete two major activities. The first involves conceptualization of the task. This conceptualization allows a plan to be created, which includes steps that need to be followed, the order of the steps, the tools that will be needed to accomplish the task, how those tools should be used, and how the body will need to move to use the tools and complete the activity (Gazzaniga et al., 2019). The second major activity of praxis involves implementation of the plan (Gazzaniga et al., 2019). Praxis is the cognitive skill behind skilled motor function and can occur and affect performance without any impairment in the motor system itself (Gazzaniga et al., 2019).

Roy and Square (1985) explained that praxis is made up of two systems: conceptual and production. The conceptual system incorporates three types of knowledge relative to motor planning: (a) knowledge of the actions and functions of objects and tools; (b) knowledge of movements independent of tools or objects, but into which tools or objects may be incorporated; and (c) knowledge about how to organize single actions into a sequence. These different types of knowledge combine to allow individuals to understand how to use objects or tools for particular activities, in addition to knowing the actions necessary for carrying out these functions (Roy & Square, 1985).

The second system described by Roy and Square (1985) is the production system of motor action. This is thought to consist of different parallel processes that may operate somewhat independently. Control may shift from one level to another with the performance of action dependent on a delicate balance between higher- and lower-level processes. Higher-level processes focus attention on the execution of the planned movement and keep the action sequence directed toward the intended goal. The lower-level system is more autonomous and involves actual execution of the motor plan (Roy & Square, 1985).

Praxis appears to make use of a pathway that starts in the left hemisphere. Motor programs, called *schemas*, are stored in the left parietal lobe (Árnadóttir, 2021). Information from this area of the brain is transmitted to the left premotor cortex and then crosses to the right hemisphere through the corpus callosum if the left side of the body needs to be incorporated into the task execution. This network enables the person to activate the schema and transmit the information to the premotor and then the motor cortices to enable movement to occur in a smooth and bilateral fashion (Árnadóttir, 2021). As a result of the nature of this pathway, damage to the left hemisphere can result in bilateral motor planning deficits rather than deficits that are seen only on the contralesional side (Árnadóttir, 2021; Gazzaniga et al., 2019; Schenkman et al., 2013).

As people grow and develop, they are thought to create many schemas in order to execute movements smoothly and quickly. Anderson and colleagues (1997) defined a schema as the fundamental unit of organized behavior necessary for the performance of everyday actions. Schemas are goal-directed actions that are triggered by situations in the external environment (Anderson et al., 1997). For example, the presence of small portable objects in the environment may trigger the schema for picking up such objects. Schemas may also be triggered by the internal environment (i.e., when a different cognitive process directs an action; Anderson et al., 1997). For example, the desire to place sugar from a sugar bowl into a coffee mug may trigger a schema that allows the person to pick up a teaspoon.

Golisz and Toglia (2003) described many skills associated with praxis separated into two major categories: cognitive formulation of movement intention and knowledge of the functional properties of objects. Cognitive formulation of movement intention requires people to have several skills, including the ability to select a goal, plan movement, and anticipate results of actions. Knowledge of the functional properties of objects requires people to know how to plan and execute actions and action sequences, attend to aspects of the objects, and integrate and interpret tactile-kinesthetic input (e.g., where the body is in space, how the parts of the body relate to each other during movement, and how the body and limbs are positioned) in order to direct movement. In turn, these skills require underlying abilities, including cognitive, language, tactile, visual, kinesthetic, and vestibular processing. For example, vestibular input provides a sense of body position, and language can help the client translate verbal commands into action (Golisz & Toglia, 2003).

ABI can lead to deficits in praxis, which can negatively affect clients' motor planning, thus limiting their ability to perform everyday activities without error (Árnadóttir, 2021; Phipps, 2018; Toglia et al., 2019). This impaired ability is termed *apraxia* and is defined as the inability to perform certain skilled purposeful movements in the absence of motor or sensory deficits. It is a cognitive disorder that involves the loss or impaired ability to program motor systems to perform purposeful skilled movements (Árnadóttir, 2021; Toglia et al., 2019). Apraxia, or motor planning problems, may be subtle or extremely obvious. Depending on the type of apraxia, the client may be unaware of the problem or highly aware and frustrated by it (Sunderland, 2000). Although there may be some spontaneous recovery from apraxia, generally some degree of impairment persists and causes a deficit that interferes with ADLs (Toglia et al., 2019).

Apraxia is commonly observed with aphasia, due to both the language center and motor planning schema being stored in the left hemisphere for most people, but aphasia does occur without apraxia and vice versa (Kobayashi & Ugawa, 2013; Phipps, 2018). Some hypothesize that praxis and language use two different, but partly overlapping, networks (Kobayashi & Ugawa, 2013). At times, aphasia may be confused with apraxia. For example, clients who do not understand verbal instructions because of aphasia may appear to have apraxia when they do not move after being given a command. The opposite may also happen when clients with apraxia are mistakenly thought to have a comprehension deficit when their failure to follow a verbal command is actually the result of an inability to produce the correct movements.

In summary, apraxia may take several different forms, with a breakdown occurring in the conceptual and/or production systems, depending on the location and extent of the damage. The major types of apraxia that may be manifest in the client with ABI include ideomotor and ideational apraxia. The definition of these categories of deficits are described in the following sections.

Ideomotor Apraxia

Ideomotor apraxia, one of the most common and widely studied forms of apraxia, is the inability to imitate gestures or perform a purposeful motor task on command, even though the client fully understands the idea or concept of the task (Árnadóttir, 2021). It happens most commonly after there is damage to the left supramarginal gyrus and the superior parietal lobe, in addition to the superior longitudinal fasciculus (Schenkman et al., 2013). In ideomotor apraxia, the breakdown in motor planning occurs at the execution stage of the activity rather than the conceptualization stage. As a result, clients with ideomotor apraxia often understand what they need to do to complete a motor action (Árnadóttir, 2021). When making errors, they are aware that they are not performing motor tasks accurately but are unable to correct themselves (Schenkman et al., 2013). In addition, these clients, although unable to perform movements on command, often retain kinesthetic memory patterns and, therefore, frequently have the ability to carry out many habitual motor tasks automatically (Phipps, 2018). For example, a client with ideomotor apraxia

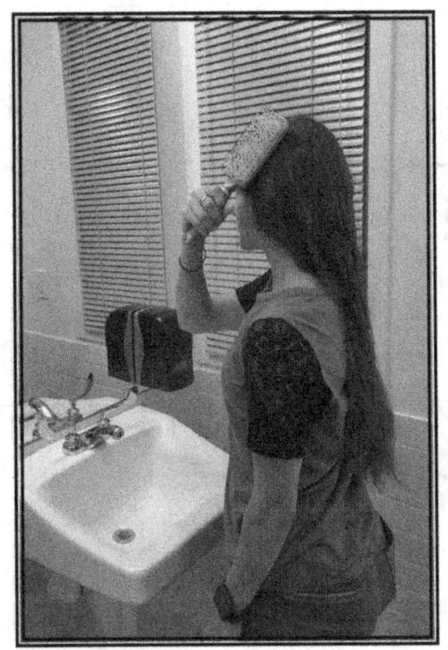

Figure 7-15. One sign of ideomotor apraxia is difficulty in orienting the body correctly for tasks. In this case, the client did not adjust hand position when she stopped brushing the right side of her hair and moved to brush the left side of her hair. As a result, the brush is positioned improperly.

may not be able to follow a series of spoken commands for moving from sitting to standing and require the assistance of two people to move from the bed to a wheelchair. However, the same person might be able to bring their legs up smoothly to rest on a mat table on their own and, when instructed with a more general, automatic command such as, "Let's go," be able to stand up and walk unassisted.

The area of function that is often most affected in ideomotor apraxia is that of pantomime, including when using gestures. These clients are unable to act out a movement without it being a part of a functional activity (Schenkman et al., 2013). For example, when asked to pantomime using a key to unlock a door, people with ideomotor apraxia are unable to simulate the action. However, if given an actual key and a locked door, they are more likely to be able to complete the task (Phipps, 2018). In addition to difficulty with pantomime, these clients also demonstrate impairments in the ability to mimic actions that another demonstrates (Schenkman et al., 2013). Other motor planning errors are also often present in clients with ideomotor apraxia. For example, these clients often display difficulties with the timing of actions. In this case, a client with ideomotor apraxia reaching for a glass of water may close their hand too early, thus knocking over the water rather than grasping the glass. Clients also demonstrate errors in positioning their limbs correctly while completing activities. For example, to brush hair, people need to use different hand and arm positions when brushing the hair on the left versus the right side of their head. People with ideomotor apraxia often demonstrate difficulty with this type of activity and continue to use the same hand and arm position even when they are not effective in completing a task (Figure 7-15). More subtle deficits may be observed as well, usually resulting in a person appearing to be clumsy (Schenkman et al., 2013).

One final consideration when observing a person with ideomotor apraxia is the need for a qualitative analysis of the client's performance. The client with ideomotor apraxia often exhibits common errors in motor performance. These errors may include the following (Árnadóttir, 2021; Golisz & Toglia, 2003):

- Difficulty in interacting with objects accurately in the physical space, as evidenced by errors such as not reaching smoothly and accurately for objects (knowledge of how to use the objects will be intact)
- Errors in positioning limbs in space, including the adjustment of positioning while completing activities

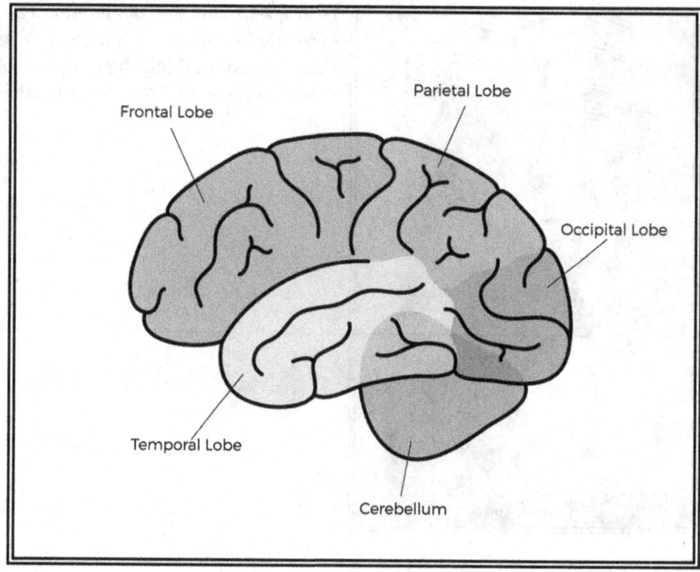

Figure 7-16. Ideational apraxia, when a person has difficulty with the conceptual portion of motor planning, can result from damage to the location where the occipital, parietal, and temporal lobes meet (i.e., the parieto-temporo-occipital junction). (Pikovit/shutterstock.com)

- Clumsy and uncoordinated movement
- Difficulty using gestures, including difficulty with mimicking others' physical actions
- Motor perseveration, which may be observed when a person fails to change from one movement pattern to another (e.g., a person may accurately use a stirring motion to mix sugar into coffee with a spoon and then demonstrate perseveration by continuing to use a stirring motion when attempting to use the spoon to eat oatmeal)
- Timing and/or motor sequencing errors, which may manifest in a number of ways, including grasping or releasing objects too early or late. For example, to successfully mail a letter, a person needs to insert the letter into the mail slot, release the letter, and then withdraw the hand; a person with ideomotor apraxia may instead insert the letter into the mail slot, withdraw the hand, and then release the letter.

Ideational Apraxia

Ideational apraxia is caused by a disruption of the *conception* rather than the *execution* of the motor act (Phipps, 2018). This type of apraxia is more common with a lesion to the left parieto-temporo-occipital junction (Schenkman et al., 2013; Figure 7-16). Unlike people with ideomotor apraxia, people with ideational apraxia do not understand how they are to move and how to interact appropriately with objects in the environment (Figure 7-17). The deficits the client with ideational apraxia display are characterized by a loss of knowledge of tool function, as well as difficulty sequencing actions involving objects (Rumiati et al., 2001). The difficulty with the selection and use of tools and utensils occurs despite normal sensation, motor power, and coordination (Phipps, 2018).

The client with ideational apraxia performs poorly with activities that require a series of movements. These clients are also at a loss when attempting activities that require the use of tools, such as using a screwdriver, unlocking a padlock, or cutting bread with a knife (Phipps, 2018). These clients cannot pretend to perform an act or describe the function of an object. For example, if given a comb and told to comb their hair, the client with ideational apraxia may instead attempt to use the comb to brush their teeth. The client will also be unable to describe the function of the comb.

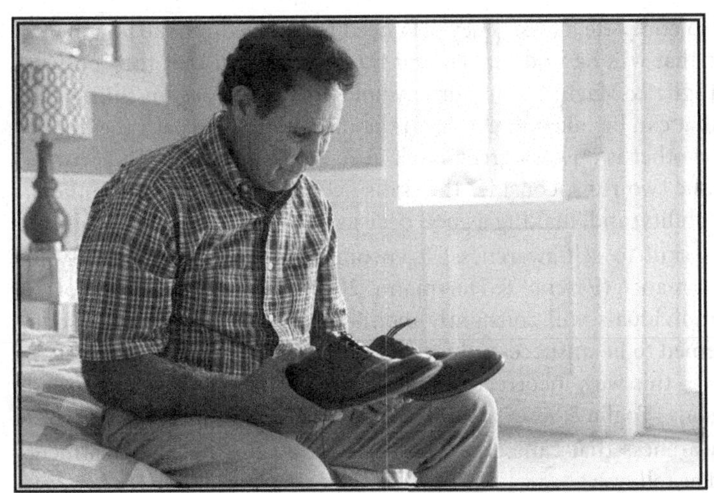

Figure 7-17. Ideational apraxia leads to disruption in conceptualizing how to complete tasks. This can be observed as difficulty with such things as initiating tasks and the appropriate use of items or tools. (Monkey Business Images/shutterstock.com)

Ideational apraxia affects performance bilaterally, resulting in the client making errors with both the ipsilesional and contralesional upper extremity (Schenkman et al., 2013). Common errors that characterize performance include the following (Schenkman et al., 2013):

- Elements of the task occur in the wrong order. For example, the client might put shoes on before putting on socks.
- Sections of the sequence are omitted. For example, the kettle is put on the stove with no water inside.
- Two or more elements may be blended together. For example, the client lifts sugar toward the cup while at the same time making a stirring motion.
- The action remains incomplete. For example, when cutting meat, a client may make a single slice and try to eat a bite even though the meat has not been completely cut.
- The action overshoots what is necessary. For example, rather than pouring a small amount of milk in a cup of tea, the client will fill the whole cup.
- Objects are used inappropriately, either for the context or overall. These errors can also be subtle or more obvious. A more subtle error may be seen if a client uses a related tool rather than an appropriate one. For example, the client may use a fork to eat soup instead of a spoon. In this case, both the fork and the spoon are eating utensils, but the fork is the wrong tool to use for the job of eating soup. A more obvious error is when a tool is used completely inappropriately. For example, a pencil might be used as a comb.
- Movements may be made in the wrong plane or wrong direction. For example, the client might "stir" tea by lifting the spoon up and down or make a pulling-away motion when trying to push in a plug.
- Errors may be perseveratory. For example, after pouring the tea from the pot into the cup, the client might then perform a similar act with the sugar bowl instead of spooning it in.

Awareness and Self-Monitoring

Effective self-awareness and self-monitoring are crucial in everyday life and have been shown to have a strong relationship to functional outcomes (Fisher et al., 2004; Toglia et al., 2019; Toglia & Maeir, 2018). To have effective self-awareness, people need to have the ability to accurately judge the abilities that will be needed to complete a task. They also need to be able to make judgments about the difficulty of the tasks that will be undertaken and the level of skill that they possess (Dirette & McCormack, 2021; Toglia & Maeir, 2018). For example, imagine a person skiing and faced with a choice of ski runs that can be taken to get down the mountain. One path is a highly difficult black diamond run. The other is an easy green circle run. A novice skier with accurate self-awareness is able to look at the two runs, consider the skills needed to safely navigate them, compare those with their skiing ability, and, making a good decision, opt for the green circle run.

Self-monitoring is a related skill to self-awareness. It encompasses individuals' ability to evaluate and regulate their performance (Parenté & Herrmann, 2010). When a plan of action is decided on and implemented, individuals will constantly monitor their performance and outcomes. If the performance is deemed to be unsuccessful for achieving a goal, the plan is adjusted, and a new plan is implemented. In this way, incorrect responses can be identified and corrected in order to achieve the desired goals (Toglia & Maeir, 2018).

There are three types of awareness that can serve as a basis for evaluation and treatment (Gillen, 2021). These are defined as follows:

1. *Intellectual awareness* is the cognitive capacity of the client to understand to some degree that a particular function is diminished from premorbid levels. Clients with intellectual awareness are able to verbally state that there is an issue. For example, a client may articulate that poor memory is a problem. The client may not, however, then recognize how the deficit might impact their future performance or that it is causing them difficulty during task performance.
2. *Emergent awareness* is the ability of clients to recognize a problem when it is actually occurring. These clients are aware of mistakes as they make them.
3. *Anticipatory awareness* refers to the ability to anticipate that a problem is going to happen because of some deficit. In the example of the novice skier described previously, the individual was able to look at the two ski run options, consider their skiing ability, and anticipate that choosing the difficult black diamond run would lead to problems because its challenges exceeded their abilities.

Some degree of intellectual awareness is considered a prerequisite for both emergent and anticipatory awareness (Radomski & Morrison, 2014), although some authors have pointed out that the types of awareness are interrelated but not hierarchical (Toglia & Kirk, 2000). Clients without intellectual awareness are unaware that deficits are present. On the other hand, clients with intellectual awareness but poor emergent awareness can describe their deficits and what should be done, but they cannot compensate when necessary because they do not recognize when problems arise. Clients with intellectual and emergent awareness who lack anticipatory awareness are able to recognize when problems arise but are unable to foresee and avoid issues. The complete understanding of the implications of one's deficits and the ability to take steps to avoid errors or compensate for the lack of skills are dependent on anticipatory awareness (Gillen, 2021).

Golisz and Toglia (2003) observed that clients at the stage of intellectual awareness are a safety risk because they do not perform within their limitations. For example, the clients at this level may realize they have a memory problem but will not make lists or use mnemonics to help them remember (Golisz & Toglia, 2003). Clients with emergent awareness may be a safety risk if they try to perform tasks outside their ability (Burgess & Shallice, 1999). Clients with anticipatory awareness are generally not a safety risk (Golisz & Toglia, 2003).

Deficits with self-awareness are common after ABI, especially when there is damage to the prefrontal cortex (Schenkman et al., 2013). Clients with issues with self-awareness can demonstrate both unawareness of the deficit itself (intellectual awareness) and unawareness of the consequences of the deficit (emergent and/or anticipatory awareness). These types of deficits can cause clients to exhibit poor social judgment and interpersonal awareness, difficulty in anticipating change, and decreased awareness for the consequences of actions (Prigatano, 2008; Toglia et al., 2019).

Clients with moderate to severe ABI often exhibit some degree of decreased awareness of the changes in their physical, cognitive, and behavioral function, resulting in an impaired understanding of their functional disabilities (Toglia & Maeir, 2018). Clients with decreased awareness may be completely unaware of blatant deficits that are obvious to those around them. Some clients deny that they have a problem to the point of becoming defensive, even hostile to those who attempt to point deficits out (Parenté & Herrmann, 2010, Prigatano, 2008). Still others may be indifferent to their limitations (Prigatano, 2008).

As previously described, decreased awareness is an inability to recognize deficits or problem circumstances caused by neurological injury (Gillen, 2021; Toglia et al., 2019). There is a failure to acknowledge impairments of cognitive and/or motor function when questioned. Because clients do not acknowledge or understand impairments, they have little motivation to compensate for them (Toglia et al., 2019; Toglia & Maeir, 2018). As a result, decreased awareness of deficits can have a profound effect on clients' behavior as well as their ability to participate in rehabilitation. In some cases, individuals will not seek out or accept treatment due to the inability to perceive a problem for which treatment is needed (Toglia et al., 2019; Toglia & Maeir, 2018).

Functional implications of decreased awareness include impulsiveness and poor safety awareness. Many studies report that clients consistently over-rate their abilities, which puts them at risk for injury because they may place themselves into situations that have demands that exceed their skills (Abreu et al., 2001). Clients also often have low frustration tolerance, which may result in anger when struggling with tasks. In addition, these clients may have difficulty correcting any errors or mistakes because they are unable to perceive those errors. As previously noted, some clients with emerging awareness of deficits may be able to perceive their errors but are unable to self-correct and regulate the quality of their behavior and performance. This is a deficit of self-monitoring and results in the inability to evaluate and regulate the quality of behavior (Toglia & Maeir, 2018).

Other Influences on Cognition

It is important to remember that people's cognitive skills do not function in isolation. Reasoning, remembering, attending, and all other cognitive skills happen when people are engaging in activities in all types of environments. These environments influence people's cognitive functioning, with busy, loud, and dynamic environments putting a greater demand on a person and making it more difficult for people to function, especially when they have cognitive deficits (American Occupational Therapy Association, 2020; Dirette & McCormack, 2021). As a result, it is essential that occupational therapy practitioners consider the impact of environment when evaluating and treating clients with cognitive impairments (Sbordone, 2001).

In addition to the environment, a person's other abilities, including sensory, perceptual, and motoric, will have an impact on their cognitive functioning (Glogoski et al., 2006). Without accurate sensory and perceptual functioning, a person may misinterpret information in the external world, which can lead to errors in judgment and decision making. For example, imagine Sakura, who has a central scotoma (blind spot) caused by macular degeneration. Her occupational therapy practitioner is having her follow a map to find the gift shop in a hospital. Because of her macular degeneration, Sakura misreads the map and ends up getting lost. The practitioner needs to cue Sakura to help her find her way. Without taking Sakura's visual impairment into account, the practitioner may conclude that Sakura has a cognitive impairment instead of a sensory disorder.

Motoric ability can also influence cognitive functioning because it is important for active exploration. This active exploration allows a person to gather information that is necessary for decision making because it enables them to interact with the environment (Glogoski et al., 2006).

As an example about how motor exploration can facilitate cognitive functioning, imagine completing a 1000-piece jigsaw puzzle without being able to move the pieces. The task would be very difficult to accomplish without being able to manipulate the pieces and rotate them to compare them with open spots in the puzzle and better visualize how the pieces can fit together. Therefore, an accurate understanding of the client's overall functioning is essential for the treating occupational therapy practitioner when conducting cognitive rehabilitation.

Conclusion

Cognitive functioning is complex. Cognitive abilities are reliant on information from other systems, such as sensory input, in addition to being highly interrelated. As a result, cognitive dysfunction can occur after any ABI, even those that appear to be mild. Deficits in cognition can have devastating and lasting consequences to occupational performance. Therefore, it is essential that cognition be evaluated and treated in order to maximize a client's ability to engage in valued occupations. Strategies for evaluating and treating clients with cognitive deficits are considered in the following chapters.

References

Abreu, B. C., Seale, G., Scheibel, R. S., Huddleston, N., Zhang, L., & Ottenbacher, K. J. (2001). Levels of self-awareness after acute brain injury: How patients' and rehabilitation specialists' perceptions compare. *Archives of Physical Medicine and Rehabilitation, 82*, 49-56. https://doi.org/10.1053/apmr.2001.9167

Alexander, M., & Stuss, P. (2000). Disorders of frontal lobe functioning. *Seminars in Neurology, 20*, 427-437. https://doi.org/10.1055/s-2000-13175

American Occupational Therapy Association. (2020). Occupational therapy practice framework: Domain and process (4th ed.). *American Journal of Occupational Therapy, 74*(Suppl. 2), 7412410010. https://doi.org/10.5014/ajot.2020.74S2001

Anderson, R. A., Snyder, L. H., Bradley, D. C., & Xing, J. (1997). Multimodal representation of space in the posterior parietal cortex and its use in planning movements. *Annual Review of Neuroscience, 20*, 303-330. https://doi.org/10.1146/annurev.neuro.20.1.303

Árnadóttir, G. (2021). Impact of neurobehavioral deficits on activities of daily living. In G. Gillen & D. M. Nilsen (Eds.), *Stroke rehabilitation: A function-based approach* (5th ed., pp. 556-592). Elsevier.

Ashley, M. J., Leal, R., Mehta, Z., Ashley, J. G., & Ashley, M. J. (2018). Remediative approaches for cognitive disorders after TBI. In M. J. Ashley & D. A. Hovda (Eds.), *Traumatic brain injury: Rehabilitation, treatment and case management* (4th ed., pp. 487-511). CRC Press.

Burgess, P., & Shallice, T. (1999). Response suppression: Initiation and strategy use following frontal lobe lesions. *Neuropsychologia, 34*, 263-273. https://doi.org/10.1016/0028-3932(95)00104-2

Cansino, S., Maquet, P., Dolan R. J., & Rugg, M. D. (2002). Brain activity underlying encoding and retrieval of source memory. *Cerebral Cortex, 12*, 1048-1056. https://doi.org/10.1093/cercor/12.10.1048

Chaku, N., & Hoyt, L. T. (2019). Developmental trajectories of executive functioning and puberty in boys and girls. *Journal of Youth and Adolescence, 48*, 1365-1378. https://doi.org/10.1007/s10964-019-01021-2

Chan, R. (2000). Attentional deficits in patients with closed head injury: A further study to the discriminative validity of the test of everyday attention. *Brain Injury, 14*, 227-236. https://doi.org/10.1080/026990500120709

Cicerone, K. D. (2002). Remediation of "working attention" in mild traumatic brain injury. *Brain Injury, 16*, 185-195. https://doi.org/10.1080/02699050110103959

Constantinidou, G., & Thomas, R. D. (2018). Principles of cognitive rehabilitation in TBI: An integrative neuroscience approach. In M. J. Ashley & D. A. Hovda (Eds.), *Traumatic brain injury: Rehabilitation, treatment and case management* (4th ed., pp. 513-539). CRC Press.

Craik, F., & Kester, J. D. (2000). Divided attention and memory: Impairment of processing or consolidation? In E. Tulving (Ed.), *Memory, consciousness, and the brain: the Tallinn conference* (pp. 38-51). Psychology Press.

Deitz, J., Tovar, V. S., Beeman, C., Thorn, D. W., & Trevisan, M. S. (1992). The test of orientation for rehabilitation patients: Test-retest reliability. *Journal of Occupational Rehabilitation, 12*, 173-185. https://doi.org/10.1177/153944929201200304

Devinsky, O., & D'Esposito, M. (2004). *Neurology of cognitive and behavioral disorders*. Oxford University Press.

Dirette, D. P., & McCormack, G. L. (2021). Cognitive assessment. In D. P. Dirette & S. A. Gutman (Eds.), *Occupational therapy for physical dysfunction* (8th ed., pp. 143-160). Wolters Kluwer.

Dorsey, J., Ehrenfried, H., Finch, D., & Jaegers, L. A. (2019). Work. In B. A. B. Schell & G. Gillen (Eds.), *Willard and Spackman's occupational therapy* (13th ed., pp. 779-804). Wolters Kluwer.

Eriksson, J., Vogel, E. K., Lansner, A., Bergström, F., & Nyberg, L. (2015). Neurocognitive architecture of working memory. *Neuron, 88*, 33-46. https://doi.org/10.1016/j.neuron.2015.09.020

Fisher, S., Gauggel, S., & Trexler, L. E. (2004). Awareness of activity limitations, goal setting and rehabilitation outcome in patients with brain injuries. *Brain Injury, 18*, 547-562. https://doi.org/10.1080/02699050310001645793

Fletcher, P. C., & Henson, R. N. A. (2001). Frontal lobes and human memory: Insights from functional neuroimaging. *Brain, 124*, 849-881. https://doi.org/10.1093/brain/124.5.849

Forde, E. M. E., & Humphries, G. W. (2000). The role of semantic knowledge and working memory in everyday tasks. *Brain and Cognition, 44*, 214-252. https://doi.org/10.1006/brcg.2000.1229

Fuster, J. M. (1998). Network memory. *Annual Review of Psychology, 49*, 451-459. https://doi.org/10.1016/S0166-2236(97)01128-4

Garcia-Rill, E. (2009). Reticular activating system. In L. R. Squire (Ed.), *Encyclopedia of neuroscience* (pp. 137-143). Elsevier.

Gazzaniga, M. S., Ivry, R. B., & Mangun, G. R. (2019). *Cognitive neuroscience: The biology of the mind* (5th ed.). W. W. Norton & Company.

Gillen, G. (2018). Evaluation and treatment of limited occupational performance secondary to cognitive dysfunction. In H. M. Pendleton & W. Schultz-Krohn (Eds.), *Pedretti's occupational therapy: Practice skills for physical dysfunction* (8th ed., pp. 645-668). Elsevier.

Gillen, G. (2021). Treatment of cognitive-perceptual deficits: A function-based approach. In G. Gillen & D. M. Nilsen (Eds.), *Stroke rehabilitation: A function-based approach* (5th ed., pp. 593-626). Elsevier.

Giovannetti, T., Libon, J. J., Buxbaum, L. J., & Schwartz, M. F. (2002). Naturalistic action impairments in dementia. *Neuropsychologia, 40*, 1220-1232. https://doi.org/10.1016/S0028-3932(01)00229-9

Glogoski C., Milligan N., & Wheatley, C., (2006). Evaluation and treatment of cognitive dysfunction. In H. M. Pendleton & W. Schultz-Krohn (Eds.), *Pedretti's occupational therapy: Practice skills for physical dysfunction* (6th ed., pp. 598-608). Mosby Elsevier.

Golisz, K., & Toglia, J. (2003). Perception and cognition. In E. Crepeau, E. S. Cohn, & B. A. B. Schell (Eds.), *Willard and Spackman's occupational therapy* (10th ed., 395-416). Lippincott, Williams and Wilkins.

Goverover, Y., & Hinojosa, J. (2002). Categorization and deductive reasoning: Predictors of instrumental activities of daily living performance in adults with brain injury. *American Journal of Occupational Therapy, 56*, 509-515. https://doi.org/10.5014/ajot.56.5.509

Hanks, A., Rapport, L. J., Millis, S. R., & Deshpande, S. A. (1999). Measures of executive functioning as predictors of functional ability and social integration in a rehabilitation sample. *Archives of Physical Medicine and Rehabilitation, 80*, 1030-1037. https://doi.org/10.1016/S0003-9993(99)90056-4

Heilman, K. M., Valenstein, E., & Watson, R. T. (2000). Neglect and related disorders. *Seminars in Neurology, 20*, 463-469. https://doi.org/10.1055/s-2000-13179

Josman, N., & Jarus, T. (2001). Construct-related validity of the Toglia Category Assessment and the Deductive Reasoning test with children who are typically developing. *American Journal of Occupational Therapy, 55*, 524-530. https://doi.org/10.5014/ajot.55.5.524

Kapur, N. (1999). Syndromes of retrograde amnesia: A conceptual and empirical synthesis. *Psychological Bulletin, 125*, 800-825. https://doi.org/10.1037/0033-2909.125.6.800

Klein, S. B., Loftus, J., & Kihlstrom, J. F. (2002). Memory and temporal experience: The effects of episodic memory loss on an amnesic patient's ability to remember the past and imagine the future. *Social Cognition, 20*, 353-379. https://doi.org/10.1521/soco.20.5.353.21125

Krellman, J. W., Tsaousides, T., & Gordon, W. A. (2018). Neuropsychological interventions following traumatic brain injury. In M. J. Ashley & D. A. Hovda (Eds.), *Traumatic brain injury: Rehabilitation, treatment and case management* (4th ed., pp. 393-409). CRC Press.

Kobayashi, S. & Ugawa, Y. (2013). Relationships between aphasia and apraxia. *Journal of Neurology & Translational Neuroscience, 2*, 1028.

Levy, L. L. (2018). Cognitive information-processing memory. In N. Katz & J. Toglia (Eds.), *Cognition, occupation, and participation across the lifespan* (4th ed., pp. 105-127). AOTA Press.

Lou, J., & Lane, S. (2005). Personal performance capabilities and their impact on occupational performance. In C. Christiansen & C. Baum (Eds.), *Occupational therapy: Performance, participation, and well-being* (3rd ed., pp. 270-296). SLACK Incorporated.

Lundy-Ekman, L. (2018). *Neuroscience: Fundamentals for rehabilitation* (5th ed.). Elsevier.

Maeir, A., & Rotenberg-Shpigelman, S. (2015). Person factors: Cognition. In C. H. Christiansen, C. M. Baum, & J. D. Bass (Eds.), *Occupational therapy performance, participation, and well-being* (4th ed., pp. 233-247). SLACK Incorporated.

Makatura, T. J., Lam, C. S., Leahy, B. J., Castillo, M. T., & Kalpakjian, C. Z. (1999). Standardized memory tests and the appraisal of everyday memory. *Brain Injury, 13*, 355-367. https://doi.org/10.1080/026990599121548

Manly, T., Hawkins, K., Evans, J., Woldt, K., & Robertson, I. H. (2002). Rehabilitation of executive function: Facilitation of effective goal management on complex tasks using periodic auditory alerts. *Neuropsychologia, 40*, 271-281. https://doi.org/10.1016/S0028-3932(01)00094-X

Markowitsch, H. J., Calabrese, P., Neufeld, H., Gehlen, W., & Durwen, H. F. (1999). Retrograde amnesia for world knowledge and preserved memory for autobiographical events. A case report. *Cortex, 35*, 243-252. https://doi.org/10.1016/S0010-9452(08)70797-4

Mateer, C. A. (2000). Attention. In S. A. Raskin, & C. A. Mateer (Eds.), *Neuropsychological management of mild traumatic brain injury* (pp. 73-92). Oxford University Press.

McAllister, T. W., Saykin, A. J., Flashman, L. A., Sparling, M. B., Johnson, S. C., Guerin, S. J., Mamourian, A. C., Weaver, J. B., & Yanofsky, N. (1999). Brain activation during working memory 1 month after mild traumatic brain injury: A functional MRI study. *Neurology, 53*, 1300-1308. https://doi.org/10.1212/WNL.53.6.1300

McDaniel, M. A., Glisky, E. L., Rubin, S. R., Guynn, M. J., & Routhieaux, B. C. (1999). Prospective memory: A neuropsychological study. *Neuropsychology, 13*, 103-110. https://doi.org/10.1037/0894-4105.13.1.103

McDonald, B. C., Flashman, L. A., & Saykin, A. J. (2000). Executive dysfunction following traumatic brain injury: Neural substrates and treatment strategies. *Neurorehabilitation, 17*, 333-344. https://doi.org/10.3233/NRE-2002-17407

Mellon, L., Brewer, L., Hall, P., Horgan, F., Williams, D., & Hickey, A. (2015). Cognitive impairment six months after ischaemic stroke: A profile from the ASPIRE-S study. *BMC Neurology, 15*, 31. https://doi.org/10.1186/s12883-015-0288-2

Nieber, E., & Koch, C. (2000). Computational architectures for attention. In R. Parasuraman (Ed.), *The attentive brain* (pp. 163-186). MIT Press.

Parenté, R., & Herrmann. D. (2010). *Retraining cognition: Techniques and applications* (3rd ed.). PRO-ED Inc.

Parker, R. S. (2012). *Concussive brain trauma: Neurobehavioral impairment and maladaptation* (2nd ed.). CRC Press.

Persel, C. S., & Persel, C. H. (2018). The use of applied behavior analysis in traumatic brain injury rehabilitation. In M. J. Ashley & D. A. Hovda (Eds.), *Traumatic brain injury: Rehabilitation, treatment and case management* (4th ed., pp. 411-450). CRC Press.

Phipps, S. (2018). Evaluation and intervention for perception dysfunction. In H. M. Pendleton & W. Schultz-Krohn (Eds.), *Pedretti's occupational therapy: Practice skills for physical dysfunction* (8th ed., pp. 631-644). Elsevier.

Prigatano, G. P. (2008). Anosognosia and the process and outcome of neurorehabilitation. In D. T. Stuss, G. Winocur, & I. H. Robertson (Eds.), *Cognitive neurorehabilitation: Evidence and application* (2nd ed., pp. 218-231). Cambridge University Press.

Radomski, M. V., & Morrison, M. T. (2014). Assessing abilities and capacities: Cognition. In M. V. Radomski & C. A. Trombly Latham (Eds.), *Occupational therapy for physical dysfunction* (7th ed., pp. 121-143). Lippincott Williams & Wilkins.

Roy, E. A., & Square, P. A. (1985). Common considerations in the study of limb, verbal and oral apraxia. In E. A. Roy (Ed.), *Neuropsychological studies of apraxia and related disorders* (pp. 111-164). North-Holland.

Rumiati, R., Zanini, S., Vorano, L., & Shallice, T. (2001). A form of ideational apraxia as a selective deficit of contention scheduling. *Cognitive Neuropsychology, 18*, 617-642. https://doi.org/10.1080/02643290126375

Sbordone, R. J. (2001). Limitations of neuropsychological testing to predict the cognitive and behavioral functioning of persons with brain injury in real-world settings. *NeuroRehabilitation, 16*, 199-201. https://doi.org/10.3233/NRE-2001-16402

Schenkman, M. L., Bowman, J. P., Gisbert, R. L., & Butler, R. B. (2013). *Clinical neuroscience for rehabilitation*. Pearson.

Sohlberg, M. M., & Mateer, C. A. (2001). *Cognitive rehabilitation: An integrative neuropsychological approach*. The Guilford Press.

Sohlberg, M. M., McLaughlin, K. A., Pavese, A., Heidrich, A., & Posner, M. I. (2000). Evaluation of attention process training and brain injury education in persons with acquired brain injury. *Journal of Clinical and Experimental Neuropsychology, 22*, 656-676. https://doi.org/10.1076/1380-3395(200010)22:5;1-9;FT656

Stuss, D. T., & Alexander, M. P. (2000). Executive functions and the frontal lobes: A conceptual view. *Psychological Research, 63*, 289-298. https://doi.org/10.1007/s004269900007

Sunderland, A. (2000). Recovery of ipsilateral dexterity after stroke. *Stroke, 31*, 430-433. https://doi.org/10.1161/01.STR.31.2.430

Toglia, J. (1993). *Contextual Memory Test.* Therapy Skill Builders.

Toglia, J. (2018). The dynamic interactional model and the multicontext approach. In N. Katz & J. Toglia (Eds.), *Cognition, occupation, and participation across the lifespan* (4th ed., pp. 355-385). AOTA Press.

Toglia, J. P., Golisz, K. M., & Goverover, Y. (2019). Cognition, perception, and occupational performance. In B. A. B. Schell & G. Gillen (Eds.), *Willard and Spackman's occupational therapy* (13th ed., pp. 901-941). Wolters Kluwer.

Toglia, J., & Katz, N. (2018). Executive functioning: Prevention and health promotion for at-risk populations and those with chronic disease. In N. Katz & J. Toglia (Eds.), *Cognition, occupation, and participation across the lifespan* (4th ed., pp. 129-141). AOTA Press.

Toglia, J., & Kirk, U. (2000). Understanding awareness deficits following brain injury. *NeuroRehabilitation, 15*, 57-70. https://doi.org/10.3233/NRE-2000-15104

Toglia, J., & Maeir, A. (2018). Self-awareness and metacognition: Effect on occupational performance and outcome across the lifespan. In N. Katz & J. Toglia (Eds.), *Cognition, occupation, and participation across the lifespan* (4th ed., pp. 143-163). AOTA Press.

Wolf, T. J., Baum, C., & Connor, L. T. (2009). Changing face of stroke: Implications for occupational therapy practice. *American Journal of Occupational Therapy, 63*, 621-625. https://doi.org/10.5014/ajot.63.5.621

Ylvisaker, M., & Szekeres, S. F. (1989). Metacognitive and executive impairment in head-injured children and adults. *Topics in Language Disorders, 9*, 34-49. https://doi.org/10.1097/00011363-198903000-00005

CHAPTER 8

Cognitive Assessment

As stated in Chapter 7, cognition is complex, made up of many different skills, such as memory, attention, problem solving, and executive functioning. It is also influenced by a variety of factors, including sensation, perception, emotional state, activity demands, and environmental influences (Dirette & McCormack, 2021; Maskill & Tempest, 2017a; Toglia, 2018). Unlike physical deficits, impairments in cognition, especially mild ones, are often difficult to detect, with assumptions made that people living with these deficits are more capable and independent than they actually are (Grieve & Gnanasekaran, 2008). In these cases, people may be discharged from rehabilitation too early, if they are ever referred for rehabilitation at all. The result is that people may function well in controlled environments with established routines, such as at home while doing their basic self-care, but struggle in complex and dynamic environments, including many work settings or with complex instrumental activities of daily living (IADLs). Cognitive impairment may also be misunderstood and mislabeled (Grieve & Gnanasekaran, 2008). People may incorrectly be seen as having behavioral issues and perceived as unmotivated, uncooperative, or, in some instances, as not giving full effort for some type of secondary gain, such as a pending financial settlement.

Cognitive impairment, even when mild, can lead to difficulties in organizing and processing incoming information. People can also have difficulty in using prior experience and knowledge in informing their decision making in the present. They may have poor insight into their cognitive functioning, which leads to overestimation of their abilities. When people do not have an accurate understanding of their abilities, they are less able to accurately predict when problems are likely to arise. They may not monitor their performance very well, failing to recognize when their plans are not working as anticipated. They are also less likely to use strategies to compensate for cognitive limitations because they do not understand why the strategies are necessary (Toglia, 2018).

All of these issues can have a devastating impact on independent living, especially when activities with higher cognitive demands, such as work and complex IADLs, need to be completed (Toglia, 2018). As a result, careful evaluation and treatment in the area of functional cognition are essential parts of occupational therapy practice (American Occupational Therapy Association [AOTA], 2019).

Kaminsky, T. A., & Powell, J. M.
Zoltan's Vision, Perception, and Cognition: Evaluation and Treatment of the Adult With Acquired Brain Injury, Fifth Edition (pp. 203-236).

As described in Chapter 2, occupational therapy practitioners are members of interdisciplinary teams that work together to treat clients, including those with cognitive and/or perceptual deficits after acquired brain injury (ABI). Other members of the team who regularly evaluate and treat clients with these deficits are speech-language pathologists and neuropsychologists. In order to gain a complete understanding of the client's deficits and how they impact functioning, in addition to avoiding duplicating services, it is important for the members of the team to coordinate, communicate, and focus their expertise on the unique characteristics of their professions (Miller et al., 2010). For occupational therapy practitioners, this means that our attention should be directed to the area of functional cognition. Giles and colleagues (2017) defined functional cognition as "the ability to use and integrate thinking and performance skills to accomplish complex everyday activities" (p. 1). Therefore, when evaluating clients with cognitive deficits after ABI, occupational therapy practitioners should attend to how cognitive functioning is specifically affecting people's ability to engage in occupation (AOTA, 2019; Giles et al., 2017).

This chapter discusses some of the main principles to consider with cognitive rehabilitation and reviews common cognitive evaluation strategies and tools used by occupational therapy practitioners. Subsequent chapters consider the specific treatment techniques for people with cognitive impairment after ABI.

Influences on Cognitive Rehabilitation

Cognitive rehabilitation involves treatment that is focused on lessening the impact of cognitive deficits to improve safety, functioning, independence, and quality of life (Haskins, 2012). As stated previously, a variety of professionals may be involved in assessing and treating the cognitive functioning of clients, including neuropsychologists, speech-language pathologists, and occupational therapy practitioners. (See Chapter 2 for further discussion of working with an interdisciplinary team.) There are a number of approaches for cognitive rehabilitation, which are discussed further in Chapters 9 and 10. Decisions about appropriate evaluation and treatment depend on a variety of factors, including the person's goals and prior abilities, caregiver concerns, the health and safety of the client, where the client is in recovery, current functioning, insight and awareness, and the type of setting (Haskins, 2012; Maskill & Tempest, 2017a).

A person's goals should always drive therapy so that treatment is targeted at what is most meaningful and relevant to that person. (The impact of decreased insight and awareness on setting goals is discussed later in this chapter.) A thorough and complete occupational profile is invaluable in helping to determine those goals (Erez & Katz, 2018). In turn, the goals will help clinicians decide on the skills that a person needs to resume prior occupations. It is also important to learn about the cultural influences that surround the person, including what the person's role was before ABI and the roles that the person will be expected to fill after discharge (Sohlberg & Turkstra, 2011). To illustrate this, let us consider two examples of clients who are being treated by occupational therapy practitioners.

Mr. Sanchez is an 82-year-old man recovering from a stroke. He is retired and lives with his adult daughter, who is a stay-at-home mother, and her family. He has a bedroom on the main floor of the house. Before his stroke, he was independent with his basic activities of daily living (ADLs), including bathing, dressing, toileting, and grooming. His daughter took care of the cooking, cleaning, grocery shopping, and other home management tasks. Mr. Sanchez was not driving any longer; he got rides from his daughter or a friend when he went out. He filled his days with quiet activities at home, including completing the crossword in the newspaper each day, watching television, going for walks in the neighborhood, and gardening. Twice each week he met friends for lunch and cards at the senior center. He also enjoyed playing board games with his teenage grandchildren.

Ms. Lin is a 45-year-old woman recovering from traumatic brain injury (TBI). Before her injury, she worked full time as a high school math teacher. She is a single mother to two children ages 10 and 13. She has primary custody of her children, and they live with her, except for every other weekend when they stay with their father. She lives in a three-story townhouse with her children. Before her injury, she was responsible for all of the household tasks, including pet care (she has two dogs), home maintenance, financial management, cooking, and cleaning. She also had child care responsibilities. She drove independently and was responsible for transporting her children to after-school activities. She had an active lifestyle, including jogging with her dogs, hiking with her children, spending time with friends, and dating.

These brief occupational profiles illustrate that the responsibilities of each of these individuals are very different. As a result, the skills that each need to return to their prior occupations are also very different. Mr. Sanchez's lifestyle places fewer demands on his cognitive functioning because his activities are regular and predictable. In contrast, Ms. Lin's lifestyle requires high levels of cognitive abilities. Many of her occupations take place in unpredictable and dynamic environments, and she needs to be able to manage many complex activities, sometimes simultaneously. The rehabilitation process for these people will need to be individualized for them, with different strategies and techniques that are most appropriate to each.

In addition to the client's goals and prior level of functioning, the concerns and abilities of caregivers need to be considered. Their availability (including where they live in relation to the client), their abilities, and their desires will all influence the skills that a person needs when returning to the community (Haskins, 2012). Regarding the examples provided earlier, Mr. Sanchez lives with his adult daughter, and she stays at home during the day. She is already completing many activities for Mr. Sanchez and is likely willing and able to assist more if needed. In contrast, Ms. Lin lives with her children, who are too young to be primary caregivers. If she needs a caregiver, arrangements would need to be made with another family member, a friend, or a paid caregiver, and the availability, willingness, and skills of those caregivers are uncertain. Included in the decision making about caregiver responsibilities is the consideration of ways to reduce the likelihood of caregiver burnout and stress. Inclusion of the caregiver early in the rehabilitation process is essential in order to make decisions about what caregivers are and are not able to manage (Haskins, 2012). A further discussion of caregiver training is included in Chapter 9.

The client's health and safety are always important to consider with any type of treatment, and cognitive rehabilitation is no exception (Maskill & Tempest, 2017b). When cognitive deficits are present, people may be at risk for injury for a variety of reasons. Judgment and safety awareness are often impaired, and clients may present with other symptoms, such as impulsivity. It is essential for treating occupational therapy practitioners to keep client safety at the forefront of their minds, although the way that client safety is addressed may vary based on factors such as the client's current level of functioning (Grieve & Gnanasekaran, 2008). For example, a client with more severe deficits and significantly impaired judgment may require extensive environmental modification, including the use of bed alarms, secured cabinets and drawers for the storage of potentially dangerous items (e.g., medication, knives), and 24-hour supervision. Clients with mild deficits who have slight memory loss may benefit from different types of environmental modification or cognitive strategies, such as an alarm to signal when medications should be taken and a log to record which medications were taken and when.

A highly important factor to consider when making decisions about appropriate evaluation and treatment strategies is the level of insight clients have into their strengths and limitations (Haskins, 2012; Toglia, 2018). Clients with little to no awareness of their strengths and limitations will be unable to accurately assess their needs, which will impact their ability to help set reasonable and realistic goals (Haskins, 2012). A lack of insight will also negatively impact some types of treatment (Toglia, 2018). For example, the use of metacognitive strategies (discussed in

Chapter 10) requires significant practice in a variety of situations, especially when working toward generalization (i.e., when the client is able to independently use strategies in numerous contexts). Clients without insight into their deficits will be less likely to see the need for the strategies and, in turn, less likely to practice those strategies. For those clients without insight into the nature of their deficits, it is important to start by building awareness and/or use treatment techniques that are less reliant on the client having insight into deficits (Toglia, 2018). Treatment techniques such as environmental modification and errorless learning may be more appropriate for these clients than metacognitive strategy training (Haskins, 2012). It is also important to remember that insight often develops over time. In the initial days after ABI, clients may not be aware of cognitive deficits, especially if those deficits are milder. Upon returning home and attempting to resume prior roles, clients may begin to realize that they do not have the skills they need to fully engage in their desired occupations (Toglia, 2018).

Finally, decisions about the approach to cognitive rehabilitation will be influenced by the type of setting because that will affect the resources that are available as well as the types of occupations that are most easily and realistically addressed (Grieve & Gnanasekaran, 2008; Maskill & Tempest, 2017b). For example, taking clients into the community is not the focus, nor is it feasible, for clinicians who work in an acute setting. Instead, the focus of acute treatment is on stabilizing clients and discharging them to a lesser level of care (e.g., home, inpatient rehabilitation, skilled nursing). In acute care settings, the focus is often on assessing independence with ADLs and determining what level of care and rehabilitation is needed after the person is medically stabilized and ready to be discharged from the acute care environment. On the other hand, practitioners working in an outpatient setting are much better able to focus treatment on community reintegration and to consider occupations such as IADLs and work.

Evaluation in Cognitive Rehabilitation

The evaluation of clients is essential in order to understand their current level of functioning and their strengths and deficits and to guide treatment decisions. Evaluation also enables practitioners to determine a client's baseline level of functioning and show progress over time (Haskins, 2012; Radomski & Morrison, 2014). The typical evaluation process includes several steps. The first involves gathering information before meeting the client. During this first step, the practitioner reviews the client's medical record and may speak to other team members who have already met with or who previously worked with the client. If possible, the occupational therapy practitioner should gather information about the client's primary language, communication abilities, education level, and medical issues (Maskill & Tempest, 2017a; Radomski & Morrison, 2014). The next step involves interviewing the client and caregivers, as appropriate and applicable, to begin to create an occupational profile and gain information about the client's goals and understanding of deficits. An instrument such as the Canadian Occupational Performance Measure can be invaluable during this portion of the evaluation in targeting areas of concern and creating client-centered goals, although it does require people to have an accurate understanding of their needs and abilities (Katz et al., 2011; Radomski & Morrison, 2014). The third step in the process is to select and administer assessments. There are numerous evaluation tools that occupational therapy practitioners can use with clients with suspected cognitive deficits. Some of these tools consider clients' occupational performance as a whole, whereas others focus on specific impairments. Both types of assessments can provide useful information to guide treatment (Dirette & McCormack, 2021; Erez & Katz, 2018).

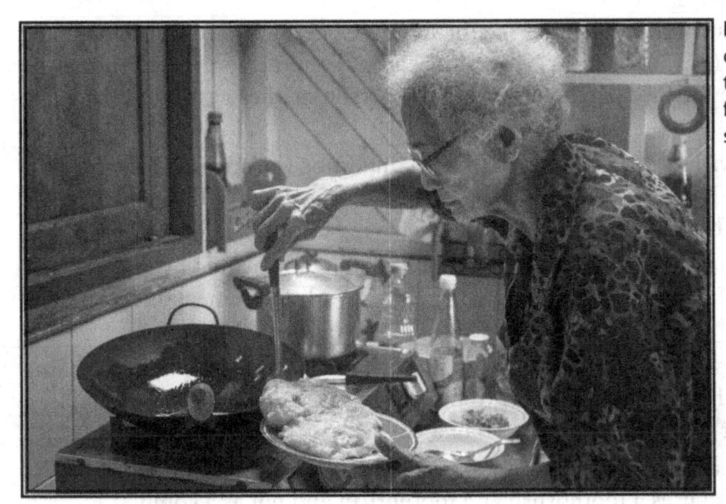

Figure 8-1. Non-standardized skilled observation of occupation can assist the clinician in seeing cognitive functioning in context. (CGN089/ shutterstock.com)

Beginning the evaluation process with a top-down approach by first considering occupational performance allows the evaluating occupational therapy practitioner to consider the client's functioning in context, enabling factors such as the impact of environmental considerations to be better identified (Weinstock-Zlotnick & Hinojosa, 2004). It is also rare for clients to have only one type of cognitive deficit. The evaluation of occupational engagement in context (i.e., functional cognition) can allow the client's cognitive functioning as a whole to be seen more easily (AOTA, 2019; Giles et al., 2017; Toglia, 2018). For example, consider a client who is preparing omelets, toast, and bacon for two people. The client is asked to prepare the meal and serve it along with beverages at a table (Figure 8-1). Numerous cognitive skills, in addition to sensory and motoric ones, are needed to successfully complete this activity within a reasonable time frame. The observation of a client completing the task enables the practitioner to consider a number of the client's abilities at once, including various types of attention, memory, problem solving, and executive functioning, and the interaction of different abilities during task performance. It also allows for the observation and identification of compensatory strategies that the client may be using. This type of assessment can be more informative than evaluation of individual skills in tabletop tasks on determining the functional impact of cognitive deficits (AOTA, 2019; Fisher & Jones, 2011; Giles et al., 2017).

Non-Standardized Skilled Observation

Non-standardized skilled observation of clients completing tasks is one of the primary means by which occupational therapy practitioners can evaluate clients' occupational performance, including determining how cognitive deficits are impacting function (Maskill & Tempest, 2017a; Radomski & Morrison, 2014). Making observations of cognitive impairment, especially more subtle deficits, during functional activities can be challenging. It is helpful if clinicians have guidance as they evaluate clients completing occupations. The fourth edition of the *Occupational Therapy Practice Framework: Domain and Process* (*OTPF-4*; AOTA, 2020) can assist in a thorough consideration of the cognitive skills that are necessary to complete functional activities. Especially important for cognition are process skills, a subset of performance skills, although it is important to remember that impairments in cognition can affect motor skills as well (AOTA, 2020). Making observations about a client's performance skills can inform the clinician about cognitive strengths and deficits and how those are influencing occupational engagement. Twenty process skills are included in the *OTPF-4* (AOTA, 2020), which were originally described in the Assessment of Motor and Process Skills (AMPS; Fisher & Jones, 2011).

1. "*Paces*: Maintains a consistent and effective rate or tempo of performance throughout the entire task performance" (AOTA, 2020, p. 45). For example, the person's pace should be consistent and appropriate for the specific task (e.g., the person neither rushes nor takes an extraordinarily long time).
2. "*Attends*: Does not look away from task performance, maintaining the ongoing task progression" (AOTA, 2020, p. 45). For example, the person is able to wipe down a dining room table without getting distracted by other household members having a conversation.
3. "*Heeds*: Carries out and completes the task originally agreed on or specified by another person" (AOTA, 2020, p. 45). For example, a person completes a work assignment as directed by their supervisor.
4. "*Chooses*: Selects necessary and appropriate type and number of objects for the task, including the task objects that one chooses or is directed to use" (AOTA, 2020, p. 45). For example, a person selecting a hammer to pound nails instead of a wrench.
5. "*Uses*: Applies task objects as they are intended . . . and in a hygienic manner" (AOTA, 2020, p. 45). For example, a person uses a toothbrush as a toothbrush and not as a comb.
6. "*Handles*: Supports or stabilizes task objects appropriately, protecting them from being damaged, slipping, moving, or falling" (AOTA, 2020, p. 45) For example, a person supports a full dustpan as it is being transported to the trash can so that the contents do not spill.
7. "*Inquires*: (1) Seeks needed verbal or written information by asking questions or reading directions or labels and (2) does not ask for information when fully oriented to the task and environment and recently aware of the answer" (AOTA, 2020, p. 45). For example, a person refers to the instructions on a box of cake mix to successfully make cupcakes.
8. "*Initiates*: Starts or begins the next task action or task step without any hesitation" (AOTA, 2020, p. 45). For example, a person follows their morning routine and puts clothing on after bathing without prompting.
9. "*Continues*: Performs single actions or steps without any interruptions so that once an action or task step is initiated, performance continues without pauses or delays until the action or step is completed" (AOTA, 2020, p. 45). For example, a person vacuums a living room carpet without stopping, such as to recall the next step of the task.
10. "*Sequences*: Performs steps in an effective or logical order and with an absence of randomness in the ordering or inappropriate repetition of steps" (AOTA, 2020, p. 46). For example, a person puts socks on before attempting to don shoes.
11. "*Terminates*: Brings to completion single actions or single steps without inappropriate persistence or premature cessation" (AOTA, 2020, p. 46). For example, a person spreads butter over an entire slice of toast rather than only in the middle.
12. "*Searches/locates*: Looks for and locates task objects in a logical manner" (AOTA, 2020, p. 46). For example, a person looks for a pair of shoes in a closet and not in the refrigerator.
13. "*Gathers*: Collects related task objects into the same work space and regathers task objects that have spilled, fallen, or been misplaced" (AOTA, 2020, p. 46). For example, a person who is making breakfast retrieves both milk and orange juice from the refrigerator and takes them to the same part of the kitchen rather than needing to repeat trips or placing items haphazardly.
14. "*Organizes*: Logically positions or spatially arranges task objects in an orderly fashion within a single work space or between multiple appropriate work spaces such that the work space is not too spread out or too crowded" (AOTA, 2020, p. 46). For example, a person places tools needed for a woodworking task within easy reach while maintaining a clear area for working.
15. "*Restores*: Puts away task objects in appropriate places and ensures that the immediate work space is restored to its original condition" (AOTA, 2020, p. 46). For example, a person returns scissors to a drawer after using them to cut wrapping paper.

16. "*Navigates*: Moves body or wheelchair without bumping into obstacles when moving through the task environment or interacting with task objects" (AOTA, 2020, p. 46). For example, a person avoids bumping into doorways and the edges of furniture while cleaning.
17. "*Notices/responds*: Responds appropriately to (1) nonverbal task-related cues (e.g., heat, movement), (2) the spatial arrangement and alignment of task objects to one another, and (3) cupboard doors or drawers that have been left open during task performance" (AOTA, 2020, p. 46). For example, a person closes a cupboard door that was left open.
18. "*Adjusts*: Overcomes problems with on-going task performance effectively by (1) going to a new workspace; (2) moving task objects out of the current workspace; or (3) adjusting knobs, dials, switches, or water taps" (AOTA, 2020, p. 46). For example, a person recognizes that the stove is too hot and that a pot of soup is in danger of boiling over, so they lower the heat on the burner.
19. "*Accommodates*: Prevents ineffective performance of all other motor and process skills and asks for assistance only when appropriate or needed" (AOTA, 2020, p. 47). For example, a person creates a list so that items are not forgotten when going grocery shopping.
20. "*Benefits*: Prevents ineffective performance of all other motor and process skills from recurring or persisting" (AOTA, 2020, p. 47). For example, a person does not repeatedly call the same wrong number.

The last four process skills listed (i.e., notice/responds, adjusts, accommodates, and benefits) all describe ways that people avoid, adjust to, and/or overcome difficulties encountered in the performance of everyday tasks. These adaptation skills are critical to the independent performance of tasks in a safe and efficient manner without undue effort (Fisher & Jones, 2011).

There are many advantages to the use of non-standardized skilled observation. It allows the evaluator to focus on the tasks that are most important and relevant to the client. Occupational performance can also be considered with a variety of familiar and unfamiliar activities, including ADLs, IADLs, social participation, and work. The use of these activities can allow clinicians to observe clients' decision making, problem solving, and ability to deal with distractions depending on the difficulty of the task and how it is set up (Radomski & Morrison, 2014; Toglia, 2018). There are also some cognitive skills, such as praxis, that are best evaluated during activity because standardized impairment-based evaluation can sometimes over- or underestimate the impact of deficits on activity engagement (Gillen, 2009). Skilled observation can be performed in context, allowing the clinician to observe the influence of environmental and task factors. It also requires no additional test-specific materials, which makes it flexible and inexpensive (Radomski & Morrison, 2014). In addition, practitioners can include dynamic assessment (i.e., when the clinician provides cues or grades the activity through task and/or environmental modification) to determine how the client's performance can be improved (Radomski & Morrison, 2014; Toglia, 2018).

Dynamic Interactional Approach

The dynamic interactional approach (DIA) is one model that can be used to help guide non-standardized skilled observation of functional activities and to help identify the types of support that help the client's performance (Toglia, 2018). There are also a couple of standardized assessments (e.g., the Executive Function Performance Test [EFPT; described later]) that use a dynamic approach. These standardized assessments include directions for cueing during the test administration to evaluate how the person responds to different types of cueing and how the client is approaching the assessment task and to identify what cueing strategies might be most effective during treatment. Central to the DIA is the concept that cognition is a product of the interaction among the individual, the environment, and the task and that aspects of all three need to be considered during the evaluation process (Toglia, 2018).

When evaluating the contributions of the individual, the clinician considers the client's processing strategies as well as the client's potential for learning (Toglia, 1991, 2018). Processing strategies can be either internal (e.g., self-reminders, mental rehearsals) or external (e.g., alarms, checklists). They can also be situational (effective only in specific tasks or environments) or nonsituational (able to be used in a wide variety of tasks and environments; Toglia, 2018). The type of processing strategy the client uses will affect how well the information is processed as well as how well it is retained. From this perspective, cognitive disability results from deficiencies in these strategies (Toglia, 2018). The DIA assumes that modifying an individual's processing strategies can improve performance and that processing strategies are not specific to any one type of cognitive deficit. Instead, the same strategies can be used by people with different underlying issues (Toglia, 2018). For example, strategies to help increase attention to detail can support performance in a variety of tasks that require attention, memory, and visual processing (Toglia, 2018).

In addition to the client's skills, the clinician considers how the client's social, physical, and cultural environment will influence performance. The social environment includes those with whom the client interacts. The physical can include the materials and objects that surround the client as well as visual or auditory distractions. Culture impacts the occupational choices a person makes in addition to the ways those occupations are completed (Toglia, 2018).

Finally, in addition to considering the individual's processing strategies/learning potential and environmental influences, task characteristics are examined, specifically the way they affect information processing and performance (Toglia, 2018). If a task or activity is too complex and is beyond the client's abilities, then efficient processing strategies cannot be used. For example, imagine Robin, a 32-year-old woman with TBI who plans to make a birthday cake for her girlfriend. At first, she wants to bake a two-layer cake from scratch and ice it with homemade frosting. This task proves to be too difficult for her, and she becomes overwhelmed and unable to approach the task in an organized and effective manner. A clinician using the DIA can change the task parameters one at a time to see what helps to improve Robin's performance. For example, the clinician could suggest that she use store-bought frosting. If that is insufficient, the clinician could then have Robin use a cake mix or make a single-layer cake. By changing the task parameters, the conditions under which performance breaks down can be identified. The clinician can also learn more about which behaviors are amenable to change and which types of assistance support the client's performance (Toglia, 2018).

Throughout the evaluation process, an individual's self-awareness of strengths, limitations, and processing strategies needs to be considered. The evaluation and treatment of deficits in the client's self-awareness are central in the DIA. Self-awareness is viewed as multidimensional and includes self-knowledge and online awareness (Toglia, 2018). Self-knowledge is the person's own understanding of cognitive strengths and limitations in general (outside the context of a particular task). Online awareness refers to the awareness of one's performance in the moment and includes metacognitive skills, such as the ability to accurately judge task demands, anticipate the likelihood of problems, and monitor, regulate, and evaluate performance within the context of an activity. Decreased self-awareness will affect the speed of performance, effective strategy use, the ability to learn from mistakes, and the ability to use feedback to modify behavior (Toglia, 2018).

Imagine the following scenario: Mrs. Patel has always described her memory as poor, stating, "I'd forget my head if it weren't attached!" This demonstrates self-knowledge of her cognitive skills (regarding memory specifically). Mrs. Patel's self-assessment of her memory is not task or context dependent; rather, she is making a judgment about her memory in general. Mrs. Patel has recently had medication changes, with her physician prescribing some new medications and changing the dosage of others. She uses her online awareness to make some decisions about how difficult the task of medication management will be for her. She considers factors such as needing to take different medications at different times (morning vs. evening) and needing to take some with food.

Using the two types of awareness together, she decides to use external processing strategies to support her performance. She creates a medication schedule and purchases several pillboxes in different colors, assigning each pillbox to a different time of the day (i.e., morning, noon, evening, and bedtime).

The DIA uses dynamic assessment to evaluate the client's self-awareness. This portion of the assessment is focused on the client's ability to (a) evaluate the level of difficulty of a particular task, (b) plan ahead, (c) select appropriate strategies, (d) predict the consequences of the actions taken, and (e) monitor performance (Toglia, 2018). There are three parts of the assessment process: (a) investigating clients' self-perceptions of their own abilities before the task by asking clients to predict their performance and success; (b) observing clients completing the task, making note of processing strategies used and facilitating change in performance through task/environment modification and/or verbal cues; and (c) investigating clients' self-perceptions of performance and strategy use after the task by asking them to reflect on both the outcome of the task and the methods they used to complete the task (Toglia, 2018).

If a client has difficulty during evaluation, the clinician makes adjustments in a systematic manner, and the client's subsequent response is examined. These changes are made in a graded fashion, starting by providing minimal support. The emphasis in DIA has shifted in recent years to a test-teach-retest model. Using this approach, a client is assessed completing a task with no assistance. The occupational therapy practitioner then works with the client by teaching the client how to approach the task through task/environmental modification or strategy use. The client is then asked to repeat the task, again with no assistance. This better enables the clinician to make some judgments about learning (Toglia, 2018). The assessment ultimately focuses on the client's ability to change behavior and the types of support that are most effective in bringing about that change (Toglia, 1991).

Standardized Occupation-Based Evaluation

Although non-standardized skilled observation of occupational performance, with or without dynamic assessment, is an essential part of the evaluation process, it does have disadvantages. The biggest disadvantage of skilled observation is that it can be subjective. It is influenced by the clinician's approach, experience, skills, and individual preferences and biases, which lead to difficulty in ensuring reliable findings with this evaluation method (Maskill & Tempest, 2017a; Radomski & Morrison, 2014). Standardized top-down occupation-based assessments have been designed to address this concern and allow reliable and valid evaluation of clients' occupational performance (Radomski & Morrison, 2014). These include the ADL-focused Occupation-based Neurobehavioral Evaluation (A-ONE), the AMPS, and the Performance Assessment of Self-Care Skills (PASS).

The ADL-focused Occupation-based Neurobehavioral Evaluation (Árnadóttir, 1990)

Description

The ADL-focused Occupation-based Neurobehavioral Evaluation (A-ONE), which was originally titled Árnadóttir OT-ADL Neurobehavioral Evaluation, is described in detail in Chapter 5. The A-ONE is used by occupational therapy practitioners to assess both the client's occupational performance in activities of daily living (ADLs) and to determine the underlying neurobehavioral impairments. Evaluators consider clients' performance in ADLs in five domains: dressing, grooming and hygiene, transfers and mobility, feeding, and communication. Evaluators report on the level of independence in ADLs, the type of assistance that is needed, and the types and severity of neurobehavioral impairment (Gardarsdóttir & Kaplan, 2002).

In addition to impairments related to perception and hemi-inattention, the A-ONE Neurobehavioral Scale includes multiple items related to cognition. Four of the 16 impairments on the Neurobehavioral Specific Impairment Scale focus on aspects of cognition (Árnadóttir, 2021). These impairments are motor apraxia, ideational apraxia, organization, and perseveration. Cognitive-related impairments make up 17 of the 30 items on the Neurobehavioral Pervasive Impairment Subscale. The cognitive-focused impairments are impaired alertness, disorientation, confusion, impaired attention, distractibility, field dependency, absentmindedness, performance latency, short-term memory, long-term memory, concrete thinking, impaired judgment, decreased insight, anosognosia, impaired initiative, and impaired motivation. Árnadóttir (2021) defines field dependency (which is not covered specifically in this text) as an individual being distracted by stimuli in the environment to the extent that they incorporate the object causing the distraction into the task that they are performing.

Procedure

As noted in Chapter 5, training is required before clinicians can use the standardized A-ONE tool. To administer the A-ONE, the examiner observes clients while they perform ADLs, such as dressing, and rates their level of independence with the task by using the Functional Independence Scale. The examiner also makes note of errors that are made during task completion and connects the errors that are made to specific neurobehavioral impairments by using the Neurobehavioral Scale (Árnadóttir, 2021).

Scoring

The general scoring strategy for the A-ONE is described in Chapter 5. The specific cognitive-related impairments of motor apraxia, ideational apraxia, and organization are all scored for the ADL domains of dressing, grooming and hygiene, transfers and mobility, and feeding on the Neurobehavioral Specific Impairment Scale. Perseveration is scored on this scale for those four ADL domains plus the communication domain. As per the other items on the Pervasive Impairment Scale, all of the cognitive-related pervasive impairments are scored once for presence or absence during the ADL observation (Árnadóttir, 2021).

Psychometric Properties

There are no psychometric studies of the A-ONE that are specific to the impairments related to the cognitive-related impairments. See Chapter 5 for additional information on research examining the tool as a whole.

Assessment of Motor and Process Skills (Fisher & Jones, 2011)

Description

The Assessment of Motor and Process Skills (AMPS) is a standardized, top-down assessment in which occupational therapy practitioners evaluate the quality of a person's performance of (ADLs) and/or instrumental activities of daily living (IADLs) through assessment of the impact of the person's physical and process abilities (additional description is provided later in this chapter) on their task performance. The assessment is appropriate to use with clients with the developmental age of 2 and up with a variety of diagnoses, including neurological disorders, who wish or need to engage in ADL/IADL tasks. It can also be used with healthy individuals and those who have a suspected illness/medical condition and who are at risk for decline. There are more than

120 standardized tasks to choose from that include tasks typically performed in 6 regions around the world: North America, United Kingdom and Republic of Ireland, Nordic countries, other European countries, Australia and New Zealand, and Asian countries. In addition to several personal ADL tasks, the AMPS includes a wide variety of IADL tasks in the areas of meal preparation, housekeeping, outdoor home management, pet and plant care, and simple vehicle maintenance. Tasks range from very easy (e.g., eating a snack with a utensil, brushing/combing hair) to much harder than average (e.g., vacuuming two rooms on different floors of a home).

A relatively new measure, the Assessment of Compared Qualities — Occupational Performance (ACQ-OP), can be used in conjunction with the AMPS to examine a client's self-awareness and insight (Fisher et al., 2017). After each AMPS task observation, the clinician uses a standardized, 5- to 10-minute semi-structured interview to determine the client's view of their task performance. The clinician compares this information to the AMPS ratings and uses scoring software to generate an ACQ-OP measure indicating the extent of any discrepancy between the client's and clinician's perspectives.

Procedure

The occupational therapy practitioner begins by completing an occupational interview to determine the client's interests and needs in performing ADL and IADL tasks. The practitioner then chooses four to five tasks from the standardized task options that are consistent with the client's interests and at an appropriate difficulty level based on clinical judgment. The client selects at least two tasks to complete from the options the practitioner presents. Before the client performs the two tasks, the practitioner familiarizes the client with the task environment and establishes a task contract. All ADL/IADL tasks are standardized with essential steps that need to be completed to help ensure that the task presents a consistent level of challenge. At the same time, the standardized task criteria allow for the client to perform the task in their usual manner, including using culturally relevant tools and materials. The total time for assessment is approximately 30 to 40 minutes.

Scoring

The occupational therapy practitioner makes careful observations of the client completing the chosen tasks and rates the client's performance on 16 motor skills and 20 process skills. Each of the motor and process skills is an observable, goal-directed action. Each is also considered universal in nature as they are used in all ADL and IADL tasks. The motor skills focus on moving oneself and objects. The process skills focus on (a) selecting, interacting with, and using tools and materials effectively; (b) using time and space efficiently; and (c) adapting and changing when challenges arise and to prevent problems.

As described previously, the 16 motor and 20 process performance skills that form the basis for the AMPS have been incorporated into the *OTPF-4*. However, there are a few key differences. Each of the AMPS skill definitions includes examples of effective, questionable, ineffective, and deficient performance to assist with scoring as described later. In some instances, the AMPS definition is more detailed, which also serves to clarify what is or is not included. For example, the definition of the performance skill *accommodates* in the *OTPF-4* is limited to "prevents ineffective performance of all other motor and process skills and asks for assistance only when appropriate or needed" (AOTA, 2020, p. 47). In contrast, the AMPS definition of effective performance for *accommodates* states that the person is observed to:

> readily and consistently modify his or her actions or the location of objects within the workspace, in anticipation of (i.e., to prevent), or in response to, problems that might arise. The person anticipates or responds to problems effectively by (a) changing the method with which he or she is performing an action sequence, (b) changing the manner in which he or she interacts with or handles tools and materials already in the workspace, and (c) asking for assistance when appropriate or needed. (Fisher & Jones, 2014, p. 362)

After the observation of the chosen tasks, the occupational therapy practitioner scores each skill using a 4-point scale (competent, questionable, deficient, or severely deficient) in relation to the performance of each of the observed tasks. Competent performance is considered free of clumsiness or increased physical effort, efficient in use or time and space, safe, and independent. The client is not scored down for effective use of compensatory devices and strategies. The examiner inputs the motor and process skill scores from the two (or more) tasks into their individualized computer-based scoring program, which converts these ordinal scores into linear ADL motor and process quality of performance measures. The final scores are adjusted based on difficulty of the task, the difficulty of each skill item, and the practitioner's own severity of ratings. The clinician-specific severity adjustment incorporated into the individualized computer-based scoring program based on how the clinician scores a series of calibration tapes during training is a critical element in addressing concerns regarding subjectivity in evaluations that are based on observation of everyday tasks.

The individualized AMPS computer program generates multiple reports. These include a Graphic Report, which shows the person's ADL motor and process ability measures (based on the combined motor and process skill scores from the tasks that were observed) in relation to the AMPS cutoff measures. These motor and process ability measures can be interpreted from three different perspectives: criterion-referenced, norm-referenced, and prediction of need for assistance to live in the community. From a criterion-referenced perspective, the person's motor and process ability measures shown on the Graphic Report are evaluated in relation to established motor and process cut-off scores to determine if ADL/IADL performance is competent. The further a person's motor ability measure score is below the motor cut-off, the more likely they are to be experiencing increased clumsiness, physical effort, or fatigue with ADL/IADL tasks. The further a person's process ability measure score is below the process cut-off, the more likely they are to be experiencing decreased efficiency in the use of time, space, or objects with ADL/IADL tasks. Motor or process ability measures below the cut-offs also indicate possible safety risk and/ or need for assistance with ADL/IADL tasks (the lower the score, the greater the concern). The Graphic Report, as well as one of the other reports that are generated, can also be used to compare the person's motor and/or process ability measures with the expected performance scores for well, typically developing individuals of the same age. Finally, the motor and process ability measures can be used to predict if an individual needs assistance to live in the community. Fisher and Jones (2011) stressed that this determination should not be made strictly on the basis of the AMPS scores but, rather, in conjunction with all other relevant information that is available.

The design of the AMPS allows the occupational therapy practitioner to compare the person's performance at different points even when different tasks are selected. It also allows for comparison of the result of AMPS assessments conducted by different clinicians. However, the underlying cause of any difficulties (if present) is not assessed with the AMPS. Rather, the focus is on evaluating the actual "doing" of a client's occupational performance. Thus, the AMPS might identify that the motor performance skill of "reaching" is severely deficient and does not support task performance. However, the AMPS cannot identify why a person's reach might be impaired. Additional assessments (e.g., strength and /or range of motion testing) would be needed to make that determination.

Psychometric Properties

In order to ensure that raters are reliable, all users of the AMPS must go through extensive training consisting of 45 hours in the classroom or the completion of an online course. Courses include a calibration process to determine individual rater severity. This information is then used to create a personalized copy of the AMPS scoring software for each rater. After completion of the course, the rater administers the AMPS to 10 people and submits scores for analysis as a check for continued reliability and validity (Fisher & Jones, 2011). The test developers report that extensive testing has been done to examine the reliability and validity of the AMPS with standardization completed using multifaceted Rasch analysis on a large sample of people from multiple countries with a wide range of ages (3 to 103 years) and diagnoses. Healthy, well people were also included. At the time of this writing, the standardization sample consisted of 148,158 persons. Ninety-two percent of the individuals in the sample demonstrated acceptable goodness of fit to the motor scale, and 90% demonstrated goodness of fit to the process scale per standard Rasch analyses with (fit mean square ≤ 1.4 and/or $z < 2$). The AMPS results for the standardization sample were provided by 13,070 occupational therapy practitioners who had all demonstrated valid and reliable testing and scoring procedures. Ninety-five percent of these practitioners demonstrated acceptable goodness of fit to the AMPS Rasch model (fit mean squares ≤ 1.4 and/or $z < 2$; Fisher & Jones, 2011).

Research findings have supported the use of the AMPS for people of different genders, from different regions of the world, and with a variety of disorders (including cortical damage to either hemisphere, dementia, multiple sclerosis, developmental disabilities, psychiatric disorders, and cerebral palsy). Other studies have shown the AMPS to be sensitive in showing change in clients' performance (Fioravanti et al., 2012; Lange et al., 2009). Testing has found that there may be a risk of cross-cultural bias because culture influences the way in which people complete ADL and IADL tasks. In response, the AMPS developers recommended that raters be aware of their own culture and potential biases and educate themselves about possible cultural influences on ADL/IADL task performance for their clients (Fisher & Jones, 2011).

Performance Assessment of Self-Care Skills (Rogers et al., 2016)

Description

The Performance Assessment of Self-Care Skills (PASS) is a standardized, occupation-based assessment. It was originally created in 2002 and has undergone several revisions since that time. At the time of this writing, 26 items were included in the assessment, each of which may be assessed on its own. There are 5 tasks focused on functional mobility, 3 tasks that evaluate basic ADLs, 14 IADL tasks with an emphasis on cognition, and 4 IADL tasks with an emphasis on physical function. There are two versions of the test, one that can be used in the clinic and one that can be used in the home. The tasks are the same in each version of the test, except for some adjustment on specific materials. Each subtest in the PASS is further broken down into subtasks. For example, one of the IADL tasks with an emphasis on cognition considers money management in a simulated shopping task (Figure 8-2). There are five subtasks for this subtest: selecting four items on a shopping list correctly, selecting the correct cash for the items, selecting the correct coupon for one of the items, giving the correct coupon and $1.00 to the examiner, and correctly identifying an error in the amount of change given. It has been used with a variety of patient populations. It has also been translated into Spanish, Hebrew, Mandarin, Farsi, Turkish, and Arabic (Chisholm et al., 2014). The test authors encourage clinicians to develop additional test items that can be used with the PASS and provide direction for this process. The PASS is available free of charge (https://www.shrs.pitt.edu/ot/about/performance-assessment-self-care-skills-pass).

Task # C8: IADL-C: Shopping (Money Management)

CLINIC CONDITIONS: Table and

1. 8 unopened cans, with local prices marked on the top of each box as follows:
   1) 1 (10 ¾ oz) can Campbell's Chicken Noodle soup
   2) 1 (8 oz) can Tomato sauce (different brand than can 7)
   3) 1 can local brand Chicken Noodle soup
   4) 1 (10 ¾ oz) can Campbell's Tomato Rice soup
   5) 1 (10 ¾ oz) can Campbell's Tomato soup
   6) 1 can local brand Tomato soup
   7) 1 (8 oz) can Tomato sauce (different brand than can 8)
   8) 1 (10 ¾ oz) can Campbell's Chicken and Rice soup
2. Envelope with 5 coupons; one coupon matches one of the local brand Tomato soup item (no other matches); matching coupon is 3rd coupon in envelope
3. Wallet with change purse, containing $12.60 in real money in the following denominations:
   In the wallet section: 5 - $1.00 bills, 1-$5.00 bill In the coin section: 4-Quarters, 10-dimes, 10-nickels, 10-pennies
4. Typed grocery list that includes:
   a. 1 can Campbell's Tomato Rice soup
   b. 1 can local brand Chicken Noodle soup
   c. 1 can Tomato sauce (brand not identified)
   d. 1 can local brand Tomato soup (coupon item)
5. Grocery receipts for the 4 items ($2.32 and $2.35, depending on Tomato sauce chosen – receipts can be printed front to back)
6. Tablet, pencil, calculator, hand held magnifier
6. Client seated at table with cans arranged from left to right in the order given in #1 above; the grocery list, wallet, and items in #6 are positioned in front of the cans.

CLINIC INSTRUCTIONS:

"Next we have a grocery shopping task for you to do."

"Here is a grocery list [Point to list]. Please select the items on the list from those on the table. Do you know what you are to do? Do you have everything that you need?" [Wait for response]

Keep selected cans in front of Client; push others aside

"Here is the grocery store receipt for the 4 items on the grocery list [Hand client appropriate receipt]. Pay me the exact amount for the groceries with the money in this wallet." [Point to wallet, then hold hand palm up and wait for response]

"The next shopping task includes coupons."

"There are several food coupons in this envelope [Hand Client envelope with coupons]. Check to see if any of the coupons match the items you purchased [Motion to 4 items]. If they do, use the coupons and this money [Hand Client $2.00] to pay for just the coupon items. I will then give you change. Do you know what you are to do? Do you have everything that you need?" [Wait for response]

[When Client gives you the local brand Tomato soup, the coupon for 10¢, and $1.00, give the Client 2 quarters and 4 pennies (54¢)...a 10¢ shortage].

"Here is your change. Did I give you the correct amount of change? [Wait for Client to count change]. How much change should I have given you?" [Wait for response]

SCORE	INDEPENDENCE	SAFETY	ADEQUACY	
			PROCESS	QUALITY
3	No assists given for task initiation, continuation, or completion	Safe practices were observed	Subtasks performed with precision & economy of effort & action	Optimal (performance matches the quality standards listed in each subtask)
2	No Level 7-9 assists given, but occasional Level 1-6 assists given	Minor risks were evident but no assistance provided	Subtasks generally performed w/ precision & economy of effort & action; occasional lack of efficiency, redundant or extraneous action; no missing steps	Acceptable (Performance, for the most part, matches or nearly matches the quality standards listed in each subtask)
1	No Level 9 assists given; or occasional Level 7 or 8 assists given; or continuous Level 1-6 assists given	Risks to safety were observed and assistance given to prevent potential harm	Subtasks generally performed w/ lack of precision and/or economy of effort & action; consistent extraneous or redundant actions; steps may be missing	Marginal (Performance, for the most part, does not match the quality standards listed in each subtask)
0	Level 9 assists given; or continuous Level 7 or 8 assists given; or unable to initiate, continue, or complete subtask or task	Risks to safety of such severity were observed that task was stopped or taken over by assessor to prevent harm	Subtasks are consistently performed w/ lack of precision and/or economy of effort & action so that task progress is unattainable	Unacceptable (Performance does not match the quality standards listed in each subtask, perhaps with few exceptions)

Figure 8-2. The shopping subtest of the PASS. (Reproduced with permission from Joan C. Rogers, PhD, OTR, FAOTA; Margo B. Holm, PhD, OTR/L, FAOTA; and Denise Chisolm, PhD, OTR/L, FAOTA.)

Procedure

Each item in the PASS has standardized instructions in the test manual that describe the materials needed, how the task should be set up, the directions that are given to the client, and the scoring criteria.

Scoring

Clients receive a score for each subtest that they complete. They are scored in three areas (independence, safety, and adequacy) using an ordinal scale. Independence is assessed using both the level of assistance and the type of assistance that is given on each subtask in the test item. To determine the assistance that is needed, a dynamic process is used in which the evaluating clinician gives the client assistance in a graded fashion. There is a hierarchy of assistances levels examiners are to use, ranging from a general verbal assist (e.g., encouragement) through total physical assistance (when the examiner completes the task for the client). An overall independence score is calculated for the subtest by taking the mean of the scores received on the subtasks. Safety is assessed by making observations of unsafe behaviors exhibited by the client during the task. Finally, adequacy is assessed by considering both the person's efficiency and the quality of the performance. To assign the adequacy score, the client's performance as a whole is considered (Figure 8-3).

Task # C8: IADL-C: Shopping (Money Management)

Assistive Technology Devices (ATDs) used during task:

1.

2.

3.

Total # of ATDs used:_____

		INDEPENDENCE DATA											SAFETY DATA	ADEQUACY DATA	
		No Assistance	Verbal Supportive (Encouragement)	Verbal Non-Directive	Verbal Directive	Gestures	Task or Environment Rearrangement	Demonstration	Physical Guidance	Physical Support	Total Assist	INDEPENDENCE subtask scores	Unsafe Observations	PROCESS: Imprecision, lack of economy, missing steps	QUALITY: Standards not met / improvement needed
	Assist level →	0	1	2	3	4	5	6	7	8	9				
Subtasks	Subtask Criteria														
1	Selects all 4 items on the shopping list correctly (requires identification of items, followed by choice of items as indicated by Ct gathering items in one location, pointing to items etc.)														
2	Selects the correct cash for the 4 grocery items (cash given matches the receipt amount)														
3	Selects the correct coupon for the matching item (sets one coupon aside; gestures to matching item; places coupon on appropriate can)														
4	Gives correct coupon & $1.00 to assessor (local brand Tomato soup coupon)														
5	Identifies correctly that change returned is wrong amount (too little) and correctly identifies the amount that should have been returned (64¢)														

SUMMARY SCORES

INDEPENDENCE MEAN SCORE →

SAFETY SCORE →

ADEQUACY SCORE →

Figure 8-3. The scoring sheet for the shopping subtest of the PASS. (Reproduced with permission from Joan C. Rogers, PhD, OTR, FAOTA; Margo B. Holm, PhD, OTR/L, FAOTA; and Denise Chisolm, PhD, OTR/L, FAOTA.)

Psychometric Properties

PASS workshops and training videos are available and recommended to improve inter-rater reliability. The authors of the PASS also recommend that each rater undergo inter-rater agreement testing with a trained and experienced assessor. The PASS has been shown to have test–retest reliability of $r = 0.92$ to 0.96 with inter-rater agreement between 89% and 97% (Holm & Rogers, 2008). Content and construct validity have also been assessed with the PASS showing good agreement with other measures, including the OARS Multidimensional Functional Assessment Questionnaire: Activities of Daily Living and the Functional Assessment Questionnaire (Chisholm, 2005).

Deficit-Specific Assessment Tools

After evaluation of the client's occupational performance, it can be useful to focus on specific cognitive skills to get a better sense of functioning of particular areas of cognition (Erez & Katz, 2018; Maskill & Tempest, 2017a; Radomski & Morrison, 2014). There are assessments that consider a wide variety of cognitive deficits. Some of these assessments have been designed by occupational therapy practitioners, and some have been created by professionals in other disciplines (e.g., neuropsychology). For a list of some of the assessments that are available, see Table 8-1. Some of the tools used more frequently by occupational therapy practitioners are described in more detail in the following sections. More information about many of these assessments, in addition to some we did not include, can be found through Stroke Engine at https://strokengine.ca/en/assessments/, the Center for Outcome Measurement in Brain Injury at https://www.tbims.org/, and the Rehabilitation Measures Database at https://www.sralab.org/rehabilitation-measures.

Table 8-1

Cognitive Assessments

NAME OF ASSESSMENT TOOL	DESCRIPTION	REFERENCE/ WEBSITE
The ADL-focused Occupation-based Neurobehavioral Evaluation	A standardized assessment of occupational performance in five domains of ADLs (dressing, grooming and hygiene, transfers and mobility, feeding, and communication). Clients are rated on two scales. The Functional Independence Scale gives ratings of independence with ADL tasks. The Neurobehavioral Impairment Scale gives information about the number and type of neurobehavioral deficits that are impacting function. There is extensive training needed to use this assessment tool.	Árnadóttir, 1990; http://www.a-one.is/index.html
Assessment of Motor and Process Skills	A standardized assessment of occupational performance in ADLs and IADLs. Clients complete 2 tasks, and clinicians rate performance on 16 motor skills and 20 process skills. Final scores give information on independence, safety, effort, and efficiency. There is extensive training needed to use this assessment tool.	Fisher & Jones, 2011; https://innovativeotsolutions.com/tools/amps
Awareness Questionnaire	A quick (10-minute) screening of a client's level of awareness of deficits. The client, a family member, and a clinician all complete a version of the questionnaire so that a client's level of insight can be assessed. There are 17 questions on the client and family versions. There are 18 on the clinician version. All questions are rated using an ordinal scale. It is available to use for free.	http://www.tbims.org/combi/aq
Cognitive Performance Test	A standardized, performance-based assessment with seven tasks titled Dress, Shop, Toast, Phone, Wash, Travel, and Medbox. Clients complete the tasks, and their performance is rated. The scores on each task are averaged to provide an overall score, which correlates with the Allen Cognitive Levels. Completion of the entire assessment takes approximately 45 minutes.	Burns, 2018

(continued)

Table 8-1 (continued)

Cognitive Assessments

NAME OF ASSESSMENT TOOL	DESCRIPTION	REFERENCE/ WEBSITE
Complex Task Performance Assessment	Newer assessment (first described in the literature in 2008). Simulates working in a library completing two work tasks: inventory control and telephone messaging. Both tasks are performed simultaneously. Manual is free online. Kit needs to be set up. Takes up to 40 minutes to complete.	https://www.ot.wustl.edu/mm/files/CTPA.zip
Contextual Memory Test	A standardized test that assesses memory, including a person's use of cognitive strategies. Self-awareness of memory and cognitive strategies are also assessed. This test has two versions (with items relating to a restaurant or morning routine). It was published in 1993.	Toglia, 1993
Executive Function Performance Test	A standardized, occupation-based test that considers a client's performance with functional tasks. A pretest (handwashing) can be given to see if the client can follow directions. There are four subtests: oatmeal preparation on a stove top, using the telephone, taking medication, and paying bills. Dynamic assessment principles are incorporated with cueing guidelines to use if the client needs assistance completing tasks. Clients are also asked to make predictions about their performance. The test manual is free online. The most recent version was published in 2013. There is also an alternate version that can be used for retesting clients. It has similar subtests to the original version: cooking noodles, filling a pillbox, using the telephone, and ordering from a catalog.	http://www.ot.wustl.edu/about/resources/executive-function-performance-test-efpt-308
Kohlman Evaluation of Living Skills, Fourth Edition	A standardized assessment that looks at basic living skills in five areas (self-care, safety and health, money management, community mobility and telephone, and employment and leisure). There are 13 tasks, and it takes approximately 45 minutes to complete in its entirety. It has been used with clients with psychiatric diagnoses as well as for those with ABI. The fourth edition was published in 2016.	Kohlman Thomson, 2016

(continued)

Table 8-1 (continued)

Cognitive Assessments

NAME OF ASSESSMENT TOOL	DESCRIPTION	REFERENCE/ WEBSITE
Loewenstein Occupational Therapy Cognitive Assessment, Second Edition	An impairment-based standardized test battery that has 6 sections: orientation, visual perception, spatial perception, motor praxis, visuomotor organization, and thinking operations. It has 26 subsections. It was originally created for people with ABI, and the first edition was published in 1990. The second edition was published in 2000.	Itzkovich et al., 2000
Montreal Cognitive Assessment	A screening tool designed for people with cognitive impairment. It takes approximately 10 minutes to administer and asks questions that consider a number of cognitive functions, including memory, orientation, and attention. People who score 26 or higher (30 points are possible) are listed as having a normal result. This cognitive screen is available online. Training and certification are required to use it. The latest version was published in 2010. It is available in numerous languages.	http://www.mocatest.org/
Moss Attention Rating Scale	A scale that is completed by a clinician on two separate occasions. It has 22 items and asks the rater to consider several types of attention. Each item is rated with a 5-point scale. The raw scores are then converted to give an overall rating of attention, with a higher score indicating better attention. It is available for free online.	http://tbims.org/combi/mars/index.html
Multiple Errands Test	A performance-based test of executive function designed for adults with ABI. In this assessment, clients are asked to complete a list of six errands within a facility (e.g., hospital, shopping mall). The client is given the list of errands and a map. The clinician follows the client and makes notes about performance. It was originally described in 1991 and has undergone revision since that time. It is available through one of the authors (although it needs to be modified to fit the specific location).	Dawson et al., 2009

(continued)

Table 8-1 (continued)

Cognitive Assessments

NAME OF ASSESSMENT TOOL	DESCRIPTION	REFERENCE/ WEBSITE
Participation Objective, Participation Subjective	An assessment with 26 items designed to gather information about participation in 5 general areas: domestic life; major life activities; transportation; interpersonal interactions and relationships; and community, recreational, and civic life. The person is asked to estimate the frequency/amount of time engaged in each activity, satisfaction with the amount of time engaged in the activity, and importance of the activity. It is available for free online.	http://tbims.org/combi/pops/index.html
Performance Assessment of Self-Care Skills	A standardized, occupation-based assessment. It has 26 items in 4 areas: functional mobility, ADLs, IADLs with an emphasis on cognition, and IADLs with an emphasis on physical function. There are two versions of the test, one that can be used at home and one for use in the clinic. Raters assess clients in the areas of independence, safety, and adequacy.	Rogers et al., 2016
Rivermead Behavioural Memory Test, Third Edition	A standardized assessment that was designed to be used with people with ABI. It strives to predict the impact of memory deficits on everyday function and to provide a way to monitor change over time. There are 10 subtests, and it takes approximately 30 minutes to administer. The third edition was published in 2008.	Wilson et al., 2008
Saint Louis University Mental Status Examination	A screening tool designed for people with cognitive impairment. It has 11 questions that consider a number of cognitive functions, including memory, orientation, and visuospatial skills. Thirty points are possible. This cognitive screen is available online.	http://aging.slu.edu/index.php?page=saint-louis-university-mental-status-slums-exam
Self-Awareness of Deficits Interview	A structured interview that evaluates clients' intellectual awareness in three areas: presence of deficits, functional implication of deficits, and ability to set realistic goals. Clinicians rate the client's level of awareness in each area using a 4-point ordinal scale.	Fleming et al., 1996

(continued)

Table 8-1 (continued)

Cognitive Assessments

NAME OF ASSESSMENT TOOL	DESCRIPTION	REFERENCE/ WEBSITE
Test of Everyday Attention	A standardized test battery that assesses various types of attention. It contains eight subtests and strives to consider different types of attention in the context of functional tasks. There are three versions to allow administration of the tests multiple times while controlling for practice effects. It was created for people with ABI, and norms have been established for different adult age groups. It was published in 1994.	Robertson et al., 1994
Test of Grocery Shopping Skills	A performance-based test of executive functions designed for adults with ABI. In this assessment, clients visit a grocery store in the community. They need to locate and select 10 items from a list, looking for the least expensive options that are in the desired amount (e.g., a 6-ounce can of tuna in water). The clinician follows the client and takes notes about performance. This assessment was published in 2009.	Brown et al., 2009
Test of Upper Limb Apraxia	An impairment-based standardized test of apraxia. It has 6 subtests with a total of 48 items looking at imitation and pantomime of meaningless, communicative, and tool-related gestures. There is a screening tool that uses a subset of 12 items that is available online.	Vanbellingen et al., 2010; http://capstoneapraxiaoccupationalfunct.weebly.com/uploads/1/9/3/3/19336053/apraxia_screen_of_tulia_ast.pdf
Weekly Calendar Planning Activity	A test of executive function designed for adolescents and adults (ages 16 and up) with mild cognitive impairment. It takes approximately 20 to 25 minutes to administer. In the test, people are asked to fill out a weekly calendar with 17 to 18 appointments (taking care not to have them conflict) while simultaneously being asked to follow rules, disregard distractions, and monitor the passage of time. It was published in 2015.	Toglia, 2015

Assessment Tools for Awareness

Self-Awareness of Deficits Interview (Fleming et al., 1996)

Description

The Self-Awareness of Deficits Interview (SADI) is a structured interview used to obtain qualitative and quantitative data on the status of self-awareness after ABI. It contains three areas of questioning: (a) self-awareness of deficits, (b) self-awareness of the functional implications of those deficits, and (c) the client's ability to set realistic goals. The specific interview questions for each of these areas are presented in Figure 8-4. Note that the questions can be adapted or reworded by the interviewer within the context of the interview.

Procedure

The test administrator interviews the client using the questions and prompts outlined in the interview guide. Clients are asked about their deficits post–brain injury, how deficits impact their function, and their goals. Interviews start with broad questions and then can continue with questions that are more direct if a client does not identify an area of concern.

Scoring

Responses are rated on a 4-point scale with 0 indicating no disorder of self-awareness and a score of 3 indicating a severe disorder of self-awareness. Specific scoring criteria for each of the three interview categories are shown in Figure 8-5.

Psychometric Properties

Inter-rater reliability among 5 interviewers and 25 clients with TBI was established through analysis of variance (ANOVA) and intraclass agreement (0.78, 0.57, and 0.78) on the three sections, respectively. The scores for the three subsections combined had an intraclass correlation coefficient (ICC) of 0.82 (Fleming et al., 1996). In validity testing, the SADI correlated with the Awareness Questionnaire (Wise et al., 2005). It also was able to distinguish between those with mild versus severe TBI (Bogod et al., 2003) and was found to be sensitive to change (Fleming et al., 2006).

Awareness Questionnaire (Sherer, 2004)

Description

The Awareness Questionnaire has three forms that are completed by three different people: (a) the client, (b) a family member or significant other who was familiar with the client before the ABI, and (c) a clinician who is familiar with the client after the ABI. The forms all focus on ratings of the client's current performance.

Procedure

The client completes a self-assessment form where they rate their functioning in physical, cognitive, behavioral, and community areas (Figure 8-6). The family member and the clinician use their forms to rate the client's functioning in the same areas. The clinician also provides a rating of their impression of the accuracy of the client's self-awareness.

Self-Awareness of Deficits Interview

SELF-AWARENESS OF DEFICITS

1. Are you any different now compared to what you were like before your accident? In what way? Do you feel that anything about you or your abilities has changed?
2. Do people who know you well notice that anything is different about you since the accident? What might they notice?
3. What do you see as your problems, if any, resulting from your injury? What is the main thing you need to work on/would like to get better?

Prompts

Physical abilities (e.g., movement of arms and legs, balance, vision, endurance)?
Memory/confusion?
Concentration?
Problem solving, decision making, organizing, and planning things?
Controlling behavior?
Communication?
Getting along with other people?
Has your personality changed?
Are there any other problems that I haven't mentioned?

SELF-AWARENESS OF FUNCTIONAL IMPLICATIONS OF DEFICITS

1. Does your head injury have any affect on your everyday life? In what way?

Prompts

Ability to live independently?
Managing finances?
Look after family/manage home?
Driving?
Work/study?
Leisure/social life?
Are there any other areas of life that you feel have changed/may change?

ABILITY TO SET REALISTIC GOALS

1. What do you hope to achieve in the next 6 months? Do you have any goals? What are they?
2. In 6 months' time, what do you think you will be doing? Where do you think you will be?
3. Do you think your head injury will still be having an effect on your life in 6 months' time?
   If yes: How?
   If no: Are you sure?

Figure 8-4. The SADI. (Reproduced with permission from Fleming, J. M., Strong, J., & Ashton, R. [1996]. Self-awareness of deficits in adults with traumatic brain injury: How best to measure? *Brain Injury, 10*[1], 14.)

Scoring Criteria for the Self-Awareness of Deficits Interview

SELF-AWARENESS OF DEFICITS

0 Cognitive/psychological problems (where relevant) reported by the client in response to general questioning or readily acknowledged in response to specific questioning.

1 Some cognitive/psychological problems reported, but others denied or minimized. Client may have a tendency to focus on relatively minor physical changes (e.g., scars) and acknowledge cognitive/psychological problems only on specific questioning about deficits.

2 Physical deficits only acknowledged; denies, minimizes, or is unsure of cognitive/psychological changes. Client may recognize problems that occurred at an earlier stage but denies existence of persisting deficits or may state that other people think there are deficits but he or she does not think so.

3 No acknowledgement of deficits (other than obvious physical deficits) can be obtained, or client will only acknowledge problems that have been imposed on him or her (e.g., not allowed to drive, not allowed to drink alcohol).

SELF-AWARENESS OF FUNCTIONAL IMPLICATIONS OF DEFICITS

0 Client accurately describes current functional status (independent living, work/study, leisure, home management, driving) and specifies how his or her head injury problems limit function (where relevant) and/or any compensatory measures adopted to overcome problems.

1 Some functional implications reported following questions or examples of problems in independent living, work, driving, leisure, etc. Client may not be sure of other likely functional problems (e.g., is unable to say because he or she has not tried an activity yet).

2 Client may acknowledge some functional implications of deficits but minimizes the importance of identified problems. Other likely functional implications may be actively denied by the client.

3 Little acknowledgement of functional consequences can be obtained; the client will not acknowledge problems, except that he or she is not allowed to perform certain tasks. The client may actively ignore medical advice and may engage in risk-taking behaviors (e.g., drinking and driving).

ABILITY TO SET REALISTIC GOALS

0 Client sets reasonably realistic goals and (where relevant) identifies that the head injury will probably continue to have an impact on some areas of functioning (i.e., goals for the future have been modified in some way since the injury).

1 Client sets goals that are somewhat unrealistic or is unable to specify a goal but recognizes that he or she will still have problems in some areas of function in the future (i.e., sees that goals for the future may need some modification even if he or she has not yet done so).

2 Client sets unrealistic goals, or is unable to specify a goal, and does not know how he or she will be functioning in 6 months' time but hopes he or she will return to pretrauma (i.e., no modification of goals has occurred).

3 Client expects without uncertainty that in 6 months' time he or she will be functioning at pretrauma level (or at a higher level).

Figure 8-5. Scoring for the SADI. (Reproduced with permission from Fleming, J. M., Strong, J., & Ashton, R. [1996]. Self-awareness of deficits in adults with traumatic brain injury: How best to measure? *Brain Injury, 10*[1], 15.)

Self-Awareness Questionnaire

ORIENTATION TO TIME AND PLACE

(Three choice format.)

Day:

Month:

Date:

Year:

Town:

What is this place?
(army) (school) (rehabilitation center)

What is the name of this place?

AWARENESS OF BRAIN INJURY

(Personalize these items for each survivor.)

What happened to you to bring you here?
(parents/relatives sent you here) (car accident/fall/blow) (volunteered to come)

Why are you here?
(to receive therapy) (punishment) (unsure)

Has your brain been injured? (Yes) (No)

When were you injured?
(at birth) (I have not been injured) (actual year)

AWARENESS OF PHYSICAL IMPAIRMENT

Can you walk?	(Yes)	(No)
Do you have difficulty moving your legs?	(Yes)	(No)
Can you move both your arms normally?	(Yes)	(No)
Do you have difficulty moving your fingers?	(Yes)	(No)

AWARENESS OF COMMUNICATION IMPAIRMENT

Can you speak normally?	(Yes)	(No)
Can you understand what people say to you?	(Yes)	(No)
Do you have difficulty reading?	(Yes)	(No)
Do you have difficulty writing?	(Yes)	(No)

Figure 8-6. The Self-Awareness Questionnaire. (Reproduced with permission from Casquoine P. G., & Gibbons, T. A. [1994]. Lack of awareness of impairment in institutionalized, severely and chronically disabled survivors of traumatic brain injury: A preliminary investigation. *Journal of Head Trauma Rehabilitation, 9*[4], 16-24.) *(continued)*

Scoring

Decreased awareness is measured by discrepancy scores between family member ratings and client self-ratings, clinician ratings and client self-ratings, and client self-ratings and standardized tests of cognitive abilities.

Self-Awareness Questionnaire

ACTIVITIES OF DAILY LIVING

Do you need help to feed yourself?	(Yes)	(No)
Can you dress yourself?	(Yes)	(No)
Do you need help to bathe yourself?	(Yes)	(No)
Can you shave/apply makeup yourself?	(Yes)	(No)

AWARENESS OF SENSORY/COGNITIVE DEFICITS

Do you have a good memory?	(Yes)	(No)
Do you have good vision?	(Yes)	(No)
Do you get fatigued/tired easily?	(Yes)	(No)
Do you have trouble thinking clearly?	(Yes)	(No)

Figure 8-6 (continued). The Self-Awareness Questionnaire. (Reproduced with permission from Casquoine P. G., & Gibbons, T. A. [1994]. Lack of awareness of impairment in institutionalized, severely and chronically disabled survivors of traumatic brain injury: A preliminary investigation. *Journal of Head Trauma Rehabilitation, 9*[4], 16-24.)

Psychometric Properties

Internal consistency of the instrument has been reported as good (0.88; Sherer et al., 1998). Test–retest and inter-rater reliability have not been established. Several studies examining validity have been completed. Scores on the Awareness Questionnaire have been shown to predict later employment status. Clients with greater discrepancies between their own ratings and family/clinician ratings were more likely to be unemployed after approximately 2 years (Sherer et al., 1998). Awareness Questionnaire scores were also correlated with the Satisfaction with Life Scale (Evans et al., 2005) and the Patient Competency Rating Scale (Sherer et al., 2003) and the SADI (Wise et al., 2005), demonstrating construct validity.

Assessment Tools for Memory

Rivermead Behavioral Memory Test, Third Edition (Wilson et al., 2008)

Description

The Rivermead Behavioral Memory Test, Third Edition (RBMT-3) is a test of everyday memory functioning. It consists of 10 subtests, some of which are repeated to assess delayed recall. Examples include recalling names, keeping appointments, recognizing pictures previously shown, recalling details of a story, and completing a novel task. The final subtest is one in which the client needs to learn a new task (e.g., putting together a puzzle in a specific way), recall it, and repeat the task. There are two parallel versions of the test to minimize practice effects due to repeated testing. Items are presented in sequences so that early items can be recalled by the client later in testing. It takes approximately 30 minutes to complete the test.

Procedure

The test manual provides specific instructions for administering each of the 10 subtests, all of which are completed with the client seated at a table.

Scoring

Clients are given a raw score for each subtest, which is converted to a scaled score based on the client's age. The scaled scores are summed and converted into a General Memory Index score, percentile rank, and confidence intervals. Standardization data were determined for the RBMT-3 by using 333 people between the ages of 16 and 89 years.

Psychometric Properties

Reliability between the two versions was calculated by using the scores of the standardization group in addition to scores from 75 people with memory deficits. Alternate forms reliability for the subtests ranged from 0.57 to 0.86. Alternate forms reliability for the General Memory Index score was 0.87. Inter-rater reliability was established with 18 participants and 2 raters with 0.9 to 1.0 agreement between both raters on all subtests, except one, when the inter-rater reliability was 0.79 (Wilson et al., 2008).

The RBMT-3 was given to clients with memory deficits and to control participants and was able to discriminate between those with and without memory loss ($p < .001$). Performance on the RBMT-3 was moderately correlated with performance on the Prospective and Retrospective Memory Questionnaire.

Contextual Memory Test (Toglia, 1993)

Description

The Contextual Memory Test (CMT) is intended as a supplement to other measures of memory and cognition. It is designed to objectively measure awareness and strategy use in adults with memory impairment and/or screen clients for memory impairment that may require further testing. Test items are functionally oriented, grouped into a set of restaurant-related items and another related to morning routine. Normative data were collected on 375 adults in the New York area ages 18 to 87 with a mean age of 46 and 217 adults in Israel ages 18 to 86 (Toglia, 2005).

Procedure

There are three areas addressed by the CMT: (a) awareness of memory capacity, (b) recall of line drawn objects, and (c) strategy use. The test manual provides detailed procedures for assessing each of the three areas that are summarized in the following.

1. Awareness of memory capacity: The test administrator asks clients general questions about their perception of their own memory. Clients are asked to predict their task performance before the test. After completion of the task, they are asked to estimate the number of items they were able to recall correctly.
2. Recall of line drawn objects: Clients are shown a set of 20 line pictures that are grouped into one of two sets: morning routine or restaurants. They are given 90 seconds to study and memorize the pictures. They are then asked for immediate and delayed recall of the pictures they were shown.
3. Strategy use: Clients are asked to describe the strategies they used to remember the pictures. If the client scored below normal limits for their age, they are shown the second set of pictures at a later session. This time, the examiner tells the client that all of the pictures in the set are related to a theme (morning routine or restaurant), thus providing the client with a strategy to use. The effect of the introduction of that strategy is examined with the administration of the subsequent portion of the test.

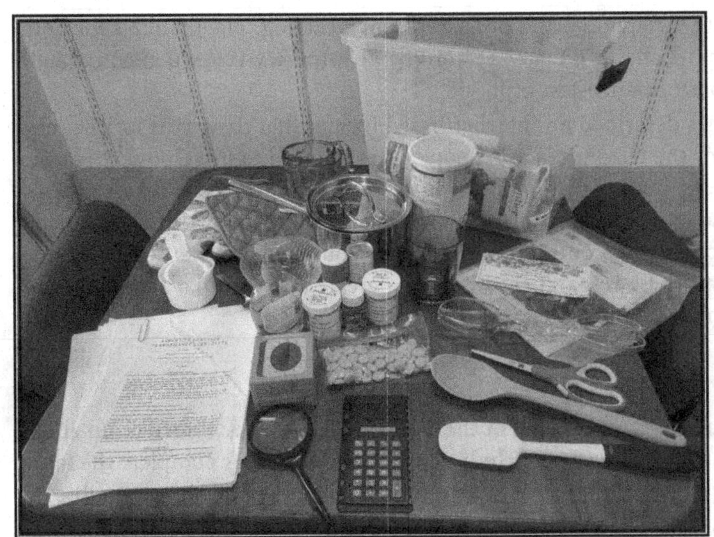

Figure 8-7. The materials of the EFPT.

Scoring

There are three recall raw scores (immediate, delayed, and total recall) that are converted to standard scores. Prediction scores are generated through comparison with the actual recall score. Strategy use is examined through the effect of context, the total strategy use, and the order of recall.

Psychometric Properties

Parallel form reliability was conducted with the two forms of the test, with reliability estimates ranging from 0.73 to 0.81. Quasi (partial) test–retest reliability ranged from 0.74 to 0.87 for the control group and from 0.85 to 0.94 for the group with brain injury (Toglia, 1993). The Rasch statistical method was utilized to generate additional reliability measures, which are covered in the test manual. Parallel form reliability for prediction and strategy scores was also generated and is described in the test manual.

One study examined concurrent validity by correlating scores of standardized cognitive measures, including the CMT, with IADL performance as measured by the AMPS. The immediate recall from the CMT had a correlation of $r = 0.59$ with IADL performance (Kizony & Katz, 2002). Concurrent validity was also determined by examining the correlation between the CMT and RBMT. Correlations ranged from 0.80 to 0.84 (Toglia, 1993). The Rasch analysis was used to chart the individual abilities and item difficulties of the controls and brain injury participants. The results are described in the test manual.

Assessment Tools for Executive Functioning

Executive Function Performance Test (Baum & Wolf, 2013)

Description

The Executive Function Performance Test (EFPT) is a standardized assessment that has four subtests: simple cooking making oatmeal on a stovetop, telephone use, medication management, and bill paying (Figure 8-7). There is also an alternate version of the EFPT available that can be used to retest clients. Like the original test, it contains four tasks: cooking noodles, filling a pillbox with three prescriptions, using the telephone, and ordering from a catalog. The manuals for both the original and alternate forms of the EFPT are free online at http://www.ot.wustl.edu/about/resources/executive-function- performance-test-efpt-308

In 2018, Rand and colleagues described an internet-based format that they used for the telephone and paying bills tasks. For the telephone task, people were allowed to use Google to locate information instead of a telephone book. For the online bill-paying task, the researchers created a bill-pay simulation that is available for use at https://www.tau.ac.il/~portnoys/Internet-based_Bill_Paying_Task.html. It is increasingly common for people to complete information gathering and bill-paying tasks online, and these researchers wanted to create subtests that retained their ecological validity with changing technologies (Rand et al., 2018).

Procedure

Clients are asked several questions at the start of the assessment to gather information about their current participation in the four activities, including whether or not they complete the tasks and how frequently. They are also asked to predict how well they will do completing the subtests. Following the pretest questions, clients complete the four tasks in this order: simple cooking, telephone, taking medication, and paying bills. All tasks should be administered. The exception is the bill-paying subtest, which may be skipped if the person does not know how to use a checkbook. The EFPT uses dynamic assessment, with the administrator providing cueing in order to achieve best performance. Cueing guidelines, in addition to more detailed instructions, are included in the manual.

Scoring

Clients are scored on each subtest separately. Clinicians score clients' performance using a 6-point scale as follows: 0 = independent, 1 = verbal guidance, 2 = gestural guidance, 3 = verbal direct instruction, 4 = physical assistance, and 5 = done for the participant. Clients receive scores for the following behaviors: initiation or beginning the task; execution, which includes three areas (organization, sequencing, and judgment/safety); and completion. In addition, the time it takes participants to complete the activity is noted. Scores for each subtest are then summarized, and the actual performance is compared to the client's prediction.

Psychometric Properties

Inter-rater reliability ratings were found to have ICC ratings for the individual subtests that ranged from 0.79 to 0.94. The inter-rater reliability of the total EFPT scoring was ICC = 0.91 (Baum et al., 2008). In the same study, the EFPT was found to have internal consistency ratings of $\alpha = 0.77$ to 0.88 for the subtests and $\alpha = 0.94$ for the total test (Baum et al., 2008). Research with the alternate form found no statistically significant differences between it and the original EFPT (Hahn et al., 2014). In other studies, researchers compared the results of the original EFPT tasks with the internet-based tasks for 15 people with a CVA and 30 adults without neurological deficits. The results showed high correlation between the internet and paper versions of the two tasks, except in the time to complete the bill-paying task with participants needing more time for the internet version. The researchers also found that there was a difference in performance between the people with CVA and those without neurological deficits on the internet bill-paying task (Rand et al., 2018).

The EFPT was also shown to correlate with other tests of executive functions, including the Trail Making Test, Logical Memory Total Recall Test, and Digit Span Backward Test (Baum et al., 2008). In addition, it correlates with the AMPS (Cederfeldt et al., 2011).

Multiple Errands Test (Dawson et al., 2009)

Description

The Multiple Errands Test (MET) is a performance-based assessment that is designed to examine executive functioning as a person completes several tasks in a shopping center/mall or a hospital. Because it is meant to be used in a community or hospital setting, a site-specific version must be created by the examiner. The client also needs to be independent with functional mobility to complete the assessment. The MET consists of four sets of tasks. These include performing six specific errands (purchasing three items, using the telephone, sending a letter, and collecting an item from an office or the examiner), obtaining four pieces of information (e.g., the closing time of a business or the number of entrances/exits available), meeting the examiner at a specific time and place, and informing the examiner when the test is complete. The client must complete these tasks while adhering to nine rules (including money spending limits, not exiting the shopping center/hospital, not speaking to the examiner, and not entering any location twice). It takes approximately 60 minutes to complete the assessment.

Procedure

The client is given a sheet of paper that outlines the tasks that are to be completed and the rules that need to be followed. The client is also given a map of the area. The examiner follows the client during test administration but does not interact with the client.

Scoring

The examiner takes notes about whether or not tasks were completed correctly, which errors were made, and whether errors were caused by efficiency or interpretation failures. The client is also timed on several of the tasks. In addition, the examiner makes notes about the strategies that the client uses during the completion of the assessment, such as making notes, checking the map, and asking for directions.

Psychometric Properties

A number of studies examining the reliability and/or validity of the MET have been performed. The MET has been found to have an internal consistency rating of $\alpha = 0.77$ (Knight et al., 2002) and inter-rater reliability ratings of ICC = 0.71 to 1.0 (Dawson et al., 2009; Knight et al., 2002).

The MET has been shown to have good discriminative validity in distinguishing between a sample of people with ABI and a sample without any diagnosed neurological deficits (Alderman et al., 2003; Dawson et al., 2009; Knight et al., 2002; Rand et al., 2009). The MET correlates with other tests of executive functioning, including the IADL questionnaire (Rand et al., 2009) and the Dysexecutive Questionnaire (Alderman et al., 2003).

Weekly Calendar Planning Activity (Toglia, 2015)

Description

The Weekly Calendar Planning Activity (WCPA) is a standardized test of executive functioning. It was designed specifically for people who are independent in ADLs but who may still have executive dysfunction that creates difficulty in more complex or novel tasks. The minimum criteria for administering this assessment are basic orientation, sustained attention for at least 10 minutes, and the ability to follow written instructions. In this assessment, clients are asked to complete a weekly schedule of 17 to 18 appointments while adhering to several rules, keeping track of time, and ignoring distractors. To accomplish the task successfully, clients need to plan ahead.

The test has normative data and can be used with people 12 years old or older. It also has alternate forms available, so it can be used to reassess performance at a later date. It takes approximately 20 to 25 minutes to complete the assessment.

Procedure

There are three levels of difficulty for the assessment. Level I is designed for people who are functioning at a lower level. Level III is designed for clients who are functioning at an exceptionally high level. Level II is the most researched and commonly used level. In all levels, clients are asked to record appointments in a calendar without allowing any conflicts. At the same time, clients are asked to adhere to five rules: (a) they are not able to cross out any appointments once they are recorded in the calendar; (b) they need to track the time and tell the examiner when it is a specific time (7 minutes after the assessment is started); (c) they need to leave 1 day free of appointments (the day specified by the examiner depending on which version of the assessment is given); (d) they need to ignore questions from the examiner; and (e) they need to tell the examiner when they are finished. After the activity, the examiner conducts an interview in which the person is asked about strategies used during the task, changes that would be helpful to make for the future, and difficulties encountered. The person is also asked to rate their performance in several areas. The test manual provides additional details.

Scoring

The examiner makes note of how long it takes the client to record the first appointment, in addition to the total time taken to complete the task. During the assessment, the examiner records whether or not the client adheres to the five rules, while also making observations about any strategies the client employs (e.g., crossing out appointments after they are put into the calendar, talking aloud, crossing out the day that is to be kept free). After administration of the test, the examiner makes note of which appointments were entered and whether or not they were accurately recorded. If errors were made, the examiner also notes whether or not the client acknowledged the error. Total scores, which are acquired by adding up the number of missing appointments, accurately logged appointments, and errors, can be converted to percentiles to allow the client's performance to be compared to normative data.

Psychometric Properties

The WCPA was shown to have inter-rater reliability of 0.98 (Toglia & Berg, 2013). It also was found to have good discriminate validity for at-risk adolescents (Toglia & Berg, 2013).

Complex Task Performance Assessment (Wolf et al., 2011)

Description

The Complex Task Performance Assessment (CTPA) is a relatively new assessment, first described in the literature in 2008 by Wolf et al. It is designed to simulate novel and complex work-related tasks in order to document dysexecutive disorder, especially for those who have more mild cognitive impairment. The assessment simulates working in a library and completing two tasks simultaneously. The first task involves inventory control, with the client calculating fines for people who are late in returning materials to the simulated library. At the same time, clients need to take messages when the telephone rings and complete different actions depending on the caller and the content of the message. In addition, the client needs to follow a series of rules, including telling the examiner when 10 minutes have passed from the start of the assessment and when they

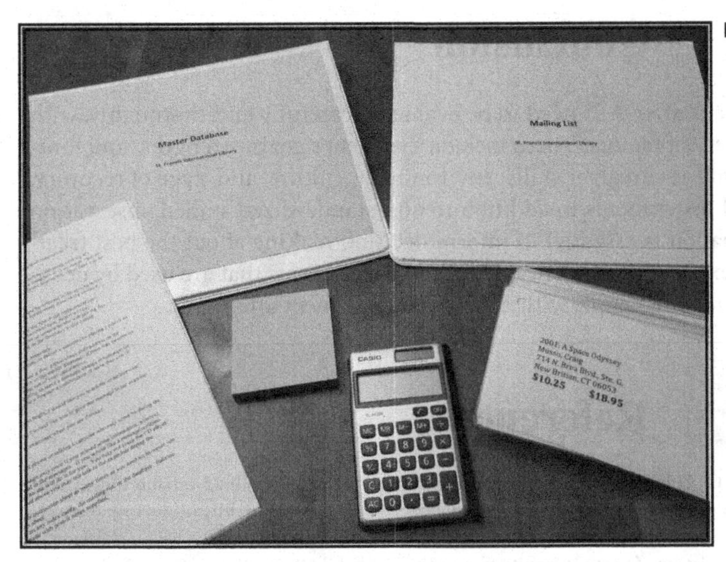

Figure 8-8. The materials of the CTPA.

have finished their tasks. Clients have up to 40 minutes to complete the activity. The manual for the CTPA is free (https://www.ot.wustl.edu/mm/files/CTPA.zip). Clinicians need to create the assessment kit (Figure 8-8).

Procedure

Before starting the assessment, clients are asked to rate their efficiency and frequency of using the telephone, completing calculations, attending appointments, and handling multiple tasks at once. At the end of the assessment, clients are asked to rate their performance. The test manual includes additional details.

Scoring

Examiners record the numbers of client errors in five areas: inefficiencies, rule breaks, interpretation failures, task failures, and inventory control accuracy. Errors from each category are summed with the task failures weighted more heavily than other categories. Qualitative observations of how people approach tasks are recorded as well, including strategies that are used.

Psychometric Properties

In a pilot study examining sensitivity of the assessment tool, researchers found significant differences in the performance of people with mild stroke ($n=6$) and healthy controls ($n=4$; Wolf et al., 2008). A larger psychometric study of the CTPA was published in 2017. These researchers found high intra-rater agreement with ICC values between 0.89 and 0.98. The ICC value for test–retest reliability was low at 0.475, indicating that participants learned how to complete the tasks between the first and second administration of the assessment. Concurrent validity was found between the Delis-Kaplan Executive Function System Color-Word Condition ($r=-.043$) and the Wechsler Test of Adult Reading ($r=-0.49$). Finally, the CTPA was able to distinguish between people who had mild dysexecutive disorder because of a CVA ($n=14$) and healthy controls ($n=20$; Wolf et al., 2017).

Conclusion

Clients with cognitive deficits after ABI need to be evaluated carefully and thoroughly, with the clinician considering a variety of factors. These include the client's goals, strengths, and limitations in addition to factors such as caregiver skills, environment, culture, and stage of recovery. A combination of standardized instruments in addition to non-standardized skilled observation of the client engaging in occupation is essential to inform decision making about the best treatment approaches to use. The next chapters describe a variety of treatments that are used by occupational therapy practitioners treating people with cognitive impairment after ABI.

References

Alderman, N., Burgess, P. W., Knight, C., & Henman, C. (2003). Ecological validity of a simplified version of the multiple errands shopping test. *Journal of the International Neuropsychological Society, 9*, 31-44. https://doi.org/10.1017/S1355617703910046

American Occupational Therapy Association. (2019). Cognition, cognitive rehabilitation, and occupational performance. *American Journal of Occupational Therapy, 73*, 7312410010. https://doi.org/10.5014/ajot.2019.73S201

American Occupational Therapy Association. (2020). Occupational therapy practice framework: Domain and process (4th ed.). *American Journal of Occupational Therapy, 74*(Suppl. 2), 7412410010. https://doi.org/10.5014/ajot.2020.74S2001

Árnadóttir, G. (1990). *The brain and behavior: Assessing cortical dysfunction through activities of daily living*. C.V. Mosby.

Árnadóttir, G. (2021). Impact of neurobehavioral deficits on activities of daily living. In G. Gillen & D. M. Nilsen (Eds.). *Stroke rehabilitation: A function-based approach* (5th ed., pp. 556-592). Elsevier.

Baum, C. M., Tabor Connor, L., Morrison, T., Hahn, M., Dromerick, A. W., & Edwards, D. F. (2008). Reliability, validity, and clinical utility of the Executive Function Performance Test: A measure of executive function in a sample of people with stroke. *American Journal of Occupational Therapy, 62*, 446-455. https://doi.org/10.5014/ajot.62.4.446

Baum, C. M., & Wolf, T. J. (2013). Executive Function Performance Test (EFPT). http://www.ot.wustl.edu/about/resources/executive-function-performance-test-efpt-308

Bogod, N. M., Mateer, C. A., & MacDonald, S. W. (2003). Self-awareness after traumatic brain injury: A comparison of measures and their relationship to executive functions. *Journal of the International Neuropsychological Society, 9*, 450-458. https://doi.org/10.1017/S1355617703930104

Brown, C., Rempfer, M., & Hamera, E. (2009). *The Test of Grocery Shopping Skills*. AOTA Press.

Burns, T. (2018). *Cognitive Performance Test (CPT)*. Maddak SP Ableware.

Cederfeldt, M., Widell, Y., Elgmark Andersson, E., Dahlin-Ivanoff, S., & Gosman-Hedstrom, G. (2011). Concurrent validity of the Executive Function Performance Test in people with mild stroke. *British Journal of Occupational Therapy, 74*, 443-449. https://doi.org/10.4276/030802211X13153015305673

Chisholm, D. (2005). *Disability in older adults with depression* [Unpublished doctoral dissertation]. University of Pittsburgh. http://d-scholarship.pitt.edu/9697/1/Chisholmd_etd2005.pdf

Chisholm, D., Toto, P., Raina, K., Holm, M., & Rogers, J. (2014). Evaluating capacity to live independently and safely in the community: Performance Assessment of Self-Care Skills. *British Journal of Occupational Therapy, 77*, 59-63. https://doi.org/10.4276/030802214X13916969447038

Dawson, D. R., Anderson, N. D., Burgess, P., Cooper, E., Krpan, K. M., & Stuss, D. T. (2009). Further development of the Multiple Errands Test: Standardized scoring, reliability, and ecological validity for the Baycrest version. *Archives of Physical Medicine and Rehabilitation, 90*, S41-51. https://doi.org/10.1016/j.apmr.2009.07.012

Dirette, D. P., & McCormack, G. L. (2021). Cognitive assessment. In D. P. Dirette & S. A. Gutman (Eds.), *Occupational therapy for physical dysfunction* (8th ed., pp. 143-160). Wolters Kluwer.

Erez, A. B.-H., & Katz, N. (2018). Cognitive functional evaluation. In N. Katz & J. Toglia (Eds.), *Cognition, occupation, and participation across the lifespan* (4th ed., pp. 69-85). AOTA Press.

Evans, C. C., Sherer, M., Nick, T. G., Nakase-Richardson, R., & Yablon, S. A. (2005). Early impaired self-awareness, depression, and subjective well-being following traumatic brain injury. *Journal of Head Trauma Rehabilitation, 20*, 488-500. https://doi.org/10.1097/00001199-200511000-00002

Fioravanti, A. M., Bordignon, C. M., Pettit, S. M., Woodhouse, L. J., & Ansley, B. J. (2012). Comparing the responsiveness of the Assessment of Motor and Process Skills and the Functional Independence Measure. *Canadian Journal of Occupational Therapy, 79*, 167-174. https://doi.org/10.2182/cjot.2012.79.3.6

Fisher, A. G., Griswold, L. A., & Kottorp, A. (2017). *Assessment of compared qualities — occupational performance (ACQ-OP) and assessment of compared qualities — social interaction (ACQ-SI)* (3rd ed.). Three Star Press.

Fisher, A. G., & Jones, K. B. (2011). *Assessment of Motor and Process Skills. Volume 1: Development, standardization, and administration manual* (7th ed., revised). Three Star Press, Inc.

Fisher, A. G., & Jones, K. B. (2014). *Assessment of Motor and Process Skill. Volume 2: User manual* (8th ed.). Three Star Press, Inc.

Fleming, J. M., Strong, J., & Ashton, R. (1996). Self-awareness of deficits in adults with traumatic brain injury: How best to measure? *Brain Injury, 10*, 1-15. https://doi.org/10.1080/026990596124674

Fleming, J. M., Winnington, H. T., McGillivray, A. J., Tatarevic, B. A., & Ownsworth, T. L. (2006). The development of self-awareness and emotional distress during early community re-integration after traumatic brain injury. *Brain Impairment, 7*, 83-94. https://doi.org/10.1375/brim.7.2.83

Gardarsdóttir, S., & Kaplan, S. (2002). Validity of the Árnadóttir OT-ADL Neurobehavioral Evaluation (A-ONE): Performance in activities of daily living and neurobehavioral impairments of persons with left and right hemisphere damage. *American Journal of Occupational Therapy, 56*, 499-508. https://doi.org/10.5014/ajot.56.5.499

Giles, G. M., Edwards, D. F., Morrison, M. T., Baum, C., & Wolf, T. J. (2017). Screening for functional cognition in post-acute care and the Improving Medicare Post-Acute Care Transformation (IMPACT) Act of 2014. *American Journal of Occupational Therapy, 71*, 7105090010. https://doi.org/10.5014/ajot.2017.715001

Gillen, G. (2009). *Cognitive and perceptual rehabilitation: Optimizing function*. Mosby.

Grieve, J., & Gnanasekaran, L. (2008). *Neuropsychology for occupational therapists: Cognition in occupational performance* (3rd ed.). Blackwell Publishing.

Hahn, B., Baum, C., Moore, J., Ehrlich-Jones, L., Spoeri, S., Doherty, M., & Wolf, T. J. (2014). Brief report—Development of additional tasks for the Executive Function Performance Test. *American Journal of Occupational Therapy, 68*, e241-e246. https://doi.org/10.5014/ajot.2014.00856

Haskins, E. C. (2012). *Cognitive rehabilitation manual: Translating evidence-based recommendations into practice*. American Congress of Rehabilitation Medicine.

Holm, M. B., & Rogers, J. C. (2008). The Performance Assessment of Self-Care Skills (PASS). In B. J. Hemphill-Pearson (Ed.), *Assessments in occupational therapy mental health* (2nd ed., pp. 73-82). SLACK Incorporated.

Itzkovich, M., Elazar, B., & Averbuch, S. (2000). *Loewenstein Occupational Therapy Cognitive Assessment (LOTCA) manual* (2nd ed.). Loewenstein Rehabilitation Hospital.

Katz, N., Baum, C. M., & Maeir, A. (2011). Introduction to cognitive intervention and cognitive functional evaluation. In N. Katz (Ed.), *Cognition, occupation, and participation across the life span: Neuroscience, neurorehabilitation, and models of intervention in occupational therapy* (3rd ed., pp. 3-12). AOTA Press.

Kizony, R., & Katz, N. (2002). Relationships between cognitive abilities and the process scale and skills of the Assessment of Motor and Process Skills (AMPS) in patients with stroke. *OTJR: Occupation, Participation, and Health, 22*, 82-92. https://doi.org/10.1177/153944920202200205

Knight, C., Alderman, N., & Burgess, P. W. (2002). Development of a simplified version of the Multiple Errands Test for use in hospital settings. *Neuropsychological Rehabilitation, 12*, 231-255. https://doi.org/10.1080/09602010244000039

Kohlman Thomson, L. (2016). *Kohlman Evaluation of Living Skills* (4th ed.). AOTA Press.

Lange, B., Spagnolo, K., & Fowler, B. (2009). Using the Assessment of Motor and Process Skills to measure functional change in adults with severe traumatic brain injury: A pilot study. *Australian Occupational Therapy Journal, 56*, 89-96. https://doi.org/10.1111/j.1440-1630.2007.00698.x

Maskill, L., & Tempest, S. (2017a). Assessment and measuring change. In L. Maskill & S. Tempest (Eds.), *Neuropsychology for occupational therapists: Cognition in occupational performance* (4th ed., pp. 17-31). Wiley Blackwell.

Maskill, L., & Tempest, S. (2017b). Intervention for cognitive impairments and evaluating outcomes. In L. Maskill & S. Tempest (Eds.), *Neuropsychology for occupational therapists: Cognition in occupational performance* (4th ed., pp. 33-49). Wiley Blackwell.

Miller, E. L., Murray, L., Richards, L, Zorowitz, R. D., Bakas, T., Clark, P., Billinger, S. A., on behalf of the American Heart Association Council on Cardiovascular Nursing and the Stroke Council. (2010). Comprehensive overview of nursing and interdisciplinary rehabilitation care of the stroke patient. *Stroke, 41*, 2402-2448. https://doi.org/10.1161/STR.0b013e3181e7512b

Radomski, M. V., & Morrison, M. T. (2014). Assessing abilities and capacities: Cognition. In M. V. Radomski & C. A. Trombly Latham (Eds.), *Occupational therapy for physical dysfunction* (7th ed., pp. 121-143). Lippincott Williams & Wilkins.

Rand, D., Ben-Haim, L., Malka, K., & Portnoy, S. (2018). Development of internet-based tasks for the Executive Function Performance Test. *American Journal of Occupational Therapy, 72*, 7202205060. https://doi.org/10.5014/ajot.2018.023598

Rand, D., Rukan, S., Weiss, P. L., & Katz, N. (2009). Validation of the Virtual MET as an assessment tool for executive functions. *Neuropsychological Rehabilitation, 19*, 583-602. https://doi.org/10.1080/09602010802469074

Robertson, I., Ward, T., Ridgeway, Y., & Nimmo-Smith, I. (1994). *Test of Everyday Attention.* Thames Valley Test.

Rogers, J. C., Holm, M. B., & Chisholm, D. (2016). *Performance Assessment of Self-Care Skills: Scoring guidelines.* University of Pittsburgh.

Sherer, M. (2004). The Awareness Questionnaire. The Center for Outcome Measurement in Brain Injury. http://www.tbims.org/combi/aq

Sherer, M., Bergloff, P., Boake, C., High, W., & Levin, E. (1998). The Awareness Questionnaire: Factor structure and internal consistency. *Brain Injury, 12*, 63-68. https://doi.org/10.1080/026990598122863

Sherer, M., Bergloff, P., Levin, E., High, W. M., Oden, K. E., & Nick, T.G. (1998). Impaired awareness and employment outcome after traumatic brain injury. *Journal of Head Trauma Rehabilitation, 13*, 52-61. https://doi.org/10.1097/00001199-199810000-00007

Sherer, M., Hart, T., & Nick, T. G. (2003). Measurement of impaired self-awareness after traumatic brain injury: A comparison of the Patient Competency Rating Scale and the Awareness Questionnaire. *Brain Injury, 17*, 25-37. https://doi.org/10.1080/0269905021000010113

Sohlberg, M. M., & Turkstra, L. S. (2011). *Optimizing cognitive rehabilitation: Effective instructional methods.* The Guilford Press.

Toglia, J. P. (1991). Generalization of treatment: A multicontext approach to cognitive perceptual impairment in adults with brain injury. *American Journal of Occupational Therapy, 45*, 505-516. https://doi.org/10.5014/ajot.45.6.505

Toglia, J. (1993). *Contextual Memory Test.* Therapy Skill Builders.

Toglia, J. P. (2005). A dynamic interactional approach to cognitive rehabilitation. In N. Katz (Ed.), *Cognition and occupation across the lifespan* (2nd ed., pp. 29-72). AOTA Press.

Toglia, J. P. (2015). *Weekly Calendar Planning Activity (WCPA): A performance test of executive function.* AOTA Press.

Toglia, J. P. (2018). The dynamic interactional model and the multicontext approach. In N. Katz & J. Toglia (Eds.), *Cognition, occupation, and participation across the lifespan* (4th ed., pp. 355-385). AOTA Press.

Toglia, J., & Berg, C. (2013). Performance-based measure of executive function: Comparison of community and at-risk youth. *American Journal of Occupational Therapy, 67*, 517-523. https://doi.org/10.5014/ajot.2013.008482

Vanbellingen, T., Kersten, B., Van Hemelrijk, B., Van de Winckel, A., Bertschi, M., Müri, R., De Weerdt, W., & Bohlhalter, S. (2010). Comprehensive assessment of gesture production: A new test of upper limb apraxia (TULIA). *European Journal of Neurology, 17*, 59-66. https://doi.org/10.1111/j.1468-1331.2009.02741.x

Weinstock-Zlotnick, G., & Hinojosa, J. (2004). The issue is: Bottom-up or top-down evaluation: Is one better than the other? *American Journal of Occupational Therapy, 58*, 594-599. https://doi.org/10.5014/ajot.58.5.594

Wilson, B. A., Greenfield, E., Clare, L., Baddeley, A., Cockburn, J., Watson, P., Tate, R., Sopena, S., & Nannery, R. (2008). *Rivermead Behavioural Memory Test—Third Edition (RBMT-3).* Pearson Assessment.

Wise, K., Ownsworth, T., & Fleming, J. (2005). Convergent validity of self-awareness measures and their association with employment outcome in adults following acquired brain injury. *Brain Injury, 19*, 765-775. https://doi.org/10.1080/0269905050019977

Wolf, T. J., Dahl, A., Auen, C., & Doherty, M. (2017). The reliability and validity of the Complex Task Performance Assessment: A performance-based assessment of executive function. *Neuropsychological Rehabilitation, 27*, 707-721. https://doi.org/10.1080/09602011.2015.1037771

Wolf, T. J., Morrison, T., & Matheson, L. (2008). Initial development of a work-related assessment of dysexecutive syndrome: The Complex Task Performance Assessment. *Work, 31*, 221-228. https://doi.org/10.1037/t71440-000

Wolf, T. J., Morrison, T., & Matheson, L. (2011). Complex Task Performance Assessment (CTPA) testing packet. https://www.ot.wustl.edu/mm/files/CTPA.zip

Chapter 9

Overview of Cognitive Treatment

As mentioned in Chapter 8, when evaluating perception and cognition for people with brain injury, there are many factors that need to be considered. Some of these factors will be assessed directly through the evaluation of the people themselves, such as their goals, their ability to learn and retain information, and the types of strategies that influence performance. Other key information, such as which aspects of a person's environment will likely support and which will likely hinder a person's occupational performance, may need to be gathered in other ways, such as through interviews with family members or observation. These same factors need to be considered when designing a treatment plan because they have a significant impact on the types of treatments that will be most appropriate for clients. This chapter provides an overview of the decision-making process occupational therapy practitioners follow in designing treatment plans for clients with perceptual and cognitive deficits after brain injury. Details of intervention strategies are described further in Chapter 10.

General Approaches to Treatment

Treatment for people with perceptual and cognitive impairments has historically fallen into one of two categories, remedial or adaptive, and some authors and researchers still discuss treatment in this way. More recently, the two approaches have been considered to be on different ends of the same continuum. Contemporary treatment often uses principles of each approach in a more blended way, with the recognition that compensation for cognitive deficits may enable people to improve their ability to use their remaining cognitive skills (Maskill & Tempest, 2017b). No matter the treatment approach, the underlying goal of the occupational therapy practitioner working in cognitive rehabilitation is to address functional cognition, which focuses on how the client's deficits impact occupational performance and how that occupational performance can be improved (Radomski & Giles, 2021).

Kaminsky, T. A., & Powell, J. M.
Zoltan's Vision, Perception, and Cognition: Evaluation and Treatment of the Adult With Acquired Brain Injury, Fifth Edition (pp. 237-262).

Remedial Approach

When practitioners use a remedial approach, they focus their interventions on attempting to improve the impairments and restore the abilities that underlie the client's occupational performance dysfunction. This approach is sometimes referred to as a *bottom-up method of rehabilitation* (Maskill & Tempest, 2017b; World Health Organization, 2008). The remedial approach is based on neuroanatomical and neurophysiological models of learning (Constantinidou & Thomas, 2018) and focuses treatment on directly changing the individual's psychological, cognitive, and neurobehavioral capabilities (Maskill & Tempest, 2017b; World Health Organization, 2008). The goal of this treatment approach in the area of cognitive/perceptual interventions is to improve the client's ability to take in, process, understand, retain, and use information, ultimately leading to increased functioning (Maskill & Tempest, 2017b; World Health Organization, 2008). The underlying belief is that the brain has the capacity to repair itself after injury by reestablishing synaptic connection, growing new synapses, or having a healthy part of the brain take over the functions of the damaged tissues. With this approach, it is believed that this healing process can be supported by directly treating the impairments themselves (Maskill & Tempest, 2017b). Research on neuroplasticity lends support to this assumption.

Traditionally, the remedial treatment approach involved repeated cognitive/perceptual exercises performed in the occupational therapy clinic. An example of this approach is the cognitive-didactic intervention used by Vanderploeg and colleagues (2008) in a randomized controlled trial that compared this approach with a functional-experiential intervention (described later). Clients receiving the cognitive-didactic treatment practiced paper-and-pencil and/or computerized cognitive tasks focused on improving attention, memory, executive functions, and pragmatic communication. (Speech-language pathologists were also part of the treatment team.) There was an emphasis on trial-and-error problem solving and building self-awareness during the treatment sessions, with practitioners helping the participants analyze their own behavior. This was accomplished through techniques such as questioning participants about their performance, including the number and types of errors, and ways that they could improve. Therapy was provided in 1:1 treatment sessions in an officelike setting. The practitioner gradually increased the difficulty of the treatment tasks based on the participant's performance.

One assumption underlying this type of approach is that the restoration of specific client factors and performance skills will generalize to actual improvement of occupational performance itself. The results of research studies testing this assumption are mixed. Vanderploeg and colleagues (2008) found that participants in the cognitive-didactic treatment group reported fewer memory problems than those in the functional-experiential group at the 1-year follow-up. The two groups had similar improvements in functional outcomes of independent living and return to work or school. Other researchers have stated that a remedial approach focusing solely on client factors has a limited direct effect on improving independence with functional activities and does not generalize well beyond the areas focused on in treatment (Cicerone et al., 2019). As a result of this concern, along with a recent shift in the occupational therapy profession toward a greater emphasis on occupation-based treatment, many occupational therapy practitioners have moved to replace worksheets and other types of cognitive/perceptual exercises with occupation-based activities in more naturalistic environments (Radomski & Giles, 2021). For example, if treating a client with visuospatial impairment who repairs computers for a living, a contemporary clinician using the remedial approach would be less likely to complete activities using parquetry blocks and copying block designs, as might have been done in the past (Figure 9-1). Instead, the practitioner would address the deficit by having the client work on repairing computers (Figure 9-2). The goal is still to facilitate visuospatial skills, but the therapy task is occupation based. The hope remains that the client's performance would more easily transfer to other, unrelated tasks. More research is needed to evaluate the effects of this shift in the remedial approach.

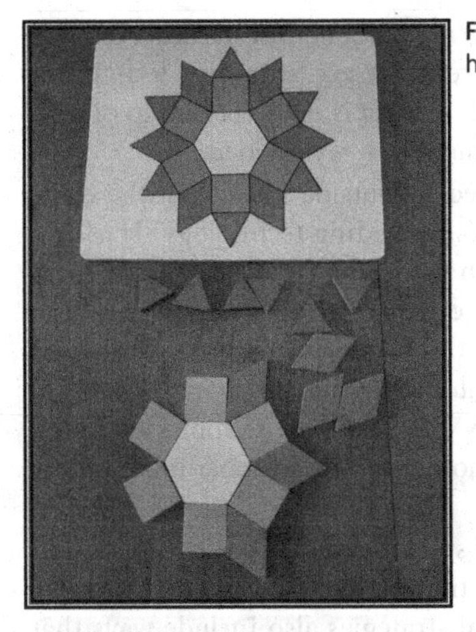

Figure 9-1. Parquetry block activity. Activities such as these have been used historically to work on remediation of skills such as spatial relations.

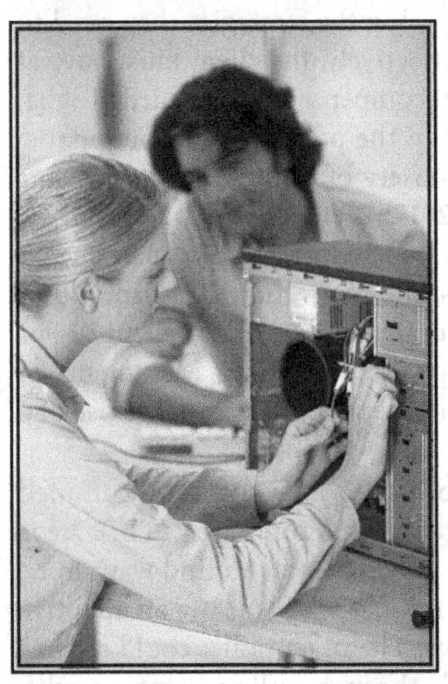

Figure 9-2. An occupationally based treatment activity, such as computer repair for individuals who engaged in this occupation pre-injury, can be used to work on visuospatial skills with clients. (Phovoir/shutterstock.com)

Adaptive, or Compensatory, Approach

The adaptive, or compensatory, approach is a top-down approach that focuses on methods that allow for effective occupational performance despite the presence of deficits and environmental and/or task demands that exceed the client's skills or abilities. When focusing on an adaptive approach, practitioners do not directly focus on remediating the person's underlying cognitive skills but are instead working to teach the person skills and/or make adaptations to the task or environment that can be used to circumvent the impact of the existing deficits (Maskill & Tempest, 2017b). An adaptive approach is appropriate in several different situations. Clinicians may use an adaptive approach at the conclusion of remedial treatment to bridge the gap between the client's occupational performance and any abilities that have not been recovered or restored completely. In other instances, clinicians may use an adaptive approach during a course of remedial treatment to make it possible for the client to perform everyday tasks while improvement in underlying impairments takes place through targeted remedial treatment and/or natural recovery (Constantinidou & Thomas, 2018). Finally, in situations when remediation is neither desired nor indicated (e.g., because of insufficient time or resources or when a client is not expected to benefit from remediation), an adaptive approach may be the sole treatment that is provided.

Compensation can be external, such as assistance provided by outside sources in the environment (people or objects and other types of assistive devices, including technology; Haskins, 2012; Radomski & Giles, 2021). These can include things such as cueing by a caregiver, timers set on smartphones, signs indicating the location of needed objects, or having a caregiver reduce the number of steps in a cooking activity. In some instances, these external compensations are temporary in nature, and, in others, there may be a permanent environmental change. External compensations can also include changes in client and/or family expectations (Radomski & Giles, 2021). An example of this would be to delegate bill paying to another family member if the task is too complex for a person who has had a stroke.

Compensation can also be internal, with the client using strategies for thinking about and approaching a task that allow them to take in and use information more effectively despite their impairments (Haskins, 2012; Radomski & Giles, 2021). Internal strategies also include ways that a client can "think about their thinking" to make sure they are using the strategies they need to be effective. In order to use internal compensation techniques effectively, the client must have at least some awareness of their existing deficits and understand that compensation is needed (Toglia, 2018). Strategies are most successful when they are overlearned to the point of being automatic. In addition, compensation strategies should be practiced in a variety of different environments to encourage the generalization of skills (Maskill & Tempest, 2017b). The choice and design of different types of compensations are based on a variety of factors, including activity analysis and client considerations, such as learning style, cognitive capabilities, and motivation. It is also helpful to consider successful strategies that the client used before the brain injury (Haskins, 2012). For example, many people now use computer-based calendars to help with scheduling. Making use of a similar system after brain injury may prove to be helpful for the client because it makes use of a familiar, premorbid strategy.

Consider this example of how the adaptive approach could be used with a client. Mohammed is a 45-year-old man with attention and memory deficits after traumatic brain injury (TBI). He is having difficulty with grocery shopping as a result of these deficits and wants to find ways to be more independent with this task. An occupational therapy practitioner who is using an adaptive approach with Mohammed could suggest a variety of possibilities. The practitioner could recommend that Mohammed change the grocery shopping task itself through online shopping with delivery or by going to the store more frequently (e.g., when he only needs to purchase 10 or fewer items) to minimize the steps he needs to complete with each shopping trip. The practitioner could focus on the physical environment and suggest that Mohammed shop at the same, small grocery store each time (preferably one that does not play loud background music) and always go at off-peak times to avoid the distraction and overstimulation of a more crowded store. The practitioner could use Mohammed's social environment and suggest that his spouse go with him each time to push the cart so Mohammed can focus on locating each item. Mohammed could also be taught to use compensatory strategies that will help him work around his attention difficulties and memory loss. One example of an external strategy would be for Mohammed to follow a written shopping list each time. The list might be even more helpful if it is created to match the layout of the store. An example of an internal strategy would be for Mohammed to take a break in the middle of his shopping trip and check the contents of the cart against his shopping list to make sure he is still on target (Figure 9-3).

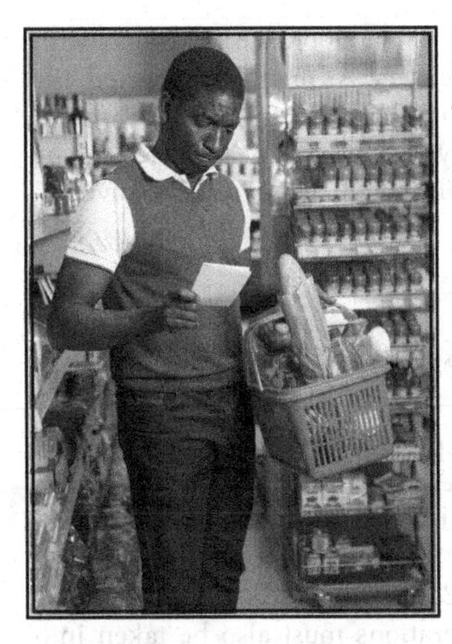

Figure 9-3. Using and double-checking a list while grocery shopping can help compensate for cognitive impairments, including impaired memory or attention. (BearFotos/shutterstock.com)

Functional Model

One of the challenges of the remediation/adaptation delineation is that the distinction between the two approaches is not always clear. As a result, they are sometimes described as parts of the same continuum (Katz, 2018; Sohlberg & Turkstra, 2011). For example, it is possible that a person who uses a compensatory strategy to overcome memory deficits (consistent with the adaptive approach) will have an improvement in memory skills themselves (the goal of the remediation approach). Another challenge is that it is rare for practitioners to use only one approach in practice. Instead, as noted previously, a hybrid approach is often used, with treatment activities from both approaches being used simultaneously or sequentially. As a result, a third approach to cognitive treatment has emerged called the *functional model of cognitive rehabilitation*, which combines treatment strategies from the remedial and adaptive approaches (Maskill & Tempest, 2017b). For example, in a review by Cicerone and colleagues (2019), the authors recommended that cognitive rehabilitation for people with attention deficits "should incorporate both direct-attention training and metacognitive training to increase task performance and promote generalization to daily functioning" (p. 1518). This recommendation includes aspects of both the remedial approach (direct attention training) and the adaptive approach (development of compensatory strategies) consistent with the functional approach to cognitive rehabilitation.

Functional-Experiential Approach

Another cognitive treatment approach, sometimes called *functional-experiential treatment*, focuses on improving a person's ability to perform valued tasks without making a distinction between remediation and compensation (Vanderploeg et al., 2008). A practitioner using a functional-experiential approach sets up each therapy session so that a client can perform a specified task with as few errors as possible. This is done through simplifying the task being trained; structuring the environment; providing external compensatory devices, such as checklists; anticipating possible errors; and giving sufficient direction and cues to keep the task performance on track (Vanderploeg et al., 2008). If the client's functional performance improves, the practitioner gradually changes the task so more complex skills are used. As described in more detail in Chapter 10, errorless learning approaches such as this assume that making errors is not beneficial to learning after brain injury. As such, it is often a primary treatment approach for clients with more severe brain injuries who do not experience substantial recovery. As might be expected, the functional-experiential approach does not include strategies to help the client gain self-awareness of the impact of their impairments or any other type of self-analysis. This type of approach can be used in both group and individual treatment with sessions typically conducted in real-life environments or environments that are as close to real-life as possible.

Factors Influencing Treatment

As discussed in Chapter 8, decisions about cognitive/perceptual rehabilitation depend on a variety of factors, including the person's goals and prior abilities, caregiver concerns, the health and safety of the client, where the client is in recovery, current functioning, insight and awareness, and the type of setting (Haskins, 2012; Maskill & Tempest, 2017a). The potential for neuroplasticity (Schenkman et al., 2013), a client's learning ability (Wolf & Josman, 2015), and capacity for retaining information (Haskins, 2012), and behavioral considerations must also be taken into account when making choices about how best to intervene because these can have a major impact on the effectiveness of treatment. In addition, the consideration of environmental influences, including those in the client's social environment, is essential during treatment because these will have an impact on the skills clients need to have in order to function at their highest potential in their everyday lives (American Occupational Therapy Association [AOTA], 2020).

Neuroplasticity

The term *neuroplasticity* refers to the nervous system's ability to change (Lundy-Ekman, 2018). Neuroplasticity provides a way for the nervous system to adjust in response to learning and also provides the means to recover, at least in part, after damage (Lundy-Ekman, 2018; Schenkman et al., 2013). In the past 50 years, there has been increasing recognition that the adult brain maintains some capacity for change and adaptation to insult. It is only recently, however, that the underlying mechanisms of this plasticity, as well as the effect rehabilitation can have on plasticity, have been better understood. Neuroplasticity has been studied through the observation of behavioral changes after injury, neuroimaging, and the examination of microscopic changes in neural tissue (Schenkman et al., 2013).

Brain plasticity appears to result from a variety of different mechanisms. On a chemical level, adjustments can be made in neurotransmitter release, with presynaptic neurons releasing greater or fewer numbers of neurotransmitters based on signaling in the brain (Schenkman et al., 2013; Figure 9-4). Several structural changes are also components of neuroplasticity. Postsynaptic neurons can change the number of receptors that are available, making the neuron more or less responsive to neurotransmitters that are present. The process by which more receptors are made available is called *upregulation*, whereas the process by which fewer receptors are available is called *downregulation* (Figure 9-5). The adjustment of receptors available on postsynaptic neurons may be temporary or more permanent (Schenkman et al., 2013). More permanent changes in the makeup of the brain require more complex changes in the structure of the neural tissues. This happens through changes in the neurons themselves. To increase responsiveness and strengthen connections, neurons can increase the numbers and length of dendrites to allow more surface area for receptors and, therefore, more responsiveness to input. The structure of the axons can also be adjusted with changes in axonal branching (Schenkman et al., 2013). For example, if a neuron is sending messages frequently, it can increase its number of axonal branches, thus enabling it to

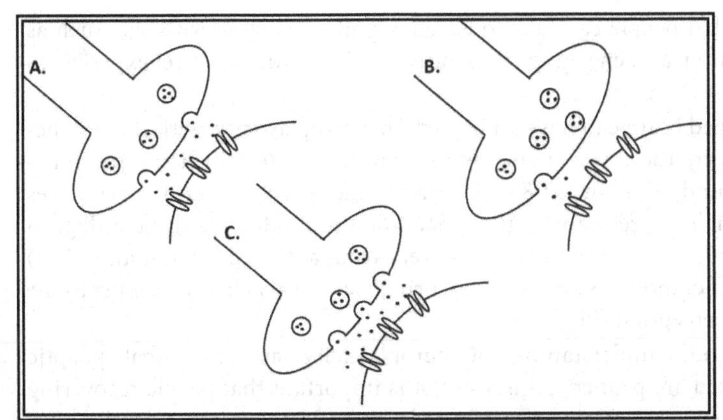

Figure 9-4. One way neurons change functioning is through changes in neurotransmitter release. From a (A) baseline level of neurotransmitter release, a neuron can release (B) less or (C) more neurotransmitters. In this case, the change in signaling comes from the presynaptic neuron.

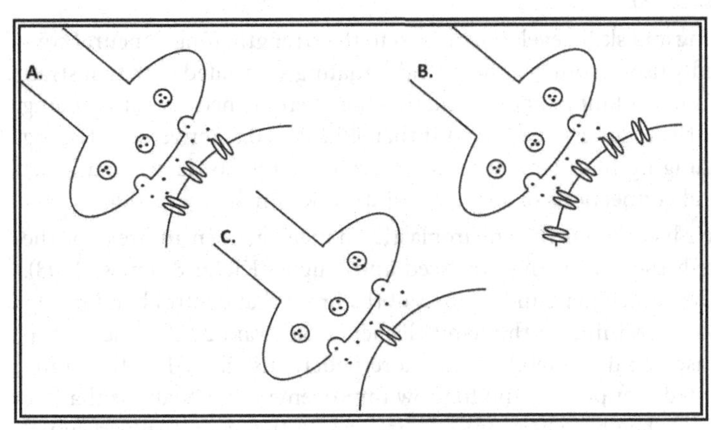

Figure 9-5. Neurons can change signaling on the postsynaptic side as well. In this case, the receiving neuron changes responsiveness from (A) baseline by changing the number of neurotransmitter receptors that are available. (B) Increasing the number of receptors will increase the postsynaptic neuron's responsiveness to the released neurotransmitter. (C) Decreasing the number of receptors will decrease responsiveness.

communicate with more postsynaptic neurons. This pattern of change to dendrites and axons results in adjustment in synaptic connectivity and is the cause of most permanent neuroplasticity (Schenkman et al., 2013). When signals are consistently sent through one set of neurons, the connections along that pathway will be increased and strengthened. This is called *long-term potentiation*. When a pathway is not used regularly, the synaptic connections are eliminated through pruning, which is also called *long-term depression* (Schenkman et al., 2013). This is the process that is described by the phrase "the neurons that fire together, wire together," which is paraphrased from an article published by Lowell and Singer in 1992.

Neuroplasticity is the phenomenon that underlies learning and memory formation. It also has an important role to play after the brain is damaged, using the same mechanisms that are used in nontraumatic neural change (Kleim & Jones, 2008; Lundy-Ekman, 2018; Schenkman et al., 2013). For example, after cortical damage, surviving neurons in a network make changes to increase their synaptic connectivity, such as by creating additional receptors on postsynaptic cells or increasing presynaptic release of neurotransmitters to compensate for lost neural input (Lundy-Ekman, 2018). Research has also demonstrated that these changes in dendritic growth after cortical injury are associated with a change in functional outcome (Kolb & Gibb, 2008). Neuroimaging studies have also shown that there is cortical reorganization after brain injury, with adjacent areas expanding into the area of damage. In this case, adjacent cortical areas can assist with functions previously accomplished by the damaged area (Grady & Kapur, 1999). Neuroplasticity occurs throughout the lifespan, although it does become less efficient as people age, which, when combined with other age-related cortical changes, slows learning and cognitive processing for older adults (Vance &

Crowe, 2006). There are steps that people can take to lessen cognitive slowing with age, such as through physical activity, nutrition, and engaging in cognitively stimulating or novel experiences (Vance & Crowe, 2006)

Rehabilitation of the damaged brain can have an impact on neuroplasticity, with the restructuring of the brain influenced by the sensory and motor experiences to which the person is exposed (Kolb & Gibb, 2008; Lundy-Ekman, 2018). Kleim and Jones (2008) described principles of neuroplasticity, many of which are relevant to the rehabilitation of adults with neurological injury. Most of the research about neuroplasticity and recovery from acquired brain injury (ABI) has focused on the rehabilitation of motor skills, but these principles are also likely to apply to the rehabilitation of cognitive and perceptual skills.

- Use it or lose it: Advances in the understanding of neuroplasticity have shown that synaptic connections that are not used are pruned. As a result, it is important that people recovering from ABI use the skills they need to retain or gain in order to build or preserve adaptive neural circuitry (Kleim & Jones, 2008).
- Use it and improve it: Training and skill development lead to the strengthening of neural connections. If a person repeatedly uses a strategy, the neural signaling associated with that strategy will be strengthened. It is important to understand that the strengthened neural signaling will occur with any skill that is regularly used even if that skill is maladaptive. Reinforcing functional skills and discouraging maladaptive ones, especially early (see later), can assist with strengthening the neural connections of adaptive abilities (Kleim & Jones, 2008).
- Specificity matters: Research has shown that neuroplastic changes happen in areas of the brain that are associated with the skill being practiced and taught (Kleim & Jones, 2008). For example, with motor recovery, changes in the areas of the brain that control hand movement are altered with dexterity training in the hand (Fisher & Sullivan, 2001). The link to cognition is less clear because cognition tends to be more widely distributed in the brain, although research has indicated that people tend to show improvement in situations that are most similar to those in which they have been trained, indicating that cognitive/perceptual rehabilitation in context may be important (Boman et al., 2004). One way in which this can be seen with cognition relates to context-dependent memory. People often have an easier time recalling information when they are in the same environment in which they formed the memory. You may have experienced this yourself if you have ever walked from your living room into your kitchen to retrieve something but find yourself struggling to recall what it was that you wanted. You may have triggered your memory by returning to the living room where the memory was initially formed. When surrounded by the context in which the memory was encoded (i.e., the living room), you are better able to remember what you wanted from the kitchen. The phenomenon of context-dependent memory has been supported by research. In 1975, Godden and Baddeley published a study describing an experiment they had performed with scuba divers. The divers were given a list of words to memorize on land and a second list to memorize underwater. When asked to recall the words, those learned on land were more easily remembered on land, whereas those learned underwater were more easily recalled underwater (Godden & Baddeley, 1975). A 2001 meta-analysis supported this finding, indicating that context does influence recall of information, although the influence of context could be lessened depending on the memory encoding strategies that were used (Smith & Vela, 2001).
- Repetition is important: Practice is essential for true neuroplasticity to occur because it is repetition, with its consistent neural firing, that enables the strengthening of signals (Kleim & Jones, 2008). It takes time and reinforcement for permanent changes in neural signaling and, therefore, synaptic connectivity to take place (Fisher & Sullivan, 2001).

- Intensity: More intense rehabilitation can promote neuroplasticity by more strongly reinforcing neural connections (Kleim & Jones, 2008). However, one caveat is that rehabilitation that is too intensive very early in recovery may cause further neurological damage. A systematic review by Coleman and colleagues (2018) reported that a couple of studies found worse outcomes for clients who had intensive therapy in the first 24 hours after stroke. There is not agreement on whether or not this is a consistent finding, and there is, in fact, research showing that early intense treatment is beneficial if started in the first 2 weeks after stroke, although caution is recommended in the first 24 hours of stroke recovery (Coleman et al., 2018). Much of the available research has focused on physically oriented interventions and outcomes. For example, one study suggested that people with a cerebrovascular accident who received more intensive therapy in the intensive care unit had positive effects on long-term outcomes, such as independence with activities of daily living (ADLs) and walking ability (Hu et al., 2010). Similar results have been found for early and intensive therapy for people with TBI, at least for physical outcomes. The impact on cognitive functioning is less clear (Cifu et al., 2003).
- Timing: Treatment given shortly after ABI onset has been shown to be more effective than that given after a delay (Kleim & Jones, 2008), with an improvement in functional outcomes for people who receive rehabilitation early in the recovery process (Cifu et al., 2003; Hu et al., 2010; Rief et al., 2021). As a result, rehabilitation should ideally start early in the recovery process to achieve maximal effect, although, as described previously, caution should be taken with highly intense therapy in the first 24 hours. An added benefit of treatment starting early is that it gives less time for maladaptive strategies to be reinforced with associated neuroplastic changes. Although maximal gains are often found early in the recovery process, it is important to note that people can still make gains with corresponding changes in neural activity in the chronic stages of brain injury, which is typically defined as more than 6 months postinjury (e.g., Carvalho et al., 2018; Ferris et al., 2018).
- Meaningfulness: Using activities that are meaningful during the rehabilitation process improves skill acquisition and retention (Kleim & Jones, 2008). A meta-analysis published by Park and colleagues in 2015 compared outcomes of cognitive rehabilitation for people with TBI when occupation-based treatment was used as opposed to more rote activities. The authors analyzed nine randomized controlled trials and found that there were statistically significantly better gains in mental function, ADLs, and psychosocial functioning (e.g., spirituality) when occupation-based treatment was used, although the effect size was small with all outcomes (Park et al., 2015) and, thus, must be interpreted with caution.
- Interference: Once a skill is learned, it can be extremely difficult to "unlearn" the skill and replace it with another because of the neural signaling pattern that has been created (Kleim & Jones, 2008). As a result, maladaptive compensatory strategies that are used after ABI can be difficult for clients to stop using, which is another reason why early rehabilitation before maladaptive skills develop is important and supports the use of errorless learning for some individuals.

It is important for the occupational therapy practitioner to have an appreciation of neuroplasticity and brain recovery in order to understand how to stimulate functional recovery. If the practitioner can understand the structural changes associated with functional recovery, including the previously discussed principles of neuroplasticity, then interventions that can promote functional skill development can be used in a way that better promotes neurorecovery.

Learning Capacity

Learning is a complex process and one that relies on numerous skills, including motor (e.g., for physically manipulating objects necessary to learn some tasks or orient one's body toward relevant input), sensory (e.g., for clearly seeing incoming information), and cognitive (e.g., for processing and remembering details) skills. The client's ability to learn is central to rehabilitation and performance outcome. In fact, learning underpins or subserves much of the recovery that occurs after brain injury (Wolf & Josman, 2015). The physical, cognitive, and sensory deficits that occur as a result of ABI often limit many of the usual mechanisms of learning (Wolf & Josman, 2015). Clients with cognitive deficits, such as decreased attention and memory, will have an especially difficult time learning and following directions during intervention because they may miss and/or fail to retain important information (Wolf & Josman, 2015). The rate at which the client is able to learn will affect how quickly rehabilitation goals are met, which will, in turn, affect the duration and cost of care (Wolf & Josman, 2015). Learning will also impact the client's independence. When thinking about learning and independence, some researchers differentiate between true learning and training (Sabari, 2011). Training results from memorization and is predictable and inflexible. It results in the same behavior every time. Training can be useful if a client is going to be performing a specific skill in a specific location, such as completing an ADL routine at home or in a residential care facility. On the other hand, learning leads to people being able to develop their own solutions to problems and apply those solutions to numerous situations. True learning results in flexibility and generalization (Sabari, 2011).

As a result of the influence of learning on rehabilitation and ultimate independence, the client's learning capacity and potential must be considered when making decisions about cognitive/perceptual rehabilitation (Wolf & Josman, 2015). To determine learning capacity and learning potential, the practitioner should have a basic understanding of specific types of learning and what may impede or facilitate the learning process. A basic overview of learning follows. A comprehensive detailed review is not within the scope of this book, and the reader is encouraged to refer to the references and seek out additional information on the topic.

There are two major types of learning: declarative and nondeclarative (Sohlberg & Mateer, 2001). Declarative learning encompasses conscious awareness and the ability to explicitly report, or declare, information that has been learned. This information may be semantic, which includes facts, or episodic, which refers to personal, autobiographical experiences. To illustrate the difference, imagine learning how to cook. Semantic learning is important for being able to measure and calculate ingredients (e.g., being able to determine which measuring cups to use when a recipe calls for 3/4 cup of flour). Episodic learning will be important for providing context to the cooking activity and for adding personal meaning, such as when learning how to make a family recipe from a grandparent. Declarative learning, both semantic and episodic, is a conscious process, and mistakes will provide valuable experiences for this type of learning (Sohlberg & Turkstra, 2011). For example, if a person learning to bake burns a batch of cookies because they were in the oven too long, they can take steps to avoid the same mistake in the future, such as by setting a timer to check the cookies earlier. Declarative memory is mediated by the hippocampus and medial temporal lobes and may be damaged in ABI (Sohlberg & Mateer, 2001; Figure 9-6). As a result, for many people with ABI, the ability to improve by using declarative learning is negatively impacted, and learning may happen better through nondeclarative learning.

Nondeclarative learning (also known as *procedural learning*) is implicit, which means that it is on a subconscious level. This type of learning results in actions and activities being performed in a more automatic or routine manner (Sohlberg & Mateer, 2001). This type of learning can be observed in many of the daily activities that people perform. For example, think about the routine you follow when you shower. You likely complete the steps of the activity in the same way each time. You may wash your hair with shampoo, rinse, put conditioner in, and then go on to soaping

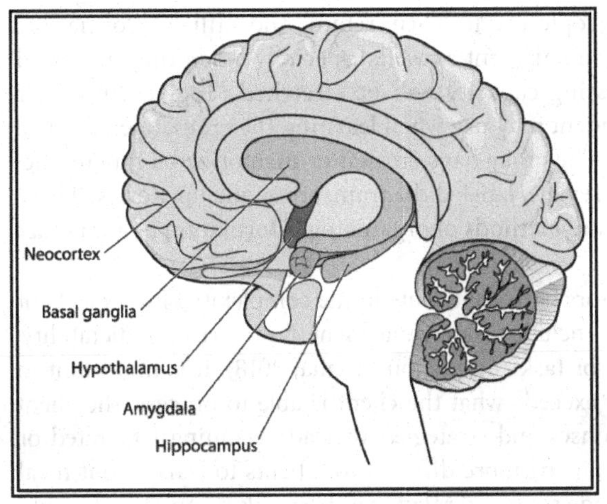

Figure 9-6. The hippocampus and medial temporal lobe are important for declarative memory. (Blamb/shutterstock.com)

your body before rinsing the conditioner back out of your hair. The completion of the activity happens on a subconscious level, which can be observed when the routine is interrupted. For example, imagine that your roommate accidently turns the bathroom light off for a moment while you are in the shower, startling you. When the light is turned back on, you may find that you are not certain where you are in your routine. This happens because your learning and, therefore, your memories of how to shower are largely implicit. Nondeclarative learning may be preserved in people with ABI even with more severe injuries. Therefore, it can be used to help improve independence for clients (Sohlberg & Mateer, 2001). Two of the strategies that can facilitate nondeclarative learning are priming (i.e., when the person's brain is prepared for incoming information; spaced retrieval is a type of priming) and errorless learning (Sohlberg & Mateer, 2001). These strategies are discussed further in Chapter 10.

There are many factors that can impede or facilitate the learning capacity of clients with ABI. Medication use, mood, anxiety, and stress can all affect the client's learning potential (Wolf & Josman, 2015). The time of day the client is asked to perform will affect learning capacity because of issues such as fatigue. Toglia (2018) identified six factors pertinent to the learning and generalization process: (a) functional processing capacity, (b) personal context, (c) self-awareness and metacognition, (d) cognitive strategies, (e) activity demands, and (f) environmental factors. She further believes that performance is the result of the interaction among these factors (Toglia, 2018).

Functional processing capacity refers to the person's ability to use their cognitive skills effectively, which will impact their ability to learn. It can be affected by numerous factors, including age and severity of ABI, task demands, and environmental factors (Toglia, 2018). This should be assessed during the occupational therapy evaluation, including determining how the person's functional cognition is influenced by the practitioner's actions (e.g., cueing). Practitioners who use the dynamic interactional approach specifically consider this interplay among different factors (Toglia, 2018). See Chapter 8 for more information about this approach.

Personal context includes aspects of clients themselves that may influence learning. These can include personality, frustration tolerance, values, and motivation, among others (Toglia, 2018). Personal factors may be premorbid or may be new after ABI. For example, behavioral issues are common after TBI and can affect learning (discussed further later).

Self-awareness and metacognition are complex phenomena that heavily influence how much people are able to learn and how what they have learned will generalize (Toglia, 2018). Self-awareness will also influence motivation. A person who is unaware of deficits and how those deficits can influence functioning may not appreciate the rationale for learning strategies or techniques to overcome deficits and, therefore, lack motivation for using those strategies.

Cognitive strategies are the tools that people use to learn, retain, and utilize information. These are used by people without cognitive impairment as well, especially when they are faced with a situation in which functional processing capacity will be stretched (Toglia, 2018). For example, think about the strategies that a student may use when learning the cranial nerves. The student likely used a variety of tools to help. They may have created or memorized a mnemonic, made flash cards to assist with repetition or review, labeled diagrams, or made up stories. These are all examples of cognitive strategies. They are methods of organizing information in a way that makes it easier to retain or learn.

Activity demands and environmental factors both contribute to the complexity of what a client needs to learn. Some of the factors to consider include task arrangement, familiarity, predictability, and the number of items and steps required for task completion (Toglia, 2018). It is important to remember that if the amount of information exceeds what the client is able to process, the client will have difficulty developing effective responses and strategies, instead becoming frustrated or overwhelmed (Toglia, 2018). For example, it may be more difficult for clients to learn about meal preparation strategies when making a homemade soup and salad in a therapy kitchen than it would be to prepare a peanut butter and jelly sandwich in their kitchen at home. The former task includes more steps, requires more equipment, and is taking place in an unfamiliar location. As a result, it will likely place more demands on the person and may result in learning being more difficult.

Strategies to Promote Learning

It is important to deliberately consider learning when designing treatment sessions for clients. The results of this deliberation will help the practitioner determine the type of therapeutic approach to use, including how and when to provide cueing and feedback. Factors to consider when designing therapy sessions include whether or not to allow errors, how to distribute (i.e., schedule) practice, and whether or not to vary stimuli in task completion (Haskins, 2012). The use of errorless learning versus a trial-and-error strategy will depend on the client's ability to retain information and the goals of therapy (Haskins, 2012). For clients with moderate to severe cognitive impairment who may have poor retention of information, the goal is often to train them to complete specific tasks to become more independent with those activities under specific circumstances and to lessen the burden on caregivers. In this case, the best approach often uses nondeclarative, or procedural, learning (Giles, 2018; Haskins, 2012; Maskill & Tempest, 2017b; Sohlberg & Turkstra, 2011; discussed further in Chapter 10). Clients who have more mild impairment and have better retention of information may benefit from a trial-and-error approach to promote learning in which they are allowed to make mistakes and use problem solving to find solutions. This type of training is also most effective for clients with insight into their deficits (Haskins, 2012; McEwen et al., 2018; Sohlberg & Turkstra, 2011).

When and how often to practice skills that are being taught should also be considered when designing treatment. Practice distribution can be massed (i.e., when a skill is practiced repeatedly in a short period of time) or distributed (i.e., when skills are practiced intermittently over a longer period of time). Research has shown that people who are in the acquisition phase (i.e., when they are first learning a skill) may benefit from massed practice (Maskill & Tempest, 2017b; Sohlberg & Turkstra, 2011). Long-term learning is encouraged when acquisition is followed up with distributed practice (Maskill & Tempest, 2017b; Sohlberg & Turkstra, 2011). For example, consider a student who is learning the ratings for manual muscle testing. When first learning what each number means, the student may review them frequently and repeatedly in a short period of time. At this point, the student is in the acquisition phase of their learning, and massed practice of the information can be helpful. As the student begins to recall the rating scale more readily, reviewing the scale periodically can help retain the information for the long term, especially if the review takes place in varied situations (e.g., with different study partners or in different locations).

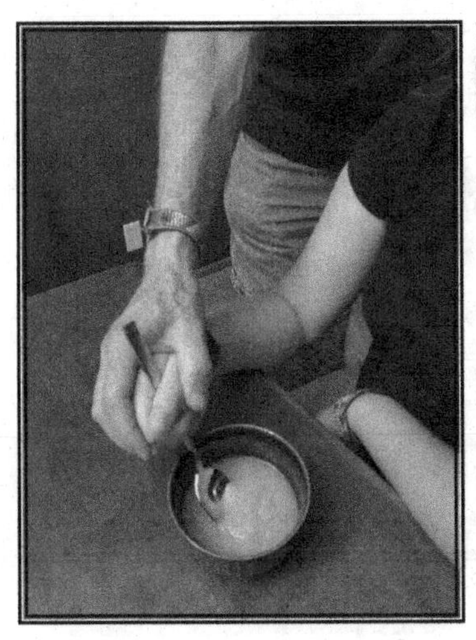

Figure 9-7. Hand-over-hand assistance is one type of physical cueing that can support a client with cognitive impairment in successfully completing activities.

Finally, the amount of stimulus variability that is used will also depend on the client's needs and goals in addition to where the client is in the learning process. When in the acquisition stage or when using nondeclarative memory, it is better to limit the amount of variation when teaching a skill. This will help to establish the skills or behaviors being taught to the client. On the other hand, introducing variation into the task will encourage long-term learning and more easily promote generalization (Sohlberg & Turkstra, 2011). For example, imagine teaching a client to use a checklist to track progress in a multistep task. When first learning how to use the checklist, the client will have an easier time if the checklist is used several times with the same task or a similar task with fewer steps. When the client begins to understand how to use the checklist, variation can be added by using a checklist with different types of activities or for activities with more steps (Toglia, 1991, 2018).

The cueing used in therapy sessions can also influence learning. Factors to consider include the type of cueing and the timing of cueing. The type of cueing used will depend on the client's needs and what works best in modifying their behavior and facilitating their acquisition of skills (Sohlberg & Turkstra, 2011). Much of this can be discovered during the evaluation process when using the dynamic interactional approach (see Chapter 8 for details). Examples of different types of cueing include physical assistance (including hand over hand; Figure 9-7), modeling, oral/spoken cues, alarms (Figure 9-8), or visual reminders (Sohlberg & Turkstra, 2011). In addition, it is important to consider the source of the cues. Cues can come from an external source, such as the practitioner. Clients can also be taught to provide their own cues and feedback (Maskill & Tempest, 2017b; Sohlberg & Turkstra, 2011). Research shows that long-term learning is facilitated when cueing and feedback come from the clients themselves (Mathiowetz et al., 2021). However, this may not be feasible for all clients. In addition to the types of cues, it is important to consider the timing of feedback, which can be given immediately or after a delay. For clients who are in the acquisition phase of learning, immediate feedback may be most helpful (Mathiowetz et al., 2021; Sohlberg & Turkstra, 2011). There is evidence that immediate feedback can be detrimental after that and can limit the client's ability to maintain and generalize skills. It also does not provide an opportunity for self-monitoring and reflection. Feedback that is given after a delay, especially when the client has a chance to reflect and analyze performance first, can support the durability of learning (Maskill & Tempest, 2017b; Mathiowetz et al., 2021; Sohlberg & Turkstra, 2011). Again, this may not be feasible or even beneficial for all clients, specifically for those with more severe cortical damage and limited insight.

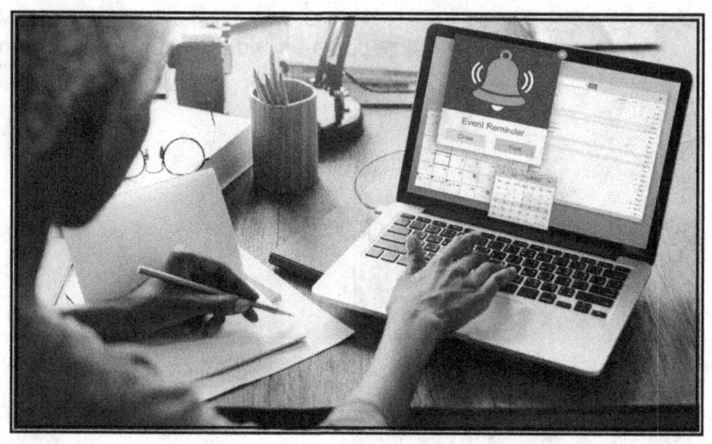

Figure 9-8. Alarms or other reminders can assist clients in compensating for memory deficits. (Rawpixel.com/shutterstock.com)

Rancho Los Amigos Levels of Cognitive Functioning Scale

One way to think about clients and their learning potential is to use a framework that describes people in different stages of recovery and with different skills. The Rancho Los Amigos Levels of Cognitive Functioning Scale (RLAS) is a widely used tool that can be helpful in classifying people with TBI. It was originally published in 1972 and had eight levels (Lin & Wroten, 2022). This version of the scale is still used, especially in acute and inpatient settings. In 1998, the RLAS was revised to the RLAS-R and includes 10 levels that categorize people who exhibit a wider range of functioning, from coma to modified independence. The revisions were made to expand on the descriptions of higher levels of functioning that may be observed more frequently in outpatient and community care settings (Lin & Wroten, 2022). Although the RLAS-R was specifically designed to be used for people with TBI, it can be a helpful tool to guide treatment of all people with ABI by considering their current level of functioning and where they fit in the RLAS-R scale. By understanding a client's capabilities, treatment can be better tailored to meet their needs and promote improvement in function. The levels in the revised 10-level scale (Lin & Wroten, 2022) are as follows:

1. Level I: No response; total assistance. At this stage, people do not respond in any observable way to stimulation, including painful input.
2. Level II: Generalized response; total assistance. At this stage, people do respond to stimulation, including painful input, but the response is generalized, meaning that people exhibit the same behavior no matter what type of input is received. The responses may include an increase or decrease in activity such as gross motor movements or vocalizations. Often the responses are delayed.
3. Level III: Localized response; total assistance. At this stage, people respond to stimulation, and the responses are becoming more specific to the input that is received, but these behaviors are still largely nonpurposeful. Examples may be withdrawal from painful stimuli, turning toward sounds, visually tracking moving objects, inconsistently following simple commands, and pulling at tubes.
4. Level IV: Confused, agitated; maximal assistance. At this stage, people are more active, but movements and actions are still not purposeful. Emotionally, people are often agitated and volatile and may be aggressive. They will also actively try to remove restraints or tubes. They have poor attention and no short-term memory. They will also not follow commands consistently, and their verbalizations are incoherent or unrelated to what is happening around them.

5. Level V: Confused, inappropriate, nonagitated; maximal assistance. At this stage, people are alert and agitation is seen less often, usually in response to overstimulation. People are able to follow simple commands, especially with support and cueing. They are better able to complete simple and familiar tasks with support. They are not able to learn new information and have severely impaired short-term memory. They are also not oriented and may wander.
6. Level VI: Confused, appropriate; moderate assistance. At this stage, people are becoming more oriented, although this is still inconsistent. Attention and memory are also improving with some ability to learn emerging, although they still need a great deal of support and assistance. They are better able to follow directions with less cueing and can participate more purposefully with activities, including self-care.
7. Level VII: Automatic, appropriate; minimal assistance for routine daily living skills. At this stage, people are able to complete many routine tasks with minimal assistance when they are in familiar situations. Orientation is improving, although they may still become confused, especially in unfamiliar surroundings. Attention is improving, as is memory, although they will continue to need support to recall new information, including minimal assistance to use memory aids. They demonstrate poor problem solving and self-awareness, often overestimating their abilities. They can also continue to have behavioral issues, becoming uncooperative with their caregivers and demonstrating poor social interactions with inappropriate behaviors.
8. Level VIII: Purposeful and appropriate; standby assistance for routine daily living skills. At this stage, people are able to initiate and complete routine tasks in familiar environments with only supervision, but they need assistance to solve problems when they arise. They are increasingly aware of their limitations, although they may still over- or underestimate their abilities. Their memory is improving, although they still need assistance, such as from external devices, to recall information. They are able to use aids with supervision. They are able to learn new skills and tasks, especially in consistent and predictable environments. Their social interaction is improving as well, and they have fewer inappropriate responses, although these can still occur. They may also demonstrate shallow irritability (i.e., when they become easily frustrated or annoyed).
9. Level IX: Purposeful and appropriate; standby assistance on request for daily living skills. At this stage, people are increasingly independent, needing occasional assistance with unfamiliar tasks or to avoid problems, especially with more complex tasks or in more complicated or dynamic environments. Their ability to complete familiar routines with ADLs, instrumental activities of daily living (IADLs), work, and leisure is vastly improved, and they can be without supervision much of the time. They may still need to use memory devices and may need occasional help with setting them up. They may still have shallow irritability but are better able to appreciate others' feelings. They can monitor their social behavior better, with only occasional assistance.
10. Level X: Purposeful and appropriate; modified independent. At this stage, people are largely independent and can live alone. They have a good understanding of their limitations and can compensate for them, including with memory devices set up independently, although they may need extra time to problem solve or complete activities. They may also become easily fatigued. Their social behavior is appropriate, and they display fewer episodes of shallow irritability unless they are ill, stressed, or tired.

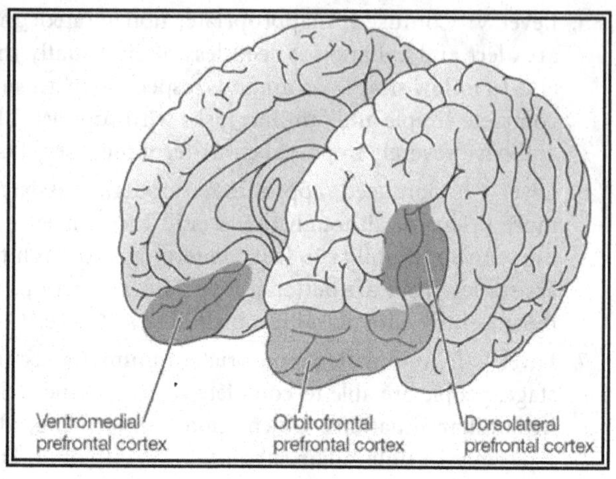

Figure 9-9. Damage to different portions of the prefrontal cortex can result in different behavioral issues. (Reproduced with permission from Bradbury, J. W., & Vehrencamp, S. L. [2011]. *Principles of animal communication* [2nd ed.]. Sinauer.)

Behavior Management

Behavioral issues after ABI, especially TBI, are common, can be long lasting, and can interfere with learning. Prevalence rates vary widely depending on the study and how the problem behaviors are defined. A review by Stéfan and Mathé (2016) looking at people with moderate to severe TBI found that aggression was present in 25% to 39% of participants and was more common after lesions affecting the orbitofrontal region of the brain. Other common behavioral issues were irritability, affecting between 29% and 71% of survivors, and apathy, affecting between 20% and 71% of people with TBI. Behavioral issues were often long lasting, with families of people who were 10 or more years postinjury reporting continuing behavioral concerns (Stéfan & Mathé, 2016). Problem behaviors can interfere with the therapeutic process and are also often difficult for staff and family to manage. The long-term consequences include an increased risk of legal issues (e.g., arrests because of inappropriate social behavior such as fighting/assault), low rates of employment, poor social participation, and lowered quality of life (Persel & Persel, 2018; Wood & Alderman, 2011; Ylvisaker et al., 2003).

The types of behavioral issues that are present can be influenced by the location of the lesion. When the brainstem is damaged, people can demonstrate disorientation, frustration, and anger. Lesions in the limbic system can result in expressions of rage. Damage to the amygdala and temporal lobes can cause people to experience fear and anxiety (Persel & Persel, 2018). When the frontal lobe is lesioned, which is often the case in TBI because of the size of the frontal lobe and the types of injuries that result in TBI, different clusters of behavior can occur. When the orbitofrontal region is impacted, people can experience behaviors such as disinhibition (including sexually), impulsivity, difficulty with anger management, and poor social judgment. When the dorsolateral or dorsomedial regions are damaged, people can have issues with initiation, apathy, inattentiveness, and emotional dullness (Ylvisaker et al., 2003; Figure 9-9).

Behavioral issues can also be influenced by the way in which people with brain injury perceive their treatment by those around them. Kivunja and colleagues (2018) completed a review of qualitative research conducted with TBI survivors, family members, and staff. The researchers reported that people with TBI stated that they were excluded from the decision-making process and felt that caregivers did not listen to them and were impatient. These perceptions can lead to frustration, anger, and desperation (Kivunja et al., 2018). Issues with awareness can also lead to an increase in behavioral issues because people with ABI may not understand why caregivers are limiting activities. As awareness improves, people may experience more frustration when they have difficulty completing tasks and compare performance to preinjury levels (Lohmann & Vas, 2021).

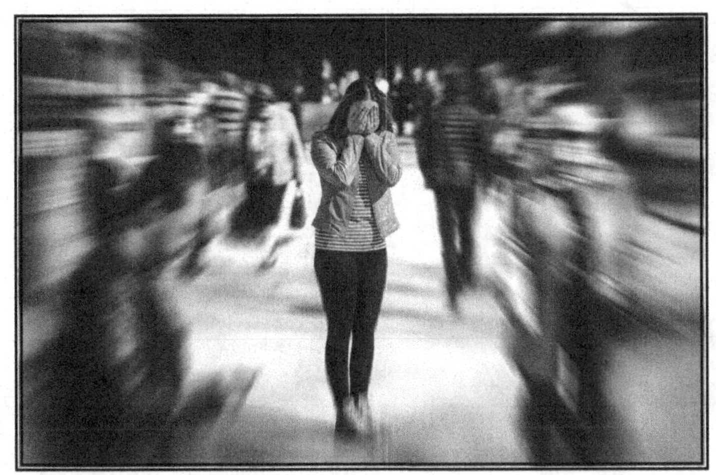

Figure 9-10. A person with brain injury can become overwhelmed with a busy environment. (Tero Vesalainen/shutterstock.com)

A complete discussion of behavior management is beyond the scope of this text, but there are some key principles that can be helpful when working with people with ABI. Researchers recommend focusing attention on antecedents to behavioral issues and identifying triggers that are linked to behavioral outbursts (Lohmann & Vas, 2021; Persel & Persel, 2018; Wood & Alderman, 2011; Ylvisaker et al., 2003). Triggers can be internal or external. Internal triggers can include issues such as pain or illness and can often only be modified through medical intervention. External triggers can be controlled by those around the individual, including health care providers, through environmental modification (Persel & Persel, 2018). For example, a person with TBI may get easily overwhelmed, especially by noisy and busy environments (Figure 9-10). Simplification of the environment for this person can include working in a quiet room to reduce extraneous noise and stimulation. This person's care team would also want to consider communication by speaking with a calm tone of voice and giving concise and simple instructions (Persel & Persel, 2018; Tipton-Burton, 2018; Ylvisaker et al., 2003). Other strategies that can help people with behavior issues include the use of predictable routines in appropriate context (e.g., completing grooming tasks at a sink rather than at bedside), working on procedural learning, providing choices, including clients in decision making as much as possible, and decreasing the chance of failure by finding the just-right challenge (Lohmann & Vas, 2021; Persel & Persel, 2018; Ylvisaker et al., 2003).

A behavioral management plan can be created to help reduce maladaptive behaviors and encourage more positive interactions. The plan should be created in partnership with the person, family, and members of the care team. Before implementing the plan, it is essential to have clear goals and expectations and to formulate those goals in a way that is culturally appropriate for the person (Kivunja et al., 2018; Persel & Persel, 2018). Behavior will also need to be clearly described, measured, and monitored so that progress can be documented (Persel & Persel, 2018). Different strategies may be used for behavior management, including positive reinforcement of wanted behaviors through praise or privileges and negative reinforcement of unwanted ones, such as through loss of attention (Persel & Persel, 2018; Wood & Alderman, 2011; Ylvisaker et al., 2003). When consequences are used, it is best if they relate naturally and logically to the behavior (Ylvisaker et al., 2003). No matter the approach that is used, it is essential for the person to get feedback about behavior and practice with skills that are being learned. Practice in a variety of contexts can encourage generalization (Ylvisaker et al., 2002, 2003). It is also important for caregivers and members of the team to always remain calm when interacting with the person with brain injury and to remember that the ultimate goal of the behavior plan is to help the person learn positive behaviors and encourage success (Persel & Persel, 2018; Ylvisaker et al., 2003).

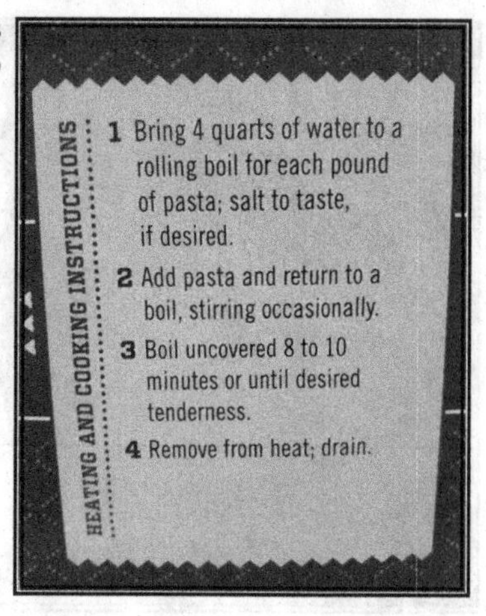

Figure 9-11. One example of instructions for cooking pasta. This format is text heavy and may be more difficult for some clients with brain injury to understand and follow.

Figure 9-12. Another example of instructions for cooking pasta. This is a pictorial format and may be easier for some clients with brain injury to understand and follow. (Irina Strelnikova/shutterstock.com)

Environment/Context

The historical view of an individual with disabilities is that any difficulties with occupational performance stem solely from the individual. When approached in this way, disability is exclusively caused by limitations in client factors, including motor, sensory, and cognitive skills. This belief does not consider how much influence the environment has on participation (White, 2019). The contemporary view of disability considers more than individual capabilities by examining task and environmental demands as well (AOTA, 2020). Through this lens, it is understood that people can perform differently in varied situations depending on what tasks they undertake and what environmental supports and barriers are present (Stark et al., 2015; White, 2019). For example, imagine that a person with cognitive impairment would like to cook pasta. There are two options for instructions on how to prepare the pasta, one on the pasta box that relies solely on text (Figure 9-11) and one that uses simple pictures (Figure 9-12). The simplified pictorial instructions may be easier for them to understand, thereby increasing the likelihood of success with this portion of meal preparation. The person's cognitive skills have not changed, but their ability to complete a pasta-cooking portion of meal preparation is different depending on the format of instructions. In this case, the factor that influences participation is the presence of an environmental support (simplified pictorial instructions) versus an environmental barrier (more complex text-heavy instructions). The *International Classification of Functioning, Disability and Health*, which is an international standard developed by the World Health Organization for describing and measuring health and disability, embraced this more holistic view of participation. It includes a mechanism to document the impact of the social and physical environment on an individual's participation (Stark et al., 2015; World Health Organization, 2008). The *Occupational Therapy Practice Framework: Domain and Process, Fourth Edition* (*OTPF-4*) also supports this concept by identifying an individual's environment as either a facilitator or barrier to occupational performance (AOTA, 2020; White, 2019).

When viewing participation in context, the practitioner considers the interplay between a person's abilities and the demands of the environments that surround the individual. Environments to be considered can include physical, social, cultural, virtual, and temporal (AOTA, 2020). Environments can be more immediate, such as the client's own home and family. They can also be broader, including both community settings and the influences on those settings, such as laws that govern the creation, upgrading, and maintenance of public spaces (White, 2019). Ultimately, clients' deficits will result in disability when they face situations in which the demands (of the task and/or the environment) exceed their skills. Therefore, the occupational therapy practitioner should consider clients as they engage in activities in a number of different situations and note which support or hinder participation. Practitioners should also make note of the environmental factors that both are and are not modifiable (AOTA, 2020; World Health Organization, 2008). These observations should then be used in treatment. Modifiable environmental factors can be adjusted to maximize the client's occupational performance (e.g., reducing the number of choices for a client with an impairment in working memory; Nalder & Fleming, 2018). For environmental factors that cannot be modified (e.g., public spaces), the client will need to be accommodated through education of both the client and their support networks (e.g., grocery shopping at non-peak times). Environmental demands also need to be considered when a practitioner works with a client on the generalization of skills because of their impact on occupational performance. People will need to practice strategies in different contexts to increase the likelihood of generalization and problem solve how to overcome environmental barriers (Toglia, 2018).

Caregivers

One specific type of environmental influence is the social environment. The *OTPF-4* labeled this as *support and relationships* with the accompanying definition of the "people or animals that provide practical physical or emotional support, nurturing, protection, assistance, and connections to other persons in the home, workplace, or school or at play or in other aspects of daily occupations" (AOTA, 2020, p. 10). Essential members of the client's social environment, as illustrated in the *OTPF-4* definition, are the people in the client's life who may be providing assistance. Care networks can have an enormous influence on clients' ability to live and participate in the community. Their presence can result in people living successfully in the community and participating fully. Their absence can result in isolation and loss of independence and health. As a result, it is essential to consider clients' family and caregivers early in the rehabilitative process.

Health care providers and researchers are increasingly realizing that ABI does not just affect the person who sustains the injury. Rather, the entire family is typically affected, and significant changes in roles for all family members result (Boschen et al., 2007; Gan et al., 2010; Powell et al., 2017). For example, imagine a man who has just retired. He and his spouse are settling into a new postemployment routine that may include greater engagement in leisure activities. Perhaps the couple planned to travel to visit family and friends who are farther away. Now imagine that the man sustained a stroke. His plans, in addition to his spouse's plans, have been interrupted. Travel arrangements are put on hold, and the focus shifts to recovery and rehabilitation. Both people

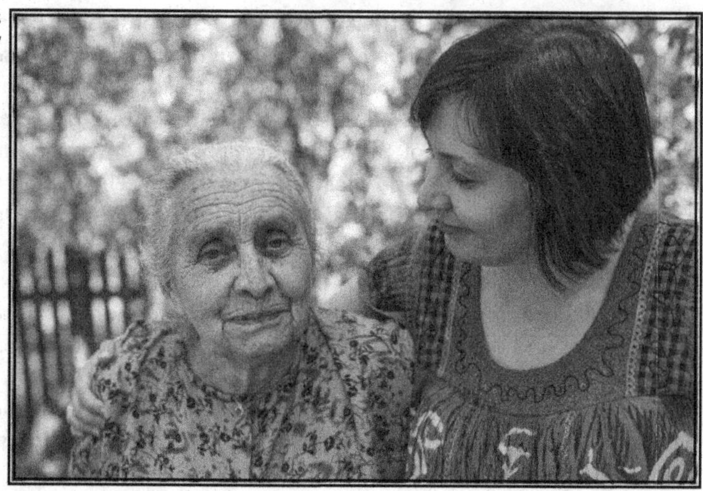

Figure 9-13. Most informal caregivers are family members. (Ocskay Mark/ shutterstock.com)

have a resulting change in roles and responsibilities. The man has become a patient and care recipient. His spouse has become a caregiver. Similarly, imagine a young woman who has recently moved out of her parents' home into her own apartment. She is living on her own for the first time, working and paying her bills independently. Now imagine that the young woman is in an automobile accident and sustains a serious TBI. After she is discharged from inpatient rehabilitation, she moves back in with her parents. All of these family members, the young woman and her parents, experience massive, and likely permanent, disruptions in their roles as a result of the brain injury.

Most caregivers of adults who receive care in the community are informal caregivers, meaning that they are unpaid. About 85% of the time, these informal caregivers are family members, but they may also be friends or neighbors (Figure 9-13). Men are increasingly involved with caregiving activities (Family Caregiver Alliance, 2016), but the majority of caregiving, especially tasks of a more personal nature (e.g., bathing, dressing, toileting), is managed by women (Family Caregiver Alliance, 2016). Caregiving encompasses assisting care recipients with a wide variety of tasks, including, but not limited to, financial management, grocery shopping, food preparation, medication management, transportation, household management, mobility, ADLs, and social participation. Informal caregivers of community-living adults (with a range of diagnoses, not just ABI) are, on average, 49.2 years old and provide an average of 24.4 hours of care per week. They may or may not live with the care recipient. The average duration of the caregiver role is 4 years, with 15% of caregivers providing care for 10 or more years (Family Caregiver Alliance, 2016).

Caregiving can lead to negative consequences for informal caregivers. Caregivers are more likely to experience family strain, emotional and mental health issues, such as depression and anxiety, feelings of burden, social isolation, loss of income, increases in substance abuse, and difficulty adjusting to their new roles, among other issues (Backhaus et al., 2010; Baker et al., 2017; Boschen et al., 2007; Gan et al., 2010). Factors that increase the likelihood of people experiencing the negative effects of caregiving are poor social networks, loneliness, and caring for a person with more severe disability including issues such as problem behaviors (Powell et al., 2017). Caregiver training may reduce the negative effects of caregiving by improving confidence with caregiving skills and quality of life (Boschen et al., 2007; Powell et al., 2016; Rivera et al., 2008). Occupational therapy practitioners have important responsibilities with caregiver training and must consider the needs of caregivers early in the rehabilitation process (Figure 9-14).

There are different ways to approach caregiver training, but research into effective caregiver training emphasizes several points that are important to consider with any approach that is taken.

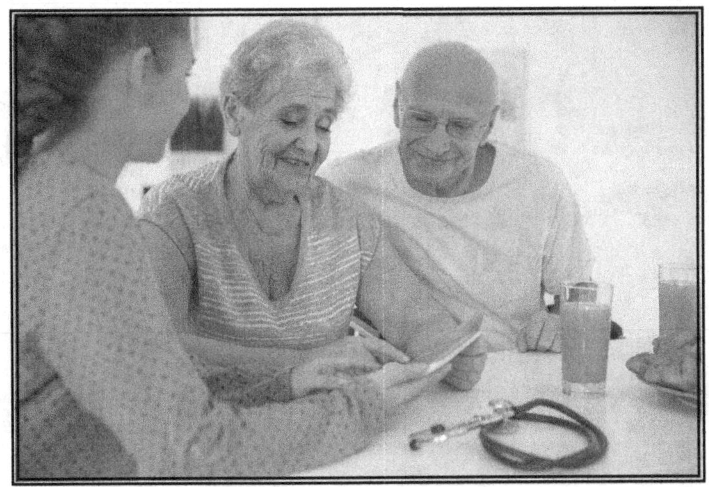

Figure 9-14. Caregiver training has been shown to improve caregiver-related outcomes, such as mood and self-efficacy. (Africa Studio/shutterstock.com)

The first is that caregiver training needs to be considered as a process rather than a single event. Caregivers need change over time, with caregivers most concerned about different things at different points in the recovery process (Damianakis et al., 2016). For example, in the early stages after ABI, caregivers tend to focus on issues such as the client's progress and chance of survival. Later in the recovery process, caregivers are often ready and interested in other aspects of the client's functioning, such as employability and behavior management. They may also have other concerns, including financial resources and respite. Ideally, caregiver training should start early and continue over the long term to help caregivers navigate different stages of the care recipient's recovery (Boschen et al., 2007; Gan et al., 2010; Powell et al., 2017). As a result of the changing needs of caregivers through the recovery process, it is important that caregiver training be driven by the caregivers themselves, with the focus of training on things that the caregivers identify as most pressing at the time (Damianakis et al., 2016; Powell et al., 2017).

A second factor to consider when approaching caregiver training is that long-term in-person access to health care providers may be difficult to achieve. This may be due to insurance not covering access to rehabilitation professionals beyond the acute and subacute stages of recovery. Caregivers may also live in areas where they do not have easy physical access to health care providers or other support networks. Increasing evidence shows that virtual support, such as web-based support groups, or telephone calls with trained support persons can assist in reducing the negative effects of caregiving (Figure 9-15). Virtual support may be something to consider when working with caregivers and considering their long-term needs (Damianakis et al., 2016; Powell et al., 2016; Rotondi et al., 2005; Sander et al., 2009).

Another important consideration for caregiver training is the accessibility of the information that is being shared. Caregivers are in a stressful situation, facing disruption of their roles and routines and an enormous amount of uncertainty about the future. It is easy for them to get overwhelmed with too much information being shared too quickly. Practitioners should consider the pace and timing of information and present material in such a way that caregivers can understand the most pertinent information at the most appropriate time (Boschen et al., 2007; Gan et al., 2010; Powell et al., 2017). It is also essential to ensure that caregivers can understand the material that they are being given. Practitioners need to be aware of the language that they are using, be careful to avoid jargon, and present material using lay terms. The reading level of printed material should also be examined, remembering that caregivers will have a wide range of literacy and education levels (Gan et al., 2010). In addition, practitioners should strive to use different types of media

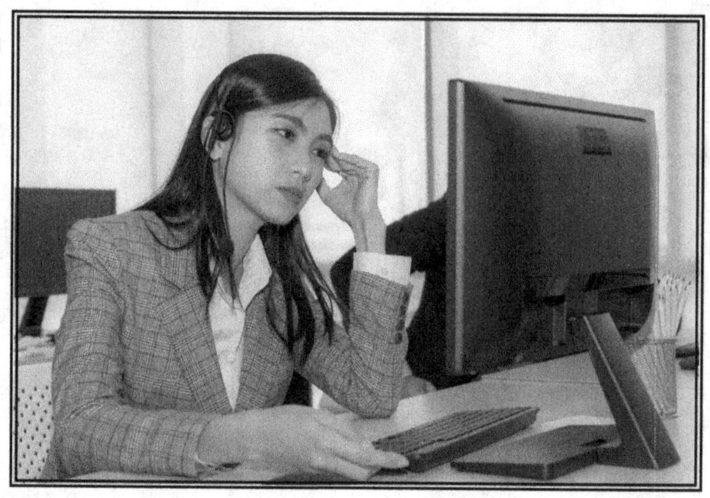

Figure 9-15. Caregiver training can be completed through different media, including virtually. Virtual support groups can also provide caregivers with resources. (Blue Planet Studio/shutterstock.com)

(written, verbal, and hands-on training) to improve access and understanding for people with different learning needs (Boschen et al., 2007).

Research does not agree on the best way to train caregivers, but the problem-solving approach is gaining empirical support. Clinicians who use the problem-solving method teach caregivers to approach issues that they face systematically by following five steps: identifying the problem, brainstorming solutions, critiquing the possible solutions, choosing and implementing one of the solutions, and evaluating the outcome (Rivera et al., 2008). When a problem-solving approach is used, the clinician acts as a mentor, assisting caregivers in learning how to navigate issues on their own rather than instructing the caregiver on specifics (Powell et al., 2016). Another advantage of the problem-solving approach is that it may help to support the client in making additional gains after therapy is discontinued. Rehabilitation may end before a person with ABI has fully mastered skills because of factors such as shorter length of stays or insurance benefits running out (Powell et al., 2016). In this case, the caregivers may be in the position of needing to support the person with ABI with continued learning and skill acquisition. The caregiver can also encourage the generalization and application of skills to a variety of real-world situations (Sander et al., 2009). Caregivers who have the ability to problem solve and identify strategies to foster the care recipients' learning may be better able to support the person with ABI in their recovery.

The problem-solving approach has shown promise with caregiver training and has been linked to a decrease in some of the negative effects of caregiving, such as depression (Backhaus et al., 2010; Baker et al., 2017; Boschen et al., 2007; Powell et al., 2017; Rivera et al., 2008). One randomized controlled trial compared an intervention in which caregivers received problem-solving training ($n = 77$) with usual care ($n = 76$). Those in the intervention group received mentorship on applying the problem-solving approach during telephone calls with one of the researchers. During the phone calls, the researcher asked open-ended questions that guided caregivers through the problem-solving process. After the intervention, there was a significant improvement in caregivers' emotional well-being compared with caregivers in the control group. Caregivers in the intervention group also reported receiving more support from family and friends and taking better care of their own health (Powell et al., 2016).

Cognitive Intervention: Decision Making

As stated previously, there are a variety of factors that guide decision making for which treatments are best suited for clients. Some important questions to ask about the client's abilities relate to their ability to follow commands, the amount of information they are able to retain, their awareness of their deficits, the types of assistance they need, and their ability to use skills and strategies in varied settings (Haskins, 2012). Much of this is captured in the RLAS-R levels, which were described earlier in this chapter. If a client's functioning can be conceptualized as fitting into one of these levels, the RLAS-R levels can serve as a framework for making decisions about intervention.

In 2012, Haskins published a decision tree that can be used to assist clinicians in making choices about their approach to treatment. According to this decision tree, the first question a clinician should answer is whether or not clients are aware of their deficits. Clinicians should then decide whether or not clients are able to use external strategies, such as memory aids. The severity of the deficit should also be considered. If a client is not aware of deficits and is not able to use external strategies, the recommendation is to work on nondeclarative/procedural learning through approaches such as errorless learning and chaining (described further in Chapter 10). Environmental adaptations and support would also be warranted. A client with this level of ability would fall approximately into RLAS-R Levels IV and V, emerging into Level VI. For people at this level of functioning, it is also important to work on trying to increase their awareness of deficits. Clients with at least some awareness of their deficits may benefit from internal strategy training in addition to external strategy use and environmental adaptation. If awareness is incomplete, such as with RLAS-R Levels VI, VII, and VIII, it would be important for the clinician to continue to work on improving understanding of deficits, strengths, and the types of strategies that can assist clients. Clients who use internalized strategies can also work on generalizing skills to promote independence in a variety of environments (Haskins, 2012). Details about each of these treatment approaches are described further in Chapter 10.

Conclusion

As occupational therapy practitioners design treatment for clients with brain injury, they will need to take into account a number of factors, including learning and retention of information, informal caregivers and their needs, and the types of occupations that are meaningful and relevant. Typically, clients with more severe injury who have poor memory and learning will benefit from procedural/nondeclarative learning with its focus on developing routines. Clients with emerging awareness of their deficits will benefit from interventions that encourage the development of insight. Clients with more mild deficits who have improved insight will benefit from metacognitive strategy training. Almost all clients benefit from environmental modification. In addition, caregiver training should be considered throughout recovery. The next chapter explains the details of different treatment approaches.

References

American Occupational Therapy Association. (2020). Occupational therapy practice framework: Domain and process (4th ed.). *American Journal of Occupational Therapy, 74*(Suppl. 2), 7412410010. https://doi.org/10.5014/ajot.2020.74S2001

Backhaus, S. L., Ibarra, S. L., Klyce, D., Trexler, L. E., & Malec, J. F. (2010). Brain injury coping skills group: A preventative intervention for patients with brain injury and their caregivers. *Archives of Physical Medicine and Rehabilitation, 91*, 840-848. https://doi.org/10.1016/j.apmr.2010.03.015

Baker, A., Barker, S., Sampson, A., & Martin, C. (2017). Caregiver outcomes and interventions: A systematic scoping review of the traumatic brain injury and spinal cord injury literature. *Clinical Rehabilitation, 31*, 45-60. https://doi.org/10.1177/0269215516639357

Boman, I.-L., Lindstedt, M., Hemminsson, H., & Bartfai, A. (2004). Cognitive training in home environment. *Brain Injury, 18*, 985-995. https://doi.org/10.1080/02699050410001672396

Boschen, K., Gargaro, J., Gan, C., Gerber, G., & Brandys, C. (2007). Family interventions after acquired brain injury and other chronic conditions: A critical appraisal of the quality of the evidence. *NeuroRehabilitation, 22*, 19-41. https://doi.org/10.3233/NRE-2007-22104

Carvalho, R., Azevedo, E., Marques, P., Dias, N., & Cerqueira, J. J. (2018). Physiotherapy based on problem-solving in upper limb function and neuroplasticity in chronic stroke patients: A case series. *Journal of Evaluation in Clinical Practice, 24*, 552-560. https://doi.org/10.1111/jep.12921

Cicerone, K. D., Goldin, Y., Ganci, K., Rosenbaum, A., Wethe, J. V., Langenbahn, D. M., Malec, J. F., Bergquist, T. F., Kingsley, K., Nagele, D., Trexler, L., Fraas, M., Bogdanova, Y., & Harley, J. P. (2019). Evidence-based cognitive rehabilitation: Systematic review of the literature from 2009 through 2014. *Archives of Physical Medicine and Rehabilitation, 100*, 1515-1533. https://doi.org/10.1016/j.apmr.2019.02.011

Cifu, D. X., Kreutzer, J. A., Kolakowsky-Hayner, S. A., Marwitz, J. H., & Englander, J. (2003). The relationship between therapy intensity and rehabilitative outcomes after traumatic brain injury: A multicenter analysis. *Archives of Physical Medicine and Rehabilitation, 84*, 1441-1448. https://doi.org/10.1016/S0003-9993(03)00272-7

Coleman, E. R., Moudgal, R., Lang, K., Hyacincth, H. I., Awosika, O. O., Kissela, B. M., & Feng, W. (2018). Early rehabilitation after stroke, a narrative review. *Current Atherosclerosis Reports, 19*, 59. https://doi.org/10.1007/s11883-017-0686-6

Constantinidou, G., & Thomas, R. D. (2018). Principles of cognitive rehabilitation in TBI: An integrative neuroscience approach. In M. J. Ashley & D. A. Hovda (Eds.), *Traumatic brain injury: Rehabilitation, treatment and case management* (4th ed., pp. 513-539). CRC Press.

Damianakis, T., Tough, A., Marziali, E., & Dawson, D. R. (2016). Therapy online: A web-based video support group for family caregivers of survivors with traumatic brain injury. *Journal of Head Trauma Rehabilitation, 31*, E12-E20. https://doi.org/10.1097/HTR.0000000000000178

Family Caregiver Alliance. (2016). Caregiver statistics: Demographics. https://www.caregiver.org/caregiver-statistics-demographics

Ferris, J. K., Neva, J. L, Francisco, B. A., & Boyd, L. A. (2018). Bilateral motor cortex plasticity in individuals with chronic stroke, induced by paired associative stimulation. *Neurorehabilitation and Neural Repair, 32*, 671-681. https://doi.org/10.1177/1545968318785043

Fisher, G. E., & Sullivan, K. J. (2001). Activity-dependent factors affecting poststroke functional outcomes. *Topics in Stroke Rehabilitation, 8*, 31-44. https://doi.org/10.1310/B3JD-NML4-V1FB-5YHG

Gan, C., Gargaro, J., Brandys, C., Gerber, G., & Boschen, K. (2010). Family caregivers' support needs after brain injury: A synthesis of perspectives from caregivers, programs, and researchers. *NeuroRehabilitation, 27*, 5-18. https://doi.org/10.3233/NRE-2010-0577

Giles, G. M. (2018). Neurofunctional approach to rehabilitation after brain injury. In N. Katz & J. Toglia (Eds.), *Cognition, occupation, and participation across the lifespan* (4th ed., pp. 419-442). AOTA Press.

Godden, D. R., & Baddeley, A. D. (1975). Context-dependent memory in two natural environments: On land and underwater. *British Journal of Psychology, 66*, 325-331. https://doi.org/10.1111/j.2044-8295.1975.tb01468.x

Grady, C., & Kapur, S. (1999). The use of neuroimaging in neurorehabilitative research. In D. Stuss, G. Winocur, & I. H. Robertson (Eds.), *Cognitive neurorehabilitation*. Cambridge University Press.

Haskins, E. C. (2012). *Cognitive rehabilitation manual: Translating evidence-based recommendations into practice.* American Congress of Rehabilitation Medicine.

Hu, M.-H., Hsu, S.-S., Yip, P.-K., Jeng, J.-S., & Wang, Y.-H. (2010). Early and intensive rehabilitation predicts good functional outcomes in patients admitted to the stroke intensive care unit. *Disability and Rehabilitation, 32*, 1251-1259. https://doi.org/10.3109/09638280903464448

Katz, N. (2018). Introduction to cognition and participation. In N. Katz & J. Toglia (Eds.), *Cognition, occupation, and participation across the lifespan* (4th ed., pp. 3-7). AOTA Press.

Kivunja, S., River, J., & Gullick, J. (2018). Experiences of giving and receiving care in traumatic brain injury: An integrative review. *Journal of Clinical Nursing, 27*, 1304-1328. https://doi.org/10.1111/jocn.14283

Kleim, J. A., & Jones, T. A. (2008). Principles of experience-dependent neural plasticity: Implications for rehabilitation after brain damage. *Journal of Speech, Language, and Hearing Research, 51*, S225-S239. https://doi.org/10.1044/1092-4388(2008/018)

Kolb, B., & Gibb, R. (2008). Principles of neuroplasticity and behavior. In D. T. Stuss, G. Winocur, & I. H. Robertson (Eds.), *Cognitive neurorehabilitation: Evidence and application* (2nd ed., pp. 6-21). Cambridge University Press.

Lin, K., & Wroten, M. (2022). Ranchos Los Amigos. StatPearls Publishing. https://www.ncbi.nlm.nih.gov/books/NBK448151/

Lohmann, A. F., & Vas, A. K. (2021). Acquired brain injury. In D. P. Dirette & S. A. Gutman (Eds.), *Occupational therapy for physical dysfunction* (8th ed., pp. 765-788). Wolters Kluwer.

Lowell, S., & Singer, W. (1992). Selection of intrinsic horizontal connections in the visual cortex by correlated neuronal activity. *Science, 255*, 209-212. https://doi.org/10.1126/science.1372754

Lundy-Ekman, L. (2018). *Neuroscience: Fundamentals for rehabilitation* (5th ed.). Elsevier.

Maskill, L., & Tempest, S. (2017a). Assessment and measuring change. In L. Maskill & S. Tempest (Eds.), *Neuropsychology for occupational therapists: Cognition in occupational performance* (4th ed., pp. 17-31). Wiley Blackwell.

Maskill, L., & Tempest, S. (2017b). Intervention for cognitive impairments and evaluating outcomes. In L. Maskill & S. Tempest (Eds.), *Neuropsychology for occupational therapists: Cognition in occupational performance* (4th ed., pp. 33-49). Wiley Blackwell.

Mathiowetz, V., Nilsen, D. M., & Gillen, G. (2021). Task-oriented approach to stroke rehabilitation. In G. Gillen & D. M. Nilsen (Eds.), *Stroke rehabilitation: A function-based approach* (5th ed., pp. 59-79). Elsevier.

McEwen, S. E., Mandich, A., & Polatajko, H. J. (2018). CO-OP Approach: A cognitive-based intervention for children and adults. In N. Katz & J. Toglia (Eds.), *Cognition, occupation, and participation across the lifespan* (4th ed., pp. 315-334). AOTA Press.

Nalder, E., & Fleming, J. (2018). Transition to community integration for people with acquired brain injury. In N. Katz & J. Toglia (Eds.), *Cognition, occupation, and participation across the lifespan* (4th ed., pp. 173-187). AOTA Press.

Park, H. Y., Maitra, K., & Martinez, K. M. (2015). The effect of occupation-based cognitive rehabilitation for traumatic brain injury: A meta-analysis of randomized controlled trials. *Occupational Therapy International, 22*, 104-116. https://doi.org/10.1002/oti.1389

Persel, C. S., & Persel, C. H. (2018). The use of applied behavior analysis in traumatic brain injury rehabilitation. In M. J. Ashley & D. A. Hovda (Eds.), *Traumatic brain injury: Rehabilitation, treatment, and case management* (4th ed., pp. 411-450). CRC Press.

Powell, J. M., Fraser, R., Brockway, J. A., Temkin, N., & Bell, K. R. (2016). A telehealth approach to caregiver self-management following traumatic brain injury: A randomized controlled trial. *Journal of Head Trauma Rehabilitation, 31*, 180-190. https://doi.org/10.1097/HTR.0000000000000167

Powell, J. M., Wise, E. K., Brockway, J. A., Fraser, R., Temkin, N., & Bell, K. R. (2017). Characteristics and concerns of caregivers of adults with traumatic brain injury. *Journal of Head Trauma Rehabilitation, 32*, E33-E41. https://doi.org/10.1097/HTR.0000000000000219

Radomski, M. V., & Giles, G. M. (2021). Cognitive intervention. In D. P. Dirette & S. A. Gutman (Eds.), *Occupational therapy for physical dysfunction* (8th ed., pp. 161-175). Lippincott Williams & Wilkins.

Rief, K., Bartels, M. N., Duffy, C. A., Beland, H. E., & Stein, J. (2021). Stroke diagnosis, acute treatment, prevention, and medical management. In G. Gillen & D. M. Nilsen (Eds.), *Stroke rehabilitation: A function-based approach* (5th ed., pp. 2-46). Elsevier.

Rivera, P. A., Elliott, T. R., Berry, J. W., & Grant, J. S. (2008). Problem-solving training for family caregivers of persons with traumatic brain injuries: A randomized controlled trial. *Archives of Physical Medicine and Rehabilitation, 89*, 931-941. https://doi.org/10.1016/j.apmr.2007.12.032

Rotondi, A. J., Sinkule, J., & Spring, M. (2005). An interactive web-based intervention for persons with TBI and their families. *Journal of Head Trauma Rehabilitation, 20*, 173-185. https://doi.org/10.1097/00001199-200503000-00005

Sabari, J. S. (2011). Activity-based intervention in stroke rehabilitation. In G. Gillen (Ed.), *Stroke rehabilitation: A function-based approach* (3rd ed., pp. 100-116). Elsevier Mosby.

Sander, A. M., Clark, A. N., Atchison, T. B., & Rueda, M. (2009). A web-based videoconferencing approach to training caregivers in rural areas to compensate for problems related to traumatic brain injury. *Journal of Head Trauma Rehabilitation, 24*, 248-261. https://doi.org/10.1097/HTR.0b013e3181ad593a

Schenkman, M. L., Bowman, J. P., Gisbert, R. L., & Butler, R. B. (2013). *Clinical neuroscience for rehabilitation*. Pearson Education, Inc.

Smith, S. M., & Vela, E. (2001). Environmental context-dependent memory: A review and meta-analysis. *Psychonomic Bulletin and Review, 8*, 203-220. https://doi.org/10.3758/BF03196157

Sohlberg, M. M., & Mateer, C. A. (2001). *Cognitive rehabilitation: An integrative neuropsychological approach.* The Guilford Press.

Sohlberg, M. M., & Turkstra, L. S. (2011). *Optimizing cognitive rehabilitation: Effective instructional methods.* The Guilford Press.

Stark, S., Sanford, J., & Keglovits, M. (2015). Environment factors: Physical and natural environment. In C. H. Christiansen, C. M. Baum, & J. D. Bass (Eds.), *Occupational therapy: Performance, participation, and well-being* (4th ed., pp. 387-420). SLACK Incorporated.

Stéfan, A., & Mathé, J. F. (2016). What are the disruptive symptoms of behavioral disorders after traumatic brain injury? A systematic review leading to recommendations for good practices. *Annals of Physical Rehabilitation Medicine, 59,* 5-17. https://doi.org/10.1016/j.rehab.2015.11.002

Tipton-Burton, M. (2018). Traumatic brain injury. In H. M. Pendleton & W. Schultz-Krohn (Eds.), *Pedretti's occupational therapy: Practice skills for physical dysfunction* (8th ed., pp. 841-870). Elsevier.

Toglia, J. (1991). Generalization of treatment: A multicontext approach to cognitive perceptual impairment in adults with brain injury. *American Journal of Occupational Therapy, 45,* 505-516. https://doi.org/10.5014/ajot.45.6.505

Toglia, J. P. (2018). The dynamic interactional model and the multicontext approach. In N. Katz & J. Toglia (Eds.), *Cognition, occupation, and participation across the lifespan* (4th ed., pp. 355-385). AOTA Press.

Vance, D. E., & Crowe, M. (2006). A proposed model of neuroplasticity and cognitive reserve in older adults. *Activities, Adaptation & Aging, 30,* 61-79. https://doi.org/10.1300/J016v30n03_04

Vanderploeg, R. D., Schwab, K., Walker, W. C., Fraser, J. A., Sigford, B. J., Date, E. S., Scott, S. G., Curtiss, G., Salazar, A. M., Warden, D. L., & the Defense and Veterans Brain Injury Center Study Group. (2008). Rehabilitation of traumatic brain injury in active duty military personnel and veterans: Defense and Veterans Brain Injury Center randomized controlled trial of two rehabilitation approaches. *Archives of Physical Medicine and Rehabilitation, 89,* 2227-2238. https://doi.org/10.1016/j.apmr.2008.06.015

White, J. A. (2019). Disability, community, culture, and identity. In B. A. B. Schell & G. Gillen (Eds.), *Willard and Spackman's occupational therapy* (13th ed., pp. 256-282). Wolters Kluwer.

Wolf, T. J., & Josman, N. (2015). A person-centered strategy using learning strategies to enable performance, participation, and well-being. In C. H. Christiansen, C. M. Baum, & J. D. Bass (Eds.), *Occupational therapy: Performance, participation, and well-being* (4th ed., pp. 485-497). SLACK Incorporated.

Wood, R., & Alderman, N. (2011). Applications of operant learning theory to the management of challenging behavior after traumatic brain injury. *Journal of Head Trauma Rehabilitation, 26,* 202-11. https://doi.org/10.1097/HTR.0b013e318217b46d

World Health Organization. (2008). *International classification of functioning, disability and health.* World Health Organization.

Ylvisaker, M., Hanks, R., & Johnson-Greene, D. (2002). Perspectives on rehabilitation of individuals with cognitive impairment after brain injury: Rationale for reconsideration of theoretical paradigms. *Journal of Head Trauma Rehabilitation, 17,* 191-209. https://doi.org/10.1097/00001199-200206000-00002

Ylvisaker, M., Jacobs, H. E., & Feeney. T. (2003). Positive supports for people who experience behavioral and cognitive disability after brain injury: A review. *Journal of Head Trauma Rehabilitation, 18,* 7-32. https://doi.org/10.1097/00001199-200301000-00005

CHAPTER 10

Details of Cognitive Treatment

Cognitive and perceptual rehabilitation has evolved rapidly in recent years, with a more robust body of evidence about the efficacy of occupational therapy treatment for cognitive and/or perceptual deficits after acquired brain injury (ABI). The evidence that has emerged increasingly shows that people can improve their occupational performance without significant changes in their scores on traditional impairment-based tests (Gillen et al., 2015; Kennedy et al., 2008). As a result, it has become more common for occupational therapy cognitive and perceptual rehabilitation to be targeted with a top-down approach in which intervention is focused on occupation rather than impairment (Gillen et al., 2015; Polatajko et al., 2011; Toglia, 2018). To be consistent with this changing view, this chapter does not discuss treatment for specific cognitive and/or perceptual deficits. Instead, it outlines different treatment approaches that can be used with all people with cognitive and/or perceptual deficits after ABI regardless of the specific impairment. We encourage practitioners to consider clients' learning ability, current performance and breakdown, occupational goals and needs, and context when making decisions about intervention approach. Many of these factors were discussed in more detail in Chapters 8 and 9. We would like to make one point that is specific to apraxia. Although apraxia manifests motorically, through conceptualization and/or execution of movement, it is a cognitive deficit (see Chapter 7 for more details). As a result, treatment of this disorder (depending on the type of apraxia) can also be addressed through the interventions we describe later in this chapter, including errorless learning and strategy training (Lidsten-McQueen et al., 2014). For readers interested in learning more about clinical treatment recommendations by impairment, including apraxia, we suggest resources such as the systematic review published by members of the Cognitive Rehabilitation Task Force of the American Congress of Rehabilitation Medicine Brain Injury Special Interest Group (Cicerone et al., 2019).

In Chapter 9, we described the revised Rancho Los Amigos Levels of Cognitive Functioning Scale (RLAS-R), which defines functioning at 10 different stages of recovery after traumatic brain injury (TBI). The RLAS-R levels provide a framework for decision making by describing the type of performance people at that level are likely to achieve in addition to learning capacity (Lin & Wroten, 2022). For example, someone at RLAS-R Level VI is starting to be able to follow

Kaminsky, T. A., & Powell, J. M.
Zoltan's Vision, Perception, and Cognition: Evaluation and Treatment of the Adult With Acquired Brain Injury, Fifth Edition (pp. 263-302).

instructions more consistently and participate more purposefully in self-care, although they will continue to need significant support from caregivers. Although the RLAS-R was created specifically for people with TBI, the levels can still provide guidance when planning for clients with other types of ABI.

In addition to the RLAS-R, there are other frameworks and models that can assist clinicians with decision making. In Chapter 9, we described a decision tree that was published by Haskins in 2012 that can serve this purpose. Using this approach, clinicians first determine clients' level of awareness about their deficits and then how performance changes with external strategies (e.g., a memory book). For clients who are not aware of their deficits and do not benefit from external strategies, Haskins (2012) recommended treatment with procedural learning (e.g., errorless learning). Clinicians can also work on assisting the client to improve awareness, which increases the likelihood of success with other interventions, including internal strategies. Clients who have or who develop at least some awareness of their deficits may benefit from internal metacognitive strategy training in addition to external strategy use and continued work on improving awareness. Clients who successfully use internalized strategies can also work on generalizing skills to promote independence in a variety of environments. People at all stages of recovery and with all types of learning capacities can benefit from environmental modification.

In this chapter, we start with a discussion of environmental modification and activity adaptation because these interventions are used by occupational therapy practitioners across the range of brain injury severity and practice settings. We next discuss awareness and interventions for awareness development because the degree to which a client is aware of (or can learn to be aware of) their deficits is a key factor in determining what treatment approach to take at a given time. We move on to errorless/procedural learning, strategy training (external and internal), and generalization. In keeping with the current thinking in occupational therapy, the focus is on occupation, with meaningful and functional activities used as treatment (Gillen et al., 2015). Throughout this chapter, we focus on how these treatment approaches can be used for people with cognitive impairment. Readers should be aware that many of these approaches are applicable to those with perceptual impairments as well, although we explicitly discuss those less frequently.

Environmental Modification and Activity Adaptation

Occupational therapy practitioners have long considered the interaction between the environment and the person's abilities. They understand that disability can decrease or increase based on the presence of supports or barriers in the environment, respectively (American Occupational Therapy Association [AOTA], 2020; Gitlin et al., 2001; Johansson et al., 2011). More recently, the broader health care community has started to recognize the interplay between skills and environment as evidenced by the inclusion of context in the World Health Organization's (2001) *International Classification of Functioning, Disability and Health*. As a result of this interaction between skills and environmental demands, a person with cognitive impairment after ABI may function relatively independently in a familiar, structured, and predictable home environment where items are recognized and routines are well established. This same person may perform poorly if asked to function in a rapidly changing environment that is novel, such as a new work or volunteer setting (Gitlin et al., 2001).

Even people without cognitive impairment and a stable set of skills perform differently in various environments. Imagine yourself driving your car home from school or work along a familiar route in the daytime. Chances are good that you would be able to drive safely even if you

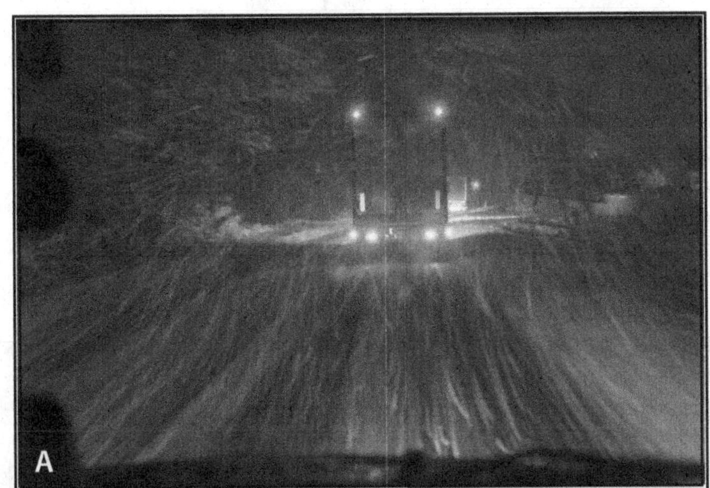

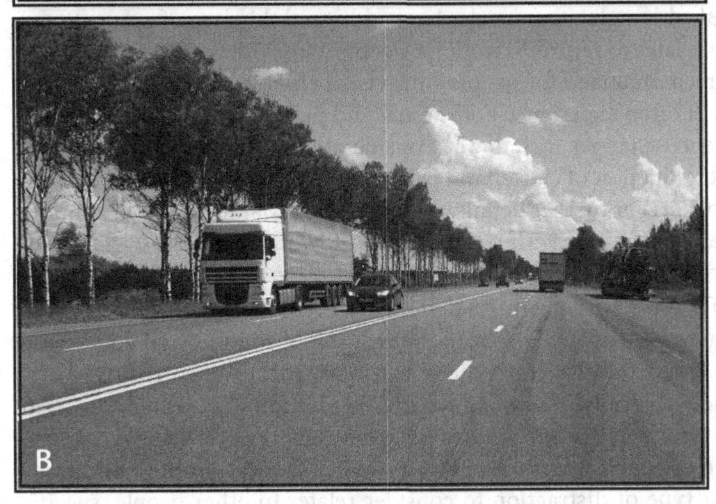

Figure 10-1. Changes in environment put different demands on people, and adjustments will need to be made to better ensure success with tasks. When driving in a snowstorm (A) at night versus (B) on a clear day, drivers will be more successful with safe driving if they slow down and reduce distractions (e.g., turning off the radio). (A: trezordia/shutterstock.com; B: Vladimir Glazkov/shutterstock.com)

had music playing or if there were other people in the car having conversations with you. Now imagine driving a rental car while looking for an unfamiliar location in an unfamiliar city at night in poor weather. It is likely that you would take steps to simplify the task for yourself, such as turning off music, asking people to cease conversation, and slowing down. By taking these steps, you make a complex task easier and increase the likelihood that you will be successful in finding your destination. You as a driver are unchanged in these scenarios. The differences lie in the environmental demands. The environmental demands in the second scenario make it more difficult for you to function, and if you do not change aspects of the task, you decrease your chances of success (Figure 10-1). This process of assessing the impact of the environment and making changes so that it better supports performance is the same for occupational therapy practitioners who are working with clients with disability, and it becomes vitally important when working with people recovering from ABI because the likelihood of a mismatch between skills and environmental/activity demands increases for this population (Wong et al., 2017).

To fully support people with cognitive deficits after ABI, the occupational therapy practitioner needs to consider the environment that surrounds the person as well as the demands of the task. The *Occupational Therapy Practice Framework: Domain and Process, Fourth Edition* (AOTA, 2020) describes four environments that should be considered in treatment: (a) natural environment and human-made changes to the environment, (b) products and technology, (c) social supports and relationships, and (d) attitudes. Natural and human-made changes to the environment, along with products and technology, make up the physical environment, which includes structures and objects as well as aspects that may not be as obvious, including types of sensory input (e.g., background noise levels) and cognitive demands (e.g., the reading level of the instruction manuals). Social supports and relationships along with attitudes make up the social environment and include those that surround the person with ABI, such as family, friends, employers, coworkers, neighbors, and others with whom the client interacts. The attitudes held by these community members (e.g., their feelings about people with disabilities) can also influence occupational engagement for the person with ABI by making the community more or less welcoming (AOTA, 2020; Cohn & Lew, 2015). It is also important to consider financial and organizational factors when approaching environmental modification, including the funds that are available to the client and the people who will be responsible for implementing and maintaining environmental changes (Cohn & Lew, 2015). Not all recommendations will be feasible and appropriate for all clients and need to be individually determined.

Little is published related to recommendations or research on the impacts of environmental modification for people with ABI, although a few articles have addressed this area of occupational therapy practice, most often as it relates to return to work for people with ABI. Some of the recommendations overlap with those recommended for people with visual changes, and it is important to remember that people with ABI often experience both visual and perceptual/cognitive deficits. These recommended environmental changes include the consideration of lighting levels, reduction of glare, increasing contrast, reduction of clutter and patterns, and emphasizing organization (Below & Lewis, 2021; Warren, 2018). (For further details, see Chapter 4.) Making the environment easier to interpret visually can assist a person with cognitive deficit by decreasing the amount of effort that is needed to process the visual scene.

Specific recommendations for those with cognitive deficits after ABI include the reduction of distractions, simplification of tasks, schedule changes and utilization of routine, and addressing others' expectations (Radomski & Giles, 2021; Wortzel & Arciniegas, 2012). When reducing distraction, it is important to consider a variety of sensory systems in addition to visual as discussed previously. Auditory distraction, such as background noise from other people's conversations, music, televisions, and more, can have an impact on a person's ability to focus on tasks and complete them successfully. Another type of distraction to consider relates to other people, specifically the number of others who are present and their proximity to the person with ABI. This is especially true in public spaces or at work (Stergiou-Kita et al., 2012). When adjusting distraction, many people benefit from quieter and less dynamic environments to maximize functioning and to allow them to focus attention more easily (Wortzel & Arciniegas, 2012; Figure 10-2). However, it is important to remember that to be fully independent people need to be able to function in a variety of situations, including those with more distraction, so it benefits the person with ABI to work in a variety of environments in occupational therapy treatment to allow the practice of skills under different circumstances when possible. Increasing or decreasing distraction is a way to grade activities in intervention sessions for those with cognitive deficits.

Task simplification principles can work in conjunction with environmental modification and can be applied to a wide variety of activities as a way to decrease their demand and the effort that is needed on the part of the person with ABI. These principles include reducing the number of steps that a person needs to complete while performing an activity, changing the tools that are used to those that are more intuitive and familiar, reducing the number of choices that need to be made, and changing setup (Wortzel & Arciniegas, 2012). For example, imagine a client named Chris, a 54-year-old man who sustained a stroke. Chris is struggling to get dressed independently. He gets overwhelmed easily and has difficulty initiating the task as a result. His occupational therapy practitioner, Duane, works with Chris and his wife to simplify the dressing task so that Chris can be more independent. One strategy they use is thinning out unnecessary clothes from

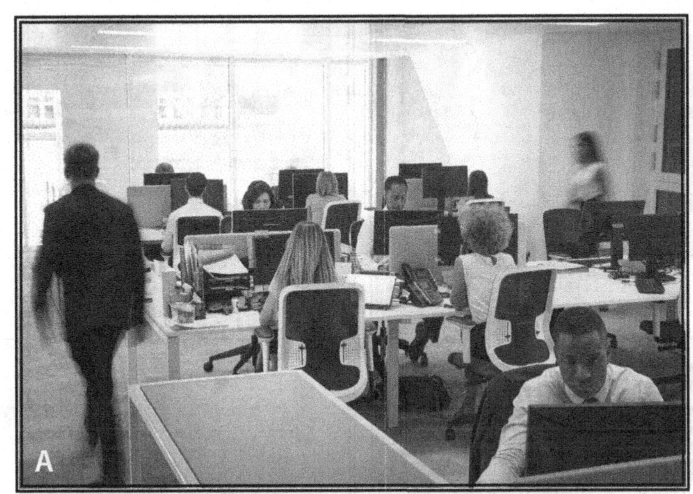

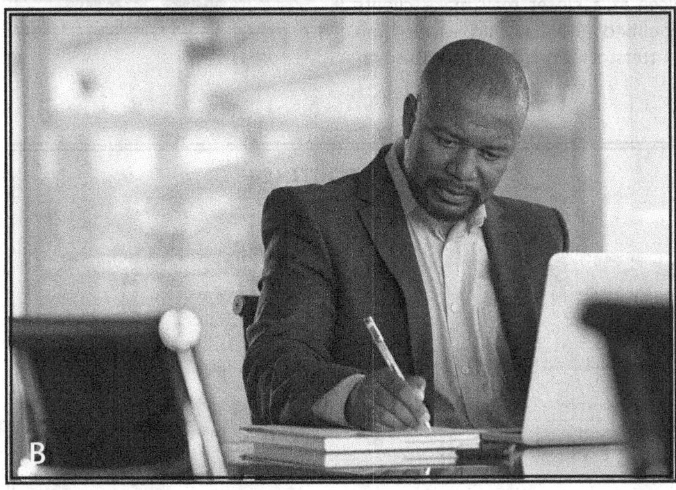

Figure 10-2. Changing the environment can improve occupational performance for people with cognitive deficits after ABI. People with ABI are often easily distracted, and (A) an open workspace plan may be too distracting for them. (B) Being able to work in a more private location with fewer distractions can improve productivity with work. (A: Monkey Business Images/shutterstock.com; B: Rido/shutterstock.com)

Chris's closet and dresser by taking out those that are not appropriate for the season and giving him fewer choices (Figure 10-3). They may need to simplify this further by having Chris's wife lay out his clothing for him, with the ultimate goal of adding the step of choosing clothes back into the task when and if Chris improves. They can also lessen the demands of the activity by simplifying the clothing itself (e.g., choosing pants with elastic waistbands rather than buttons and zippers or T-shirts rather than button-down shirts).

Schedules and routines are important to consider for those with cognitive deficits after ABI. It often takes longer for these individuals to process information, and they often need to have extra time to complete tasks. Cognitive fatigue after ABI is also extremely common and has a big impact on the person's ability to concentrate and attend to tasks (Matérne et al., 2017). These issues can impact all areas of occupation but may be especially problematic if the person wants to return to work. Flexibility with scheduling is an essential accommodation to consider, including having the person work reduced hours, adjusting work times to match when the person is well rested and most alert (e.g., working from midmorning to midafternoon only), and providing longer and more frequent breaks (Matérne et al., 2017).

In addition to considering scheduling, it is essential to set up established routines whenever possible, not only at work but at home as well. People with ABI benefit from predictability and organization (Figure 10-4). It takes longer for this population to learn new routines or to adjust

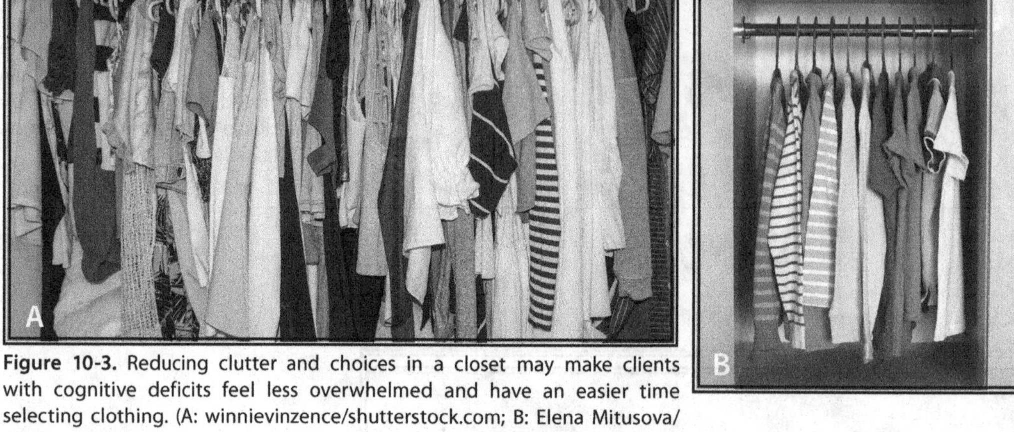

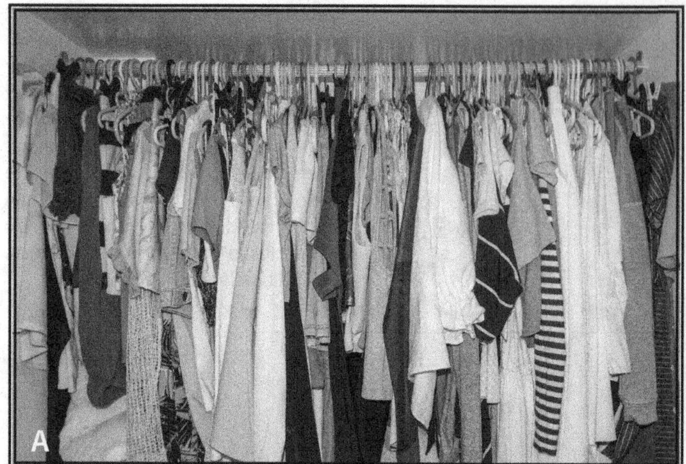

Figure 10-3. Reducing clutter and choices in a closet may make clients with cognitive deficits feel less overwhelmed and have an easier time selecting clothing. (A: winnievinzence/shutterstock.com; B: Elena Mitusova/shutterstock.com)

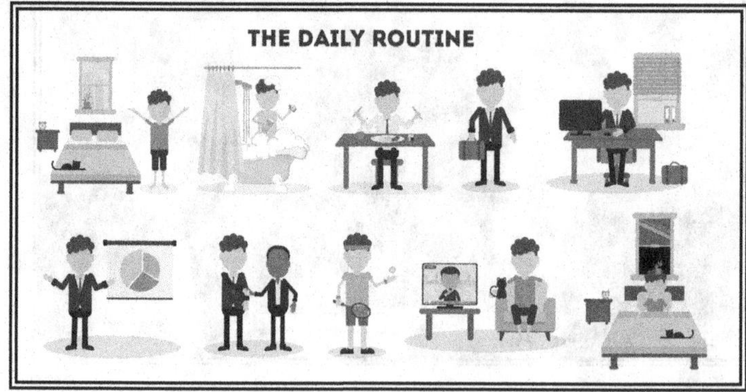

Figure 10-4. Consistent routines can help provide structure and predictability for people with cognitive impairment after ABI. (Inspiring/shutterstock.com)

after changes are made (Matérne et al., 2017). As a result, keeping home and work environments organized and using regular routines for as many everyday tasks as possible can improve a person's functioning. Examples of how organization and routines can be used include having dedicated storage for items used for activities of daily living (ADLs; e.g., returning grooming items to the same location after use; Figure 10-5) and grocery shopping in the same store every week.

Although caregiver education was discussed at length in Chapter 9, it is important to address the role of caregivers and other community members when considering environmental modification. These are the people who make up the social environment, which can have an enormous impact on functioning for people with disability (Wong et al., 2017). In many cases, caregivers will need to assist people in making and maintaining modifications in addition to other types of interventions discussed in this chapter. As a result, it is essential for caregivers to fully understand the person's functional level along with what types of cues, strategies, or modifications maximize occupational performance. A therapist who completes a thorough evaluation, including using dynamic assessment, will be able to guide caregivers most effectively (Toglia, 2018). In addition to educating caregivers who provide assistance to survivors with ABI in daily activities and home environments, training may need to be completed with other members of ABI survivors' community, including employers and coworkers, who will need to understand that people with ABI

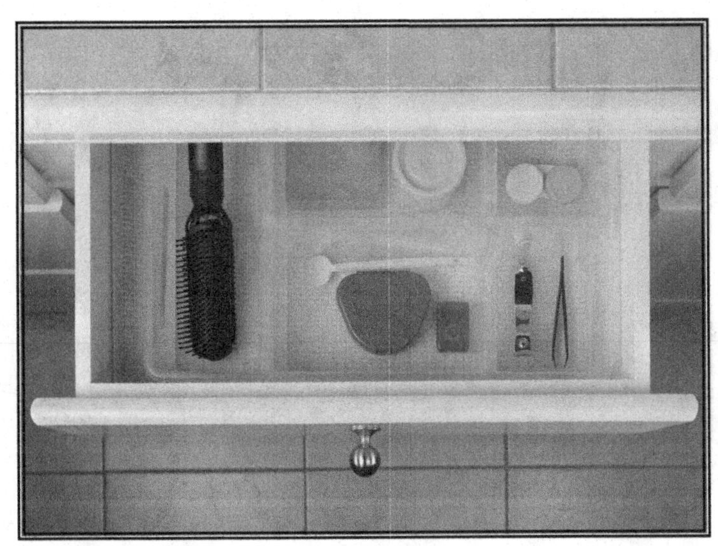

Figure 10-5. Clear organization and consistency can improve occupational performance for people with cognitive deficits after ABI. (tab62/shutterstock.com)

will need more time to complete tasks and respond to requests (Stergiou-Kita et al., 2012; Wortzel & Arciniegas, 2012). People with ABI who return to work reported that success or failure in the workplace was greatly influenced by the attitudes of others in the work environment (Matérne et al., 2017). Advocacy with the broader community, including with policy makers, to encourage universal design that takes cognition into account may also help improve community engagement for people recovering from ABI.

Although little research has been published on the impact of environmental modification for people with ABI, a great deal of research has been conducted with people with dementia. Dementia and the types of ABI considered in this text (i.e., TBI and cerebrovascular accident) differ in a variety of ways, including incidence, underlying mechanisms, and disease course, but there are similarities as well, specifically related to the presence of cognitive deficits and the increased demand on caregivers. As a result of these similarities, some of the recommendations in the literature considering environmental modification for those with dementia may be applicable to those with cognitive deficits after ABI, although it is important to recognize that not all of these have been empirically studied with the latter population. One article of interest described the following principles that can be followed when modifying the environment to maximize occupational performance and safety for people with dementia (Fleming et al., 2017):

- Unobtrusively reduce risks: People with cognitive impairment are at risk for injury, partly because of their reduced ability to recognize dangerous situations and hazards. People may wander off and get lost or access unsafe environments, such as a garage with power tools within reach. They may not recognize or remember how to use hazardous substances and other dangerous materials, such as medications and household cleansers. At the same time, they may misinterpret measures taken to ensure their safety as unnecessary and/or demeaning, which can result in anger and/or agitation. Safety measures that are more unobtrusive in nature can help give the individual as much freedom in their environment as possible while ensuring safety. For example, if a person with cognitive deficits is at risk for not recognizing materials as hazardous or not using them in a safe manner, dangerous items can be secured and stored out of sight (van Hoof et al., 2010; Figure 10-6).

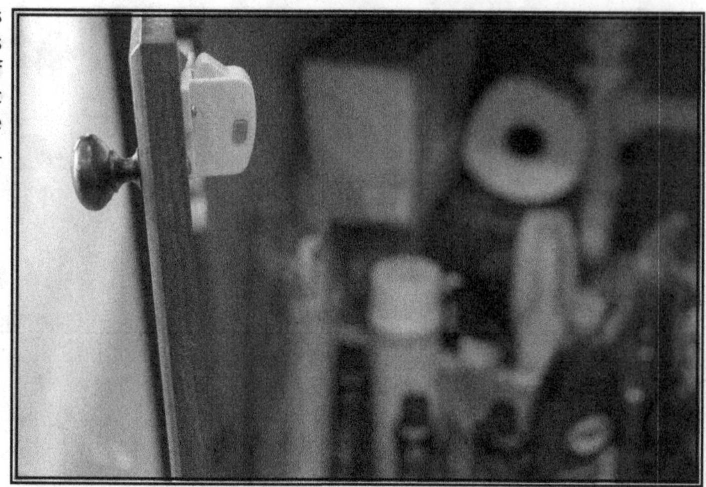

Figure 10-6. Securing hazardous household substances, such as cleaners, is important for safety if people with cognitive impairment struggle to accurately identify these items as dangerous. (Lost_in_the_Midwest/shutterstock.com)

- Manage the level of stimulation: As stated previously, it is important to consider all sensory systems when assessing the level of stimulation that is present in a setting to ensure that the environment is not overwhelming and causing sensory overload. Avoiding sensory overload is important because it can reduce the ability of the person with a brain injury to cope. Sensory overload typically results in decreased performance and can cause the person to become agitated. The authors also emphasize that the environment should not be so simplified that the person experiences sensory deprivation. Finding middle ground is important (Fleming et al., 2017; van Hoof et al., 2010) as is flexibility in making adjustments because the person's ability to cope in a particular environment can change from one time to another based on a number of factors (e.g., fatigue level; presence of an illness, such as a cold; degree of stimulation earlier in the day). Caregivers should be prepared to reduce stimulation in any given environment or to leave the setting if sufficient adjustments cannot be made. It is almost always better to err on the side of avoiding sensory overload rather than hoping the person will be able to cope or that the level of stimulation will decrease.
- Assist with orientation and provide familiar tools and materials: Setting up the environment to cue and orient a person is well described in the literature on environmental modification. The context that surrounds the person can help them in initiating routines and with locating needed items (Fleming et al., 2017; van Hoof et al., 2010). Some examples of these types of modifications include using labels to indicate what is stored in cupboards or drawers, keeping materials that are needed for a task visible, having calendars and clocks in prominent locations, and posting schedules (Padilla, 2011; Figure 10-7). It is also helpful if the tools that the person uses are familiar. Whenever possible, a person's own tools should be used. When adaptation is necessary, it is best to consider options that are more intuitive in nature. For example, replacing a round doorknob with a lever handle can improve ease with opening doors, and lever handles are intuitive to use. However, using a tool such as a buttonhook is not intuitive and will likely prove challenging for a person with cognitive impairment to use (Padilla, 2011).

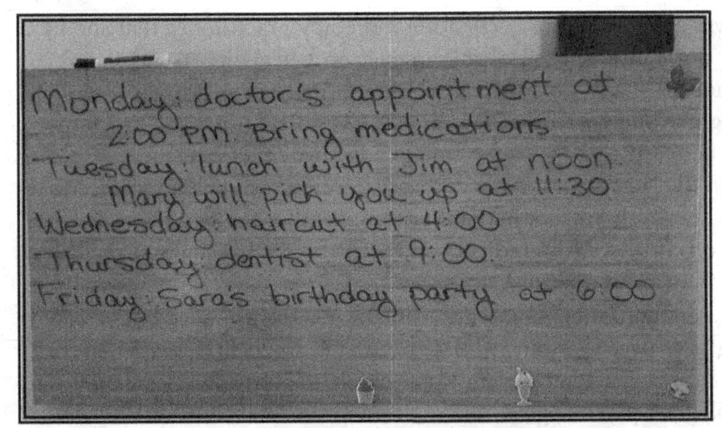

Monday: doctor's appointment at
2:00 PM. Bring medications
Tuesday: lunch with Jim at noon
Mary will pick you up at 11:30
Wednesday: haircut at 4:00
Thursday: dentist at 9:00
Friday: Sara's birthday party at 6:00

Figure 10-7. Having calendars and schedules posted in centralized and visible locations can assist with orientation and serve as reminders about appointments or other events.

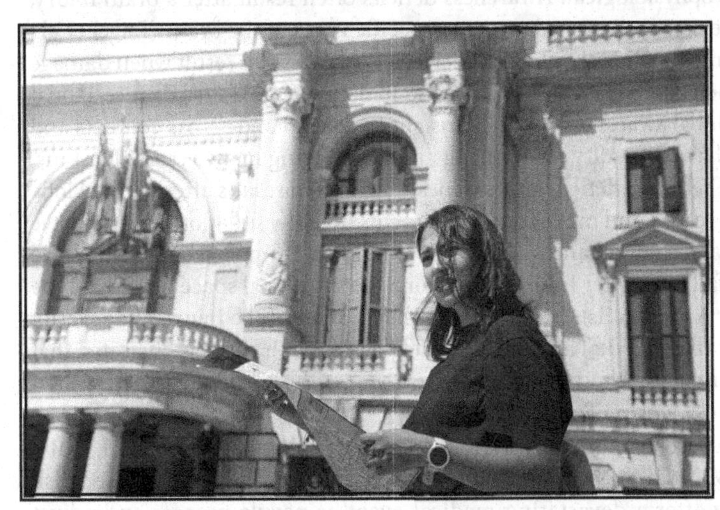

Figure 10-8. The awareness of performance and when mistakes have been made are necessary for independent functioning. In this case, this woman recognizes that she is lost (emergent awareness) and uses a strategy (looking at a map) to solve the problem. (Rizar el pixel/shutterstock.com)

Awareness Training

Awareness is critical in the recovery of people with ABI because it gives people the ability to recognize the presence and scope of deficits, to recognize the functional implications of deficits, and to anticipate situations in which deficits will create issues that need to be overcome. Awareness is oftentimes described as having three levels—intellectual, emergent, and anticipatory—although some researchers challenge a hierarchical conceptualization of these types of awareness (Toglia & Kirk, 2000). Intellectual awareness, the most basic level, is the recognition of the presence of deficits with people able to verbalize that they have deficits but have not necessarily made adjustments to accommodate their deficits. Emergent awareness is the ability to recognize that errors are occurring when they are made, allowing people to self-monitor performance during tasks and take steps to adjust their approach when needed (Figure 10-8). Anticipatory awareness, the most advanced level, is the ability to predict the impact of deficits on performance, allowing people to choose tasks that match their skills and identify and use strategies that will increase the likelihood of success (Toglia & Kirk, 2000; Toglia & Maeir, 2018). The level of awareness that is reached varies, with some individuals never reaching intellectual awareness and others developing a high level of anticipatory awareness. For example, imagine Josefina, a woman with memory impairment after a stroke, baking cookies. In the early stages of her recovery, Josefina reached the level of intellectual awareness. She was able to tell her occupational therapy practitioner that she had a memory impairment but did not consider the possible impact on her ability to bake cookies and did not recognize errors that she made. As Josefina recovered further and gained emergent awareness, she was able to recognize and correct mistakes, such as realizing that she had forgotten to retrieve sugar from the cupboard when it came time to add sugar to the recipe. After she gained anticipatory awareness in the later stages of her recovery, Josefina was able to foresee that her memory impairment could negatively impact her ability to remember the various aspects of baking cookies, so she made a careful list of ingredients and steps before baking and regularly referred to her list during the task to avoid making errors.

Impaired awareness is very common after ABI, with estimates for the presence of decreased awareness in those with TBI ranging between 76% and 97% (Goverover et al., 2007). However, the origin of impaired awareness is not fully understood. Several contributors to poor awareness have been proposed, including neurophysiological, psychological, and socioenvironmental (Haskins, 2012).

The first contributor is neurophysiological. Awareness deficits often result after a brain injury, and decreased awareness is more common after damage to specific areas of the brain (Engel et al., 2017; Haskins, 2012; Toglia & Kirk, 2000). More global deficits in awareness can result when damage occurs in the frontal lobe and when damage is more widespread in nature (e.g., from a diffuse axonal injury). People with deficits in global awareness will lack insight in general and across contexts and situations. As a result, they will have difficulty recognizing and overcoming many errors (Haskins, 2012). People can also have more selective deficits in awareness. This often results after parietal lobe damage. These clients are able to reason and make sound judgments in many situations but will have deficits in awareness under certain circumstances (Haskins, 2012). For example, people who have hemi-inattention in which they fail to register information from contralesional space have this type of awareness deficit (see Chapter 6 for details). In addition to the location of the injury, the severity of the injury will also modify the likelihood of an awareness deficit. Research has demonstrated that people with a more severe brain injury are more likely to have issues with impaired awareness than those who have more mild injuries (Morton & Barker, 2010).

The second contributor to awareness for some individuals is psychological (Engel et al., 2017; Haskins, 2012). People with ABI often experience changes in affect, including an increased risk of depression. There is grieving after a devastating medical event as people process and adjust to changes in their bodily functions, functional skills, roles, and routines. One of the things that people may experience is denial. Denial is a psychological condition that helps to protect a person from experiencing stress (Engel et al., 2017; Toglia & Kirk, 2000). In practice, clients may experience both decreases in awareness and denial, and it can be difficult to differentiate between the two (Medley & Powell, 2010; Toglia & Kirk, 2000). Psychological denial is best treated by a psychologist (Haskins, 2012), although denial may also lessen as the person goes through the rehabilitation process.

Socioenvironmental factors make up the final contributor to awareness (Engel et al., 2017; Haskins, 2012). People develop awareness of their strengths and limitations based on their experiences and the feedback they get when they attempt tasks (Engel et al., 2017; Haskins, 2012). When people have sustained a new ABI, they do not yet have experience with their new level of physical, sensory, and cognitive functioning. As a result, they often overestimate their abilities because they are making judgments based on their premorbid level of functioning (Haskins, 2012). Clinicians may also observe differences in the level of awareness people have for different types of deficits. Often people are more aware of physical deficits than those that are sensory, perceptual, or cognitive in nature (Toglia & Kirk, 2000). As people gain experiences, they may naturally develop more awareness of deficits, especially as they return to more complex tasks (Haskins, 2012).

Research has shown that a deficit with awareness has an impact on both the rehabilitation process and functional independence (Engel et al., 2017; Goverover et al., 2007; Toglia & Kirk, 2000; Toglia & Maeir, 2018). People with poor awareness of their deficits are less likely to participate fully in rehabilitation because they do not understand the need for intervention when they are unable to appreciate the presence of impairments (Medley & Powell, 2010; Toglia & Kirk, 2000). They are also less likely to implement therapeutic recommendations (e.g., the use of the metacognitive strategies described later) if they do not think there is a need for them (Medley & Powell, 2010; Toglia & Maeir, 2018).

In addition to having less motivation for participation in the rehabilitation process, people with deficits in awareness are also less likely to be independent with functional activities, including ADLs, instrumental activities of daily living (IADLs), and work. They often fail to recognize and correct errors and may have difficulty adjusting plans when those plans fail to work (Toglia & Kirk, 2000; Toglia & Maeir, 2018). Clients also often overestimate their abilities and fail to use techniques and strategies that are needed to overcome their deficits. In fact, there is a reciprocal relationship between self-awareness and the use of processing strategies (Toglia & Kirk, 2000). Self-awareness will influence the likelihood of strategies being used and the types of strategies that will be used. In turn, the use of strategies can increase awareness because the person is able to better understand what is and is not working (Toglia & Maeir, 2018).

In addition to decreased motivation for rehabilitation and less independence, overestimation of abilities also can lead to safety issues. These safety issues occur because people are less likely to ask for needed assistance and may engage in activity that is beyond their capabilities (Toglia & Kirk, 2000; Toglia & Maeir, 2018). For example, imagine Kele, a man with memory deficits and executive dysfunction after a TBI. Kele has been told that he is unsafe to drive because of his cognitive deficits, but he has poor awareness of his deficits and believes that he is a safe driver. Because of this discrepancy between Kele's beliefs about his capabilities and his skills, he is at risk for driving his car and failing at the task, putting himself and members of his community at risk. People may even continue to drive after multiple car crashes and without a current driver's license because they do not realize how their impaired abilities are affecting their ability to drive safely.

Addressing awareness of deficits is an important component of cognitive and perceptual rehabilitation and one that often requires multiple types of intervention because of the multiple factors that influence awareness described previously (neurophysiological [e.g., location and severity of injury], psychological, and socioenvironmental; Engel et al., 2017). Awareness of deficits is a key determining factor in what type of intervention approach to use. With increasing awareness comes improved safety and independence with functional tasks, including a better ability to use metacognitive or other compensatory strategies (described in more detail later in this chapter). People who do not develop awareness of their deficits will likely need to have continued supervision and assistance and will benefit most from environmental modification and the procedural learning strategies described later (Glogoski et al., 2006; Haskins, 2012). Given the importance of awareness for engagement in rehabilitation and recovery of independence in functional performance, efforts to improve awareness are a key component of rehabilitation after ABI. When working to improve awareness in their clients, occupational therapy practitioners should consider several possible approaches. These include allowing errors, self-discovery, and utilizing a collaborative approach.

Allowing Errors

As described earlier in the discussion of socioenvironmental influences, awareness of one's ability is partly influenced by the experiences a person has. People with more acute ABI often overestimate their abilities, partly because they are basing their judgment on their premorbid skills (Toglia & Kirk, 2000). As a result, it is important for people to gain experience with their abilities after injury. Allowing them to make mistakes and to learn from those mistakes is one way clinicians can encourage the development of accurate awareness of skills (Toglia & Kirk, 2000; Toglia & Maeir, 2018). When mistakes occur, people get feedback that what they are doing is not working. This can help them understand the presence and extent of their deficits (Toglia & Kirk, 2000; Toglia & Maeir, 2018). However, learning from errors does require people to be able to recognize their mistakes, which can be difficult for some people with a brain injury (Toglia & Kirk, 2000). Practitioners can guide patients' analysis of their performance and the results of their work to encourage error recognition (discussed further later in this chapter). Through error recognition and analysis of skills, people with a brain injury may start to develop a more accurate understanding of their abilities. In this way, allowing errors can be useful (Radomski & Giles, 2021). It is important to recognize that this strategy would not be used if practitioners are working to develop routines and procedural skills through errorless learning (described later). The goals of errorless learning and of allowing errors are quite different. Determining which approach to use will be based on the clinician's judgment about the needs of the client, the potential for recovery, and the goals of therapy.

Self-Discovery

In many instances, people who are working to develop better awareness of their deficits will benefit more from feedback that is internally driven than externally provided. Feedback from another person, especially from a clinician who did not know the client before the brain injury, can be difficult to receive. Patients may become defensive when receiving feedback about errors, especially if the clinician's assessment contradicts the client's own appraisal of performance. Feedback about cognitive skills, as opposed to physical ability, can be especially difficult for people to hear because cognitive skills are often associated with a person's identity and feelings of self-worth. Therefore, feedback about cognitive deficits can be interpreted as an attack on the person's identity itself (Toglia & Kirk, 2000). In some cases, feedback that is interpreted as confrontational has been shown to increase agitation in people with a brain injury (Goverover et al., 2007). As a result, it is preferable if feedback is more internally driven, with clients analyzing their own performance and results to determine where deficits occur. Because of the brain injury, however, it may be difficult for self-discovery to occur without guidance from the practitioner. As a result, the clinician needs to work in a collaborative manner with the client to assist in discovering deficits rather than simply telling the client what went wrong (Haskins, 2012).

Collaborative Approach

When working with clients with awareness deficits, it can be helpful to use some of the principles of motivational interviewing, which is a way of communicating that is designed to encourage and motivate people (Medley & Powell, 2010). Those who utilize motivational interviewing approach interactions with clients with the understanding that decision making in therapy should be collaborative as a partnership between the clinician and client and that the client is autonomous, meaning that therapy should be client centered and always focused on the client's goals

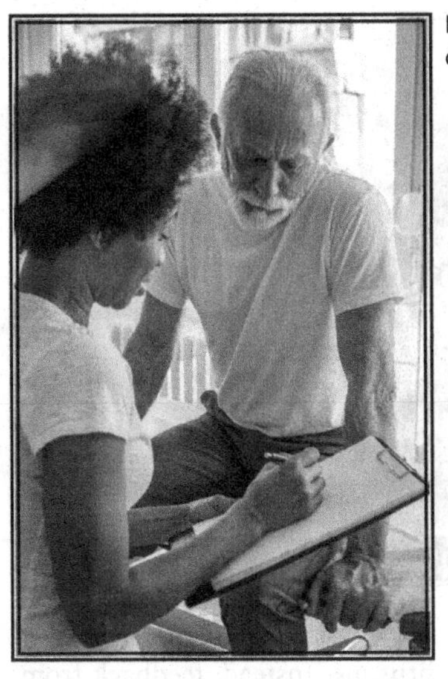

Figure 10-9. Active listening is essential for establishing a therapeutic and collaborative relationship with clients. (Mladen Zivkovic/shutterstock.com)

rather than the clinician's (Medley & Powell, 2010). There are several principles associated with motivational interviewing that can prove useful when interacting with clients with a brain injury and working with them on increasing their awareness of deficits.

The first is to express empathy. It is important for the client to view the practitioner as helpful rather than punitive. Practitioners who express empathy utilize reflective and active listening strategies and convey that they are there to work collaboratively and establish a healthy therapeutic relationship (Medley & Powell, 2010; Figure 10-9). The second principle is to avoid arguing with the client (Haskins, 2012; Radomski & Giles, 2021). A client who is displaying resistance during therapy sessions is signaling to the clinician that a different approach is needed. This may be accomplished by changing the communication style (Medley & Powell, 2010). For example, rather than dictating what needs to happen (e.g., "You need to do this"), the practitioner can work as a partner in problem solving (e.g., "This does not seem to be working; what do you think you can try instead?"). The final principle in motivational interviewing is to work toward helping the person develop self-confidence (Medley & Powell, 2010). Working at a just-right challenge and recognizing successes are important in helping the client achieve self-confidence (Toglia & Maeir, 2018). A just-right challenge also helps people to be better able to improve their awareness. If a task is too easy, they will be less likely to make errors from which they need to learn. If the task is too difficult, the person is less likely to be able to understand their own performance and be able to integrate the changes that need to be made (Goverover et al., 2007; Toglia, 2018). Recognizing success and setting a difficulty level that enables people to succeed can encourage participation in therapy and beyond. People who only see failures and do not experience successes are at risk of avoiding participation in activity, which can have major implications for subsequent occupational engagement and quality of life (Medley & Powell, 2010).

Treatment Strategies for Improving Awareness

There are two main treatment strategies to use with people who are working to develop awareness. The first is to use feedback in guiding the person toward being able to recognize errors and deficits (Cicerone et al., 2019). As stated previously, feedback needs to be carefully used when working with clients with a brain injury. Direct feedback from practitioners may not

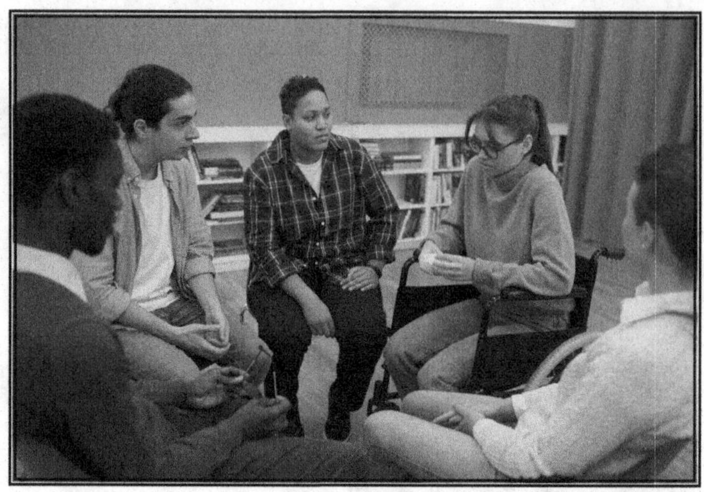

Figure 10-10. Some clients may find it easier to receive feedback about their performance from peers than from practitioners. Group treatment is one place where peer feedback may be elicited. (SeventyFour/shutterstock.com)

always be well received, especially if it is given in a way that is brusque. Instead, feedback from clinicians needs to be given in a collaborative and empathetic manner (Haskins, 2012; Radomski & Giles, 2021). Feedback can also be provided through other means. Some research has been conducted with clients receiving cognitive rehabilitation in group settings. Feedback that comes from peers who are experiencing similar challenges can be helpful and positively received by clients (Goverover et al., 2007; Figure 10-10). An added benefit to encouraging feedback in a group setting is that giving constructive feedback to another person may help people recognize similar deficits in themselves. The latter rationale underlies role reversal, another technique that can be used with clients who lack insight. In role reversal, a practitioner performs a task for a client while the client watches and critiques the practitioner's performance. The practitioner makes mistakes that are similar to those the client makes to see if the client is able to recognize errors when they are made by someone else (Toglia, 2018). An additional method to use when providing feedback is to have clients critique their own performance from a video recording of them completing tasks. This strategy enables clients to watch and critique their own performance and may allow them to recognize errors they missed while originally performing the activity (Toglia, 2018).

The most frequently used and studied treatment technique for improving awareness is a formalized process of self-discovery of deficits in which a person predicts and then reflects on their performance. This treatment technique has two main steps: prediction and reflection of performance and outcomes (Haskins, 2012; Radomski & Giles, 2021; Toglia, 2018; Toglia & Maeir, 2018). Clients may also stop to check performance in the middle of completing activities if the practitioner thinks it would be beneficial (Radomski & Giles, 2021; Toglia, 2018). It is best if this treatment technique is used with functional activity, especially those that are familiar to the person because that will enable them to compare their current performance with their premorbid levels (Goverover et al., 2007; Toglia, 2018).

- Predict performance and outcomes: Before completing an activity, a client is asked to predict both performance on the task and the outcome. The practitioner should ask the client if any issues are anticipated and what strategies will be used if problems occur (Haskins, 2012; Toglia, 2018). The client may also be asked to rate the expected difficulty of the task (Toglia, 2018).

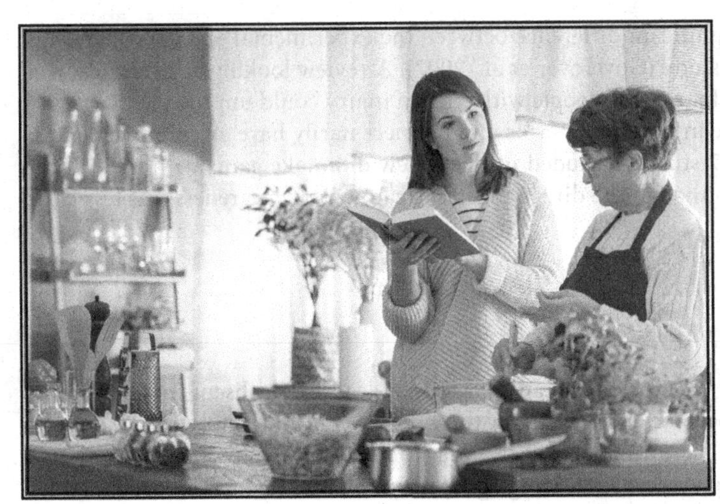

Figure 10-11. Pausing during an activity to assess performance and results is one way to teach people to monitor for errors and take steps to correct mistakes. (Photographee.eu/shutterstock.com)

- Reflect on performance and outcomes: After the task is completed, the client is asked to reflect on both the performance of the task and the outcome. Clients are asked if they used any strategies to complete the activity. If they recognize errors that were made, they are asked what they could do if a similar error is made in the future. Clients can also be asked what they would do the same or differently the next time they complete the activity (Haskins, 2012; Toglia, 2018). This step can be combined with the feedback strategies described earlier, including feedback from practitioners, peers, or self-critique from watching recordings. Reflection can also incorporate the use of a journal so that the client can track progress over time (Haskins, 2012; Toglia, 2018; Toglia & Maeir, 2018).
- Additional checks: Additional checks can be added in the middle of the process if the practitioner determines that the client would benefit from them. During this step, clients are asked to pause in the middle of their performance to analyze how performance is progressing. The clients are asked whether or not they are still on track and if anything needs to be adjusted in order to complete the task successfully (Toglia et al., 2012).

To visualize prediction and reflection within a treatment session, imagine a client named Barbara, a 72-year-old woman with a TBI. Her occupational therapy practitioner, Tanya, is working with her on improving her awareness of her abilities. In the session, Barbara prepares pasta with tomato sauce and a salad. Before starting the activity, Tanya asks Barbara to predict how she will do with the activity. Some of the questions she could ask include whether or not Barbara thinks she will be successful in making the meal, if she foresees any problems that could arise, how she thinks her performance will compare to what she would have been able to do before her injury, and if she will need to use any strategies or tools to support herself in completing the task. As Barbara completes the activity, Tanya will watch to see if Barbara is able to recognize and self-correct any errors and what, if any, strategies she uses. Tanya may ask Barbara to stop partway through her meal preparation to review how things are going and if she needs to do anything differently (Figure 10-11). At the end of the task, Tanya will ask Barbara to reflect on her performance, asking if she is satisfied with the outcome of her meal preparation, if things went as she expected, what went well for her that she could do again, and if she would make any changes the next time she prepares a meal.

Research with the prediction and reflection technique has demonstrated that some individuals can improve their performance in functional activities with this treatment approach. The direct impact on awareness itself is less clear. In one study with 20 adults with ABI, people who received therapy using the prediction/reflection strategy had significantly better self-regulation skills, although there was no significant difference between the experimental and control groups on awareness at the end of the study (Goverover et al., 2007). A review looking at the efficacy of an awareness intervention also found that people with a brain injury could improve with activity participation and independence in functional tasks and not necessarily have an improvement in awareness. Participants in all 17 studies included in the review did make gains with their occupational therapy outcomes even though the direct effect of treatment on awareness was less clear (Engel et al., 2017).

Awareness and Affect

Practitioners should know that increasing awareness may lead to a subsequent increase in emotional distress. As people become more aware of their deficits and the impact those deficits are having on their occupational performance and everyday life, they may enter into a more active state of grieving. Clinicians may observe increasing agitation or signs of depression or anxiety as a result (Toglia & Maeir, 2018). However, this is not always true for clients. In a review of 17 studies of the efficacy of the awareness intervention, no negative impact on affect was found in any of the studies. In fact, one study found that there was an improvement in life satisfaction, possibly because the research participants simultaneously improved their performance in functional activity as their awareness of deficits increased (Engel et al., 2017). Toglia and Maeir (2018) emphasized that self-efficacy should be addressed during awareness training as well to decrease the likelihood of negative affect as awareness improves.

Errorless Learning

Errorless learning is a treatment approach that is frequently used in cognitive rehabilitation. Errorless learning allows people with more severe injuries to gain the ability to perform routine tasks that have little variation (Giles, 2018). It is often the most appropriate approach for individuals with more severe memory impairment who lack awareness of their deficits and when improved awareness is not one of the expected outcomes of treatment (Ownsworth et al., 2017). In errorless learning, practitioners work to prevent clients from making errors while learning new skills (Gillen, 2018, 2021; Radomski & Giles, 2021). The goal in errorless learning is for the client to encode information, including didactic information (e.g., names) or procedures, in an accurate manner. Errors are prevented so that the person with ABI does not encode the errors (Gillen, 2018, 2021; Radomski & Giles, 2021). The belief is that errors are easier to recall, possibly because of the emotions felt when making them (Cohen et al., 2010), so to avoid encoding errors, the person is prevented, as much as possible, from making mistakes (Gillen, 2018, 2021). Another theory is that errors may not be recognized as incorrect because the explicit memory system contributes heavily to identifying and helping to correct errors. When the explicit memory system is damaged, which is frequent after ABI, errors may not be recognized and are encoded by the implicit memory system during learning (Kessels & de Haan, 2003; Pitel et al., 2006).

The neurological reason errorless learning is effective is not fully understood. Some believe it works by allowing a person to create new procedural or implicit memories, which are often relatively preserved compared with explicit memories (Campbell et al., 2007; Evans et al., 2000; Gazzaniga et al., 2019; Mount et al., 2007). (See Chapter 7 for details about different types of memory.) Others believe that errorless learning makes use of residual explicit memory even when that memory system is damaged after ABI (Campbell et al., 2007; Mount et al., 2007). Whatever the underlying mechanism, there is a significant body of research showing that errorless learning

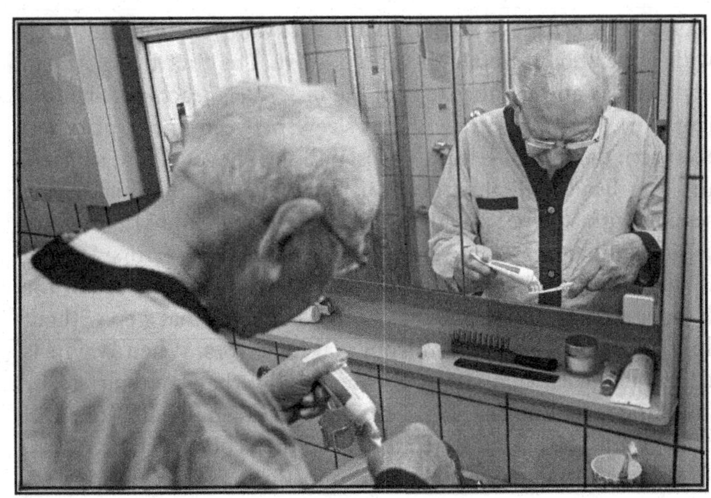

Figure 10-12. Completing activities with familiar objects and in familiar locations (e.g., when grooming with one's own tools in one's own bathroom) can improve occupational performance by making use of established routines. (Ingo Bartussek/shutterstock.com)

is helpful for teaching everyday tasks to people with ABI. It is especially useful for tasks that rely more heavily on procedural or implicit memory, namely tasks that are relatively unchanging and that take place in consistent environments (Evans et al., 2000; Gillen, 2021; Ownsworth et al., 2017). Skills that require more generalization or flexibility are not typically appropriate to teach with errorless learning because research has shown that the technique does not usually promote generalization (Cicerone et al., 2019; Cohen et al., 2010; Lidsten-McQueen et al., 2014; Ownsworth et al., 2017).

When a client's goals include learning a skill or routine that will be relatively constant (e.g., many ADLs), errorless learning is a treatment approach to consider (Ownsworth et al., 2017). It will be best for the training to occur within context as much as possible because the environment that surrounds the client can be used to help cue the person to start and progress though the routine (Cohen et al., 2010). For example, if teaching a person to be more independent with grooming activities, the practitioner will want to conduct errorless learning in the bathroom, ideally the client's own bathroom, with the tools that will be used in the task (e.g., the client's own toothbrush, razor, hairbrush; Figure 10-12). During the training, the practitioner will teach the skill or task to the client using verbal instructions, visual demonstration, or physical guidance, including hand-over-hand assistance (Cohen et al., 2010; Radomski & Giles, 2021). As the person learns the task, the cues are gradually faded (Radomski & Giles, 2021). Practitioners who use errorless learning can also use a number of treatment strategies in therapy sessions to provide additional structure to the training. Some of the more common strategies are backward chaining, forward chaining, and spaced retrieval (Campbell et al., 2007; Kelly & Nikopoulos, 2010).

Backward chaining can be used when teaching a person a multistep skill or routine. To use this strategy, the practitioner guides the client through each step of the skill or routine using verbal instruction, demonstration, or physical guidance. The next time the client attempts the routine or skill, the practitioner will guide them through each step until the last one. The client will perform the final step without assistance, although the practitioner will step in if the client cannot remember the step or starts to make an error. After the client is able to consistently perform the final step without assistance, the practitioner will guide the client through all of the steps until the second to last one; the client is asked to perform the final two steps without assistance. The process is continued, with the practitioner gradually asking the client to complete more of the skill or routine without assistance (Evans et al., 2000). To illustrate this strategy, imagine an occupational therapy practitioner named Aliyah working with Wayne, a 25-year-old man who sustained a TBI. In addition to cognitive impairment, Wayne has left hemiparesis and needs to learn one-handed dressing strategies. Aliyah decides to use errorless learning with backward chaining to teach Wayne the new skill, starting with upper body dressing with a T-shirt. The first thing Aliyah must do is to complete an activity analysis and list the steps of the task she is teaching. She lists the following: retrieve shirt, orient shirt, position shirt with left sleeve between knees, place left arm in sleeve, lean forward with left arm dangling between knees, pull sleeve over elbow, sit back, put right arm in sleeve, pull shirt over head, pull shirt down in back, and finish straightening shirt. During her first training session with Wayne, Aliyah guides him through all of the steps of the task using verbal cues and physical guidance and preventing him from making errors. During the next training session, Aliyah verbally and physically guides Wayne through all steps of the task until the last one (i.e., finish straightening shirt). She asks him to complete that step without assistance, although she will help if needed to prevent him from making errors. When Wayne is able to consistently complete the final step without assistance, Aliyah will verbally and physically guide him through the steps up until the second to last step (i.e., pull shirt down in back). She will ask him to complete the final two steps until he has mastered them and then continue the process, having him complete the final three steps without assistance and so forth.

Forward chaining uses the same general strategy as backward chaining, except that the practitioner will have the client start by completing the first step of the task without assistance rather than the final step. The practitioner will then guide the client through the remaining steps, being careful to ensure that the client does not make any mistakes (Evans et al., 2000). Using the scenario described previously, if Aliyah wants to use errorless learning with forward chaining to teach Wayne one-handed upper body dressing with a T-shirt, her first task is the same, which is to complete an activity analysis and list the steps of the activity she wants to teach to Wayne. She will then verbally and physically guide him through all steps of the activity, working to ensure that he does not make errors. In her next treatment session, Aliyah will ask Wayne to complete the first step of the upper body dressing task (i.e., retrieve shirt) without assistance as much as possible, although she will help if needed to avoid errors. She will then verbally and physically guide him through the remaining steps of the task. When Wayne masters the first step, Aliyah will ask him to perform the first two steps before assisting him and so forth until he has mastered all of the steps of the activity.

Spaced retrieval aims to systematically increase the amount of time between when a person is taught information and when that person needs to remember the information (Cohen et al., 2010). When using this approach, practitioners teach clients information and ask immediately for the information to be repeated. The practitioner will then teach the information again and allow a little time to pass before asking the client to repeat the information. If the client is accurate in recalling the information, the amount of time between the presentation of the information and the request for recall is increased. Returning to the example provided earlier, imagine that Aliyah wants to use spaced retrieval when teaching Wayne one-handed dressing. Aliyah tells Wayne that the first step is to retrieve his shirt. She then immediately asks him what the first step of upper body dressing is. If Wayne is accurate in repeating the information, Aliyah will praise him and move on. The next time she teaches Wayne upper body dressing, she will tell him that the first step is to retrieve his shirt. She will then wait for a short period of time before asking him what the first step is with upper body dressing. The amount of time between her instruction and his recall of the step will increase as long as he is still accurate in remembering the information.

One of the critiques of errorless learning is that it is time intensive and requires significant involvement from the practitioner. The creation of new procedural memories takes time. One review reported that training people to complete a task took between 2 and 5 weeks (Lidsten-McQueen et al., 2014). In addition, the avoidance of errors requires another person to be present at all times during training in order to guide the client through correct completion of activities, which can put a lot of demand on clinicians (Ownsworth et al., 2017). Some research has been performed to examine whether or not the training needed with errorless learning can be completed by people other than a practitioner. One case study looked at the use of errorless learning with a man 6 years post-TBI with residual impairment. Errorless learning was used to teach him to use his memory notebook and to walk his dog independently. His mother completed much of the training with the participant with support from the therapy team, mostly through the telephone. The participant had good outcomes with gaining independence in the trained tasks and was able to maintain his performance for at least 18 months postintervention (Campbell et al., 2007). Similar findings were reported in another case study with a woman with severe and persistent memory deficits after stroke. In this case, her family was trained with errorless learning as a way to teach daily living routines, including diabetes management. The family was able to successfully implement training with the participant at home and supported living environments with effective completion of trained tasks at close to 100% accuracy (Ferland et al., 2013). A case series with four people with severe chronic TBI had similar results when care staff implemented errorless learning under the supervision of occupational therapy practitioners. All four participants had improvement in ADL or IADL tasks (Parish & Oddy, 2007). As a result of the time and consistency that are needed for errorless learning to be effective, researchers recommended that the approach be one that is used by the entire team rather than one clinician (Pitel et al., 2006).

Errorless learning has been used with a variety of populations, including those with ABI, dementia, and schizophrenia (Ehlhardt et al., 2008). Much of the past research on errorless learning has been conducted with teaching people word lists or other semantic information (Middleton & Schwartz, 2012). More recently, people have been taught procedures for functional activities or routines. Some of the study interventions have focused on ADLs (e.g., dressing, grooming tasks), IADLs (e.g., cooking, pet care), programming devices, and using memory books (Ferland et al., 2013; Ownsworth et al., 2017). There is increasing evidence that errorless learning is effective in helping people with ABI in gaining knowledge and independence with trained tasks, especially those that are relatively unchanging (Kessels & de Haan, 2003; Ownsworth et al., 2017). This technique has been found to be helpful for people with different levels of severity with memory impairment but is most often recommended for people with more severe deficits (Cicerone et al., 2019; Cohen et al., 2010; Ferland et al., 2013; Giles, 2018; Ownsworth et al., 2017; Pitel et al., 2006; Radomski & Giles, 2021), although that may be an overgeneralization. For example, Vanderploeg and colleagues (2008) completed a randomized controlled trial with 360 active duty military personnel and veterans with moderate to severe TBI. In the study, the researchers compared two treatments. The first was a cognitive-didactic approach in which participants received impairment-focused remediation for cognitive deficits in addition to activity completion in therapy, which they completed through a trial-and-error approach. The other treatment was a functional-experiential approach in which participants completed real-life tasks in simulated and natural environments within a hospital setting using errorless learning. One year after study completion, the two groups had similar performance with independent living and employment status (or school enrollment). When subgroups were examined more closely, the researchers found that people in the functional-experimental treatment group who were over 30 years old and more highly educated had higher rates of independent living compared with participants of a similar age and education level in the cognitive-didactic group. They also found that younger participants (i.e., 30 years or younger) in the cognitive-didactic treatment group had higher rates of working or return to school than younger participants in the functional-experiential group. The researchers hypothesized that the younger participants may have benefitted from the higher level of structure and opportunities to use problem-solving strategies in the cognitive-didactic treatment sessions, whereas the older or more educated participants may have already developed those abilities preinjury and may have been able to benefit more from the direct living skills training. The researchers cautioned that the results of these subgroup comparisons should be interpreted with caution as with all ad hoc analyses that are not part of the original research question or data analysis plan.

Errorless learning may also be especially helpful in acute stages of recovery. One study examined the efficacy of errorless learning with 104 people who were experiencing post-traumatic amnesia (PTA) after TBI (Trevena-Peters et al., 2018). Researchers were curious about whether or not gains could be made if ADL retraining was started while people were still experiencing PTA, as is often done in the United States, versus waiting until people had fully emerged from PTA, which is done in other countries, including the authors' home of Australia. The researchers found that people who had received ADL retraining using errorless learning while still experiencing PTA ($n = 49$) had significantly faster improvement with ADL independence ($p = .001$). A concern with starting ADL retraining early in the recovery process was that it could increase agitation, but that was not found to be the case in this study (Trevena-Peters et al., 2018).

Strategy Training

Many people, whether they have a brain injury or not, use cognitive strategies to improve performance and successfully complete activities by bridging gaps between their abilities and the demands of the tasks they are completing (Polatajko et al., 2011). This is especially true when the task is more challenging, such as when trying to multitask or retain larger amounts of information (Toglia et al., 2012). For example, imagine Diego going to the store to shop for his weekly groceries for his family of four. He has a lot of items that he needs to pick up from all areas of the store. To make sure he gets all of the necessary items, he uses a list. Sometimes he uses one that is written, and sometimes he uses one on an app on his smartphone. He may also use his phone to text his partner to ask if an ingredient they need for a recipe is at home or if he needs to purchase more of it. He will also try to pick up items in a systematic way, moving from one side of the store to the other and gathering all of the items he needs from different sections of the store, such as produce, at once. This will minimize the number of times he needs to backtrack to get items. He may stop and check his list periodically to make sure he has not forgotten anything. All of these techniques (i.e., list making, pausing to check progress and for errors, checking in with others to confirm information, and organizing a task to maximize efficiency) are cognitive strategies and fall under the domain of metacognition, which is necessary to successfully complete many occupations, especially more complex tasks (Glogoski et al., 2006; Sohlberg & Turkstra, 2011).

Metacognition encompasses high-level cognitive skills that enable people to make judgments, plan, assess performance, correct errors, and adjust plans as needed. Metacognition also allows people to make accurate decisions about when to use cognitive strategies to help themselves in learning or improving occupational performance, a skill that requires an accurate understanding of both their own skills and the task demands (Glogoski et al., 2006; Sohlberg & Turkstra, 2011). For example, occupational therapy practitioners and students can think back to learning anatomy. As you faced the task of memorizing the structures of the hand, you made some decisions based on your own experience with your memory and similar tasks. You likely considered a variety of factors, some consciously and some unconsciously. Are you a person for whom memorizing is relatively easy or is it something that is more difficult for you? How did learning information about the hand compare with activities you had done before that had also required extensive memorization? What had you done in the past to help yourself remember information? How did that work for you? Would those techniques work for you this time or would you need to do something differently? Your ability to answer these questions relies on metacognition and your own understanding of your cognitive capabilities, specifically as they relate to memory. Your answers to the questions also enabled you to make decisions about how to approach the task of learning anatomy and the strategies that would help you succeed (Figure 10-13).

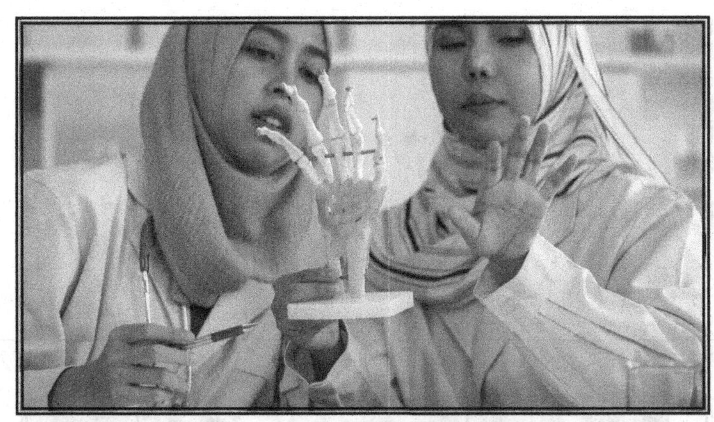

Figure 10-13. Metacognition allows people to make accurate judgments about their ability to complete tasks (e.g., learning the structures of the hand in an anatomy class) and steps they need to take to be successful (e.g., which study techniques will be most useful). (May_Chanikran/shutterstock.com)

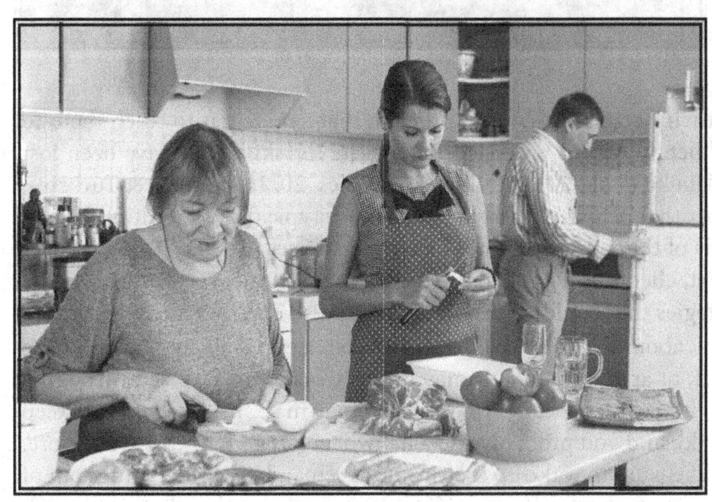

Figure 10-14. The difficulty of tasks will change the ways in which people need to approach them. Planning and cooking for a large dinner party require more planning and problem solving than preparing a simple meal for one person. (BearFotos/shutterstock.com)

Much of the time, the ability to set goals, make plans, implement plans, monitor for errors, and make adjustments happens automatically. When faced with more difficult or novel tasks, this process may become more deliberate (Fong & Howie, 2009; Sohlberg & Turkstra, 2011). Imagine making dinner for just yourself. Chances are good that it will be a fairly simple process with little effort required. It is a task that you have done countless times before, and the decision making you need is minimal. However, your metacognitive processing will continue as you complete the task and will become more apparent to you if you come across a problem (Kennedy et al., 2008). For example, if you find that you are out of an ingredient that you need, you will adjust your plan by finding a substitute, deciding the dish will be fine without the ingredient, making something else, or going to the store to pick up the needed item. Now imagine that you are planning a dinner party for six. This is a much more difficult task, requiring extensive planning and organization (Figure 10-14). Your metacognitive processing will be more effortful, and you will likely need to use strategies that you did not need when you were preparing dinner for just yourself. In both cases, you are creating goals, making plans, implementing plans, monitoring for errors, and adjusting. The effort is different, however, with the second task requiring more from you.

For many people with ABI, metacognition is impaired (Fong & Howie, 2009). This manifests as difficulty with decision making, poor awareness of deficits, inflexibility in thinking, impaired problem solving, and difficulty with error recognition (Fong & Howie, 2009; Haskins, 2012; Manly et al., 2002; Sohlberg & Turkstra, 2011). As a result, people with ABI are typically

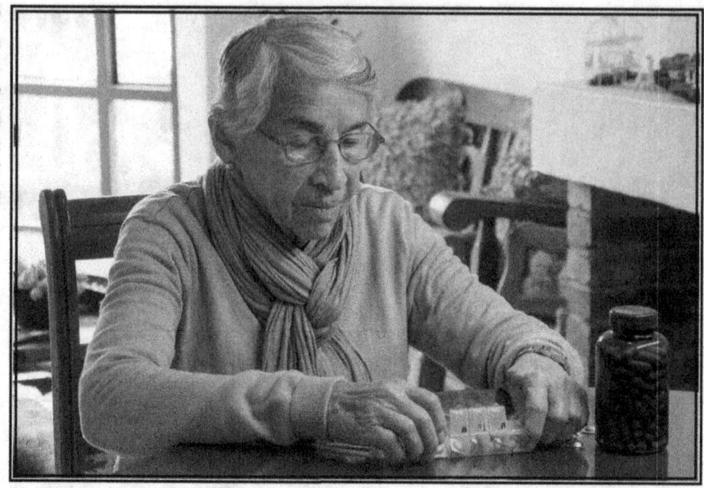

Figure 10-15. External cognitive strategies exist outside the person. This woman is using an external strategy (i.e., a pillbox) to assist her with medication management and increase her likelihood of success with the task. (Anamaria Mejia/ shutterstock.com)

less independent with many of their occupations. One approach that can help is to teach them to use cognitive strategies in a deliberate way in order to compensate for skills that have been lost or impaired (Haskins, 2012; Polatajko et al., 2011; Radomski & Giles, 2021; Sohlberg & Turkstra, 2011). It is important to remember that people without a brain injury typically use multiple cognitive strategies based on the needs of the individual and the circumstances (Toglia, 2018; Toglia et al., 2012). To be fully independent, clients will need to be flexible in the strategies they use and be able to identify a variety of strategies that could be useful (Toglia, 2018; Toglia et al., 2012).

To illustrate this point, think about the cognitive strategies you use. It is likely that you have a calendar to help you keep track of appointments. It may be electronic and accessed through a smartphone and/or computer or it may be paper based. You also may make lists to help you keep track of things that you need to do, and you probably use a list when you go to the grocery store. Alarms are also something you likely use to wake up on time or to remember to take things out of the oven. You may also set reminders for yourself to notify you when you need to do things, such as making calls to set up appointments, taking medications, or buying tickets to see your favorite band as soon as they go on sale. When working with people with cognitive deficits, strategies like these can be very helpful to improve their occupational performance (Gillen et al., 2015; Radomski & Giles, 2021). When making choices about which strategies to use with clients, practitioners need to consider a variety of factors, including a person's level of insight and ability to learn, occupations they need to complete, resources that are available to them, and caregiver support (Haskins, 2012; Toglia et al., 2012). It can also be extremely useful to learn about the types of strategies the client used before the injury. By using strategies that are familiar to people, clinicians can take advantage of already established procedural learning. These strategies will also be something clients are more likely to recognize as helpful and accept as a treatment modality (Haskins, 2012). When considering cognitive strategies, there are several categories of options.

- External strategies exist outside the person. They can be seen and heard by others (Haskins, 2012; Radomski & Giles, 2021). Examples include checklists, memory notebooks, applications on smartphones, alarms, signs, and spoken cues (Figure 10-15). For more examples of external strategies, see Table 10-1 (note that it is not exhaustive).
- Internal strategies are self-generated and cannot be observed or manipulated by other people (Haskins, 2012). Examples include using mnemonics to memorize something, self-talk when completing tasks, and double-checking work (Figure 10-16). For more examples of internal strategies, see Table 10-1 (note that it is not exhaustive).

Table 10-1

Examples of External and Internal Cognitive Strategies

External strategies: These are located outside of the person. They can be seen and/or heard by another. They may be set up and maintained by the client or by the practitioner/caregiver. These may make use of technology (e.g., smartphones). For further details about technology and people with perceptual and cognitive deficits after ABI, see Chapter 11.

STRATEGY	DESCRIPTION
Alarms	Set as a reminder for a future event, such as to remember an appointment or to take medication, or as an alert, such as if the refrigerator was left open.
Calendars	Used for organization and recall of both past and future events and appointments. When calendars are placed in prominent locations, they can assist with orientation as well.
Checklists	May be used in a variety of ways, such as making a to-do list of tasks that need to be completed. May also be used to sequence multistep activities and to help establish routines.
Memory logs	Used to help the client remember events from the day. The exact entries that are used are dependent on the person and their needs. Some common entries include appointments that occurred and any follow-up that is needed, social visits, and therapy activities that were completed (e.g., exercises, cognitive training homework). Memory logs do not need to use only written entries. For example, some clients may prefer to use photography or a combination of methods.
Signs	May be posted in a variety of places to share different types of information, including emergency numbers near a telephone, a daily schedule in the kitchen, reminders about medications on a coffee maker, and so forth.

Internal strategies: These are located within the person. They cannot be seen and/or heard by another unless the client speaks aloud. Many are used to help with remembering information, although they can be used for other activities as well.

STRATEGY	DESCRIPTION
Association	Information that needs to be remembered is linked to other things in the person's mind. For example, to remember to put trash out for pickup on Monday morning, a person may link taking out the trash to a Sunday evening television show. Immediately after the show ends, the trash is taken out.
Elaboration	The person expands on information to improve the ease of remembering it. For example, when being introduced to someone for the first time, the person may create a story or a rhyme, such as by thinking of "Gayle" and "green-eyed Gayle." In this case, the new person's name is linked to a physical feature.
Mnemonics	Use of a phrase or an acronym to remember something. For example, using "Oh, oh, oh, to touch and feel very good velvet. Such heaven!" to remember cranial nerves (Olfactory, Optic, Oculomotor, Trochlear, Trigeminal, Abducens, Facial, Vestibulocochlear, Glossopharyngeal, Vagus, Spinal accessory, Hypoglossal).

(continued)

Table 10-1 (continued)

Examples of External and Internal Cognitive Strategies

Rehearsal	Information that needs to be remembered or learned is repeated multiple times. Returning to the example of meeting Gayle, the person may repeat Gayle's name multiple times in order to remember it better.
Self-checking	Pausing in the middle of an activity to check progress. While paused, the person checks for errors and makes sure they are still on track with the task. For example, when cooking, they may pause to double-check the recipe to make sure no ingredients were missed. Self-checking can also be used to check if the person is using an identified strategy.
Self-talk	The person talks through the steps of an activity as a way to check that all steps are completed and that errors are not being made. For example, when leaving the house for work, the person may talk through the things that need to be packed up for the day. "I need to take my lunch and my wallet and my house keys. I need to take my coat and cellphone. I need to check my phone's charge before I leave the house and take a charger with me if the battery is low."

Please note that this list is not exhaustive.

Data sources: Radomski, M. V., & Giles, G. M. (2021). Cognitive intervention. In D. P. Dirette & S. A. Gutman (Eds.), *Occupational therapy for physical dysfunction* (8th ed., pp. 161-175). Wolters Kluwer and Toglia, J. P., Rodger, S. A., & Polatajko, H. J. (2012). Anatomy of cognitive strategies: A therapist's primer for enabling occupational performance. *Canadian Journal of Occupational Therapy, 79*, 225-236. https://doi.org/10.2182/cjot.2012.79.4.4

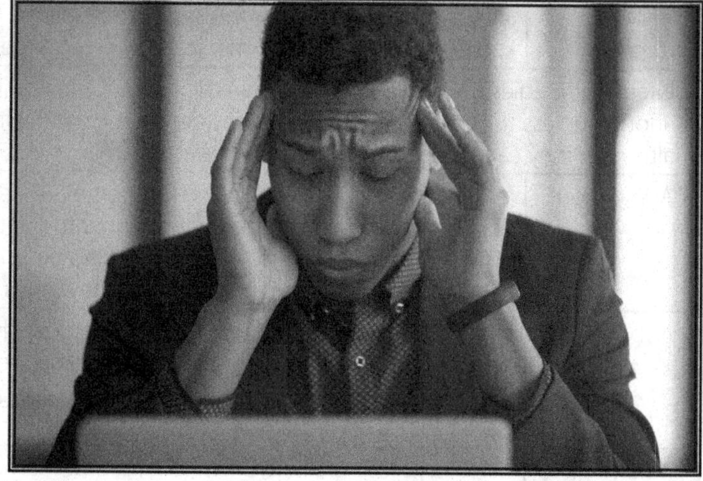

Figure 10-16. Internal strategies exist within the person. They include self-talk and pausing to check for errors during tasks. This man is using internal strategies to help with emotional regulation when feeling stressed (i.e., taking a break and using deep breathing). (fizkes/shutterstock.com)

- Domain- or task-specific strategies can be either internal or external. These strategies cannot be widely applied to all tasks. Rather, they are designed for use with certain activities under certain circumstances (Haskins, 2012; Polatajko et al., 2011; Radomski & Giles, 2021; Skidmore et al., 2017; Sohlberg & Turkstra, 2011). For example, using a recipe in a cookbook to remember the ingredients and steps to bake gingerbread cookies is an external task-specific strategy. The recipe will only work for baking gingerbread cookies, not for any other activity. Another example of an internal task-specific strategy is a person with ABI who is easily overwhelmed in crowded environments choosing to go grocery shopping midmorning on a weekday when the store is likely to be less busy.
- Global strategies, also called metacognitive strategies, are broad and can be used in a wide variety of circumstances. A global strategy provides people with a general framework that they can use to come up with more specific strategies that allow them to overcome problems they encounter (or foresee) as they engage in their occupations (Haskins, 2012; Polatajko et al., 2011; Radomski & Giles, 2021; Skidmore et al., 2017; Sohlberg & Turkstra, 2011). Global strategies have the same general framework regardless of which one is used.
  1. First, people are asked to identify problems, set goals that they want to achieve, and come up with possible solutions to the problems they have identified that will enable them to achieve their goals.
  2. People are then asked to choose a solution (or solutions) to try to create a plan for implementing that solution.
  3. People then execute their plan.
  4. Finally, people monitor their performance and respond to feedback (both internal and external).
  5. If needed, people adjust their plans when things are not going as expected and may need to start the process over again if things have gone badly astray (Haskins, 2012; Sohlberg & Turkstra, 2011).

An example of a global strategy that can be taught to people after ABI is Goal-Plan-Do-Check, which is used in the Cognitive Orientation to Daily Occupational Performance (CO-OP) Approach™ (Polatajko et al., 2011; Skidmore et al., 2017). The CO-OP Approach™ is discussed in more detail later in this chapter.

Cognitive Strategies and Phases of Learning

There are three phases people go through as they are learning new skills, including when learning to use cognitive strategies (Haskins, 2012; Radomski & Giles, 2021). The first phase is *acquisitional.* In the acquisitional phase, people are introduced to the skill they will learn, including the purpose of the skill, such as being able to compensate for cognitive deficits. It is important for people to understand the rationale behind using a skill, especially one that will be used independently, such as internal metacognitive strategies. In this phase of treatment, intervention approaches that focus on procedural learning may be helpful, including using massed practice (i.e., when the person repeatedly uses the new skill). This means that the occupational therapy practitioner plays a more active role in this phase, setting up treatment time to provide sufficient practice and repetition as people develop their abilities in using the skill (Haskins, 2012; Radomski & Giles, 2021).

The utility of using errorless learning in this initial acquisition phase of learning was reported in 2015 by Bertens and colleagues. In this study, 60 adults with cognitive deficits after a brain injury were randomized into one of two groups. The control group received metacognitive strategy training and were allowed to make errors from the beginning. The participants in the experimental group were taught the same metacognitive strategy, but errorless learning was used in the acquisition stage when people were learning to apply the metacognitive strategy to tasks. The researchers found that both groups showed improvement on their occupational performance but that those in the experimental group performed significantly better than the control group (43% of the experimental group versus 13% of the control group achieved a clinically significant improvement in their functioning on everyday tasks). The authors noted that the effect size was moderate to large (Bertens et al., 2015). A follow-up study examining transfer of learning with these same participants demonstrated no difference in the groups' abilities to transfer learning (Bertens et al., 2016).

The second phase of learning new skills is called the *application phase*. In this phase, the person begins to apply the skill in the context of activity, primarily within treatment sessions. The practitioner serves as a coach in this phase of treatment, guiding the person in using the skill, checking progress, and providing feedback. The focus in this phase of treatment is internalization, which is achieved when the person is able to apply the skill with less external assistance. This requires that the person get plenty of opportunities to practice the skill with decreasing levels of assistance from the care team, including clinicians and family caregivers (Haskins, 2012; Radomski & Giles, 2021).

The final phase of learning is called the *adaptation phase*. People who reach this stage of learning focus on using their new skills in numerous situations outside of the clinic. The goal for this phase of treatment is to facilitate generalization and transfer, enabling the client to achieve more independence as a result of using the skill in more contexts. As a result, it is essential that the client practice using the skill outside of therapy time. Clinicians can give homework assignments to clients to complete between treatment sessions. Clinicians can also encourage clients to journal, making note of times when the skill was used along with observations of what went well and what did not. Not all people with ABI will be able to reach the adaptation phase of treatment, although there are steps clinicians can take to increase the likelihood of generalization and transfer (Haskins, 2012; Radomski & Giles, 2021). These are discussed in the Generalization and Transfer section.

To illustrate the three phases in the context of intervention, imagine an occupational therapy practitioner named David working with Samara, a 62-year-old woman who sustained a stroke and has memory deficits. Samara has difficulty remembering steps to a variety of tasks, including one-handed dressing and simple meal preparation activities. David wants to teach Samara how to use a checklist as a cognitive strategy. In the acquisitional phase, David introduces the checklist to Samara and her family and explains its purpose (i.e., to compensate for memory deficits and to help Samara remember steps in tasks). In this phase, David will work with Samara on her understanding of her deficits and areas of performance breakdown. He will also start having Samara use checklists in therapy sessions, providing a lot of feedback and support as she learns to use this new strategy. In the application phase, Samara will continue to use checklists in therapy sessions as David reduces the amount of assistance he provides. He will still guide Samara in this phase by giving her feedback on her performance but will reduce the number of cues he uses as she begins to internalize the use of checklists as a strategy that can help her remember steps in tasks. He will gradually give more of the responsibility for using the cognitive strategy to Samara, including having her create her own checklists. In the adaptation phase of treatment, David will ask Samara to complete homework outside of therapy times using the checklist with activities they have not necessarily worked on in their therapy sessions. David will check in with Samara and her family if appropriate about how the use of the checklist is going and what her observations about its use outside of therapy have been. In moving through these phases, therapy shifts from being more clinician driven to client driven, with clients taking an increasingly active role in their recovery.

Teaching the use of cognitive strategies can be time consuming, especially when the goal is for the person to use strategies outside of the activities that have been addressed in therapy (Radomski & Giles, 2021). Depending on the strategy that is being taught and used, it will often also require different therapy techniques than those that are used with other treatment approaches. One of the most important ways to enable people to become skilled with using many cognitive strategies, especially those that are internal and global, is to allow them to make mistakes in the course of treatment (Sohlberg & Turkstra, 2011). This is a different approach than is used when working on procedural knowledge and routines when errorless learning can be successful (see discussion earlier). When people make errors, they can improve the robustness of their learning, especially when that learning needs to be applied to situations that are different from those that have been a focus of therapy sessions. One of the biggest reasons is that people can get feedback from the errors themselves, which enables people to recognize when strategies are not working. Making mistakes also encourages people to problem solve solutions to the issues they encounter (Ownsworth et al., 2017; Polatajko et al., 2011; Skidmore et al., 2017). As stated previously, for errors to be effective as learning tools, people need to be able to recognize their errors. Error recognition can be negatively impacted by a brain injury, but practitioners can guide people in the path of self-discovery by asking questions and having people stop to check progress as they complete activities. Strategies such as journaling and completing homework can also assist people by giving them additional opportunities to analyze their performance (Polatajko et al., 2011; Skidmore et al., 2017).

Metacognitive strategies are the most complex of the cognitive strategies. People who are taught to use metacognitive strategies learn to become their own problem solvers and to come up with their own solutions to problems they face (Polatajko et al., 2011; Radomski & Giles, 2021). To use these strategies most effectively, people need to have some awareness of their deficits and the types of occupational performance errors they make so that they can problem solve solutions; if they cannot identify issues, it will be more difficult for them to overcome them (Polatajko et al., 2011; Skidmore et al., 2017; Toglia et al., 2012). In addition to improving functioning on tasks they work on with clinicians within therapy, metacognitive strategies strive to improve people's performance on tasks that are untrained. The ability to transfer learned skills to new situations has enormous implications for independence because it means that people can learn to function at their best in novel situations even after the formal rehabilitation process has ceased (Houldin et al., 2018; McEwen & Houldin, 2017; Polatajko et al., 2011; Skidmore et al., 2017). Metacognition strategy training has been increasingly studied in recent years and is now recommended as a practice standard for people with cognitive deficits after a brain injury, especially those with executive dysfunction (Cicerone et al., 2019; Kennedy et al., 2008), including by prestigious organizations, such as the Brain Injury Interdisciplinary Special Interest Group from the American Congress of Rehabilitation Medicine (Cicerone et al., 2019; Haskins, 2012) and INCOG, which is a working group made up of international experts on cognition (Tate et al., 2014).

Cognitive Orientation to Daily Occupational Performance Approach (CO-OP Approach™)

One approach using metacognitive strategy training that has gained in prominence and popularity in cognitive rehabilitation administered by occupational therapy practitioners is the CO-OP Approach™. The CO-OP Approach™ was first used with children but has expanded to be used with adults, including those with stroke and TBI (Polatajko, 2017). It is a goal-based and occupation-focused intervention that teaches clients a general metacognitive strategy to help improve occupational performance. There are seven key features in the CO-OP Approach™, five of which are considered essential to treatment and must be present for the CO-OP Approach™ to be administered correctly. Those five are client-centered and occupation-focused goals, dynamic performance analysis, cognitive strategy use, guided discovery, and enabling principles. The other two key features are caregiver support and intervention format (Polatajko et al., 2011; Skidmore et al., 2017).

Client-Centered and Occupation-Focused Goals

The creators of the CO-OP Approach™ repeatedly emphasize that the goals addressed in therapy must be focused on occupation. Goals are identified by the client, although the practitioner can assist in guiding the client in determining feasible goals for treatment, especially if goals are determined to be unsafe or are impractical to achieve in the available treatment time (Polatajko et al., 2011; Skidmore et al., 2017). For example, many clients wish to return to driving after sustaining injury, which may not be feasible or safe. In this case, practitioners can work with clients to identify types of activities that use some of the same skills that driving does and have those occupations be the basis of the therapeutic goals. In order to both create and measure performance on occupation-based goals, practitioners using the CO-OP Approach™ are encouraged to use the Canadian Occupational Performance Measure (COPM) with clients (Skidmore et al., 2017).

Dynamic Performance Analysis

The CO-OP Approach™ is a top-down treatment, meaning that the focus is on the person's performance rather than on impairments. As a result, the clinician and the client will look for performance issues during the completion of activities and consider possible strategies that can address the issues that are observed. This is an ongoing process that is used throughout treatment rather than only at the beginning. It is also one that involves the client, who is asked to reflect on their performance and where problems arise (Polatajko et al., 2011; Skidmore et al., 2017). For example, imagine Carlos, a 24-year-old man with a TBI. One of his goals is to be independent in washing and waxing his car. During one of his outpatient sessions, he and his occupational therapy practitioner go out to the clinic parking lot, and Carlos washes his caregiver's car. After the activity, Carlos and the practitioner discuss his performance and note that Carlos washed some windows twice and did not wash other windows at all. He also did not empty the soap bucket or rinse out the sponge. They then discuss strategies he could try to use the next time he washes a car. Note that the problems that Carlos and the practitioner identified were focused on the performance level (missing steps in the task and inconsistently completing portions of the activity) rather than the impairment level (e.g., memory and/or planning deficits).

Cognitive Strategy Use

Practitioners using the CO-OP Approach™ teach clients a global/metacognitive strategy that is used throughout the therapeutic process called *Goal-Plan-Do-Check*. The practitioner teaches this global strategy to the client in the first session and revisits it in every subsequent session. It is a broad strategy that can be used in many different contexts and with many different tasks, and it is what people are taught to return to with every occupation that they approach, both within and outside of therapy. Through the use of the global strategy, people will problem solve how to overcome the performance difficulties they have and come up with domain- or task-specific approaches to use with their occupations. These latter strategies are more specific and are for use only in certain circumstances or with certain activities (Polatajko et al., 2011; Skidmore et al., 2017). For example, consider Carlos, who wants to be more independent with washing his car. Carlos and the practitioner can use the Goal-Plan-Do-Check approach the next time he washes a car in therapy. Before starting the task, Carlos sets his *goal*, which is to successfully wash a car with fewer to no errors. Guided by the occupational therapy practitioner, he creates a *plan* to overcome the problems noted during his previous performance in washing a car. He remembers that he skipped steps and repeated others. Carlos decides that he will try using a self-talk strategy in which he talks aloud as he completes the activity to see if that helps him stay on track better. The self-talk strategy is an example of a domain-specific strategy. It will work with some tasks but not with all. Carlos will then *do* the plan he created and *check* his performance to see if the strategy he identified was useful or not.

Guided Discovery

With the CO-OP Approach™, the clinician acts in the role of coach, helping the client to develop the skills needed to use the global strategy of Goal-Plan-Do-Check and come up with domain-specific strategies to use with occupation. This is different from other treatment approaches in which the practitioner may decide for clients which strategies or techniques they will use. With the CO-OP Approach™, the practitioner guides the client toward self-discovery. Practitioners use a variety of methods to assist clients in the process, including modeling, giving feedback, and providing hints. One of the most helpful ways that clinicians can coach clients is by asking questions or using guiding statements. This allows clients to come up with their own solutions to performance problems (Polatajko et al., 2011; Skidmore et al., 2017). For example, imagine Carlos's occupational therapy practitioner using guided discovery after he washed the car for the first time.

Practitioner: How did it go washing the car?

Carlos: Ok, I guess.

Practitioner: Did you notice any issues arise?

Carlos, looking more closely at the car: I don't know if I washed the windows on the passenger side. They don't look very clean.

Practitioner: So you missed some parts of the task?

Carlos: I think so.

Practitioner: Do you notice anything else? Anything you may not have finished completely?

Carlos: I don't think so.

Practitioner: What about the bucket?

Carlos: Oh, I forgot to empty the bucket and put it back.

Practitioner: Do you have any ideas about what you could do next time to avoid those issues?

The two would then continue the discussion with the practitioner guiding Carlos in brainstorming solutions that he could use the next time he approaches the task. Note that the practitioner starts with more general questions and moves to more specific ones as needed. By moving from general to specific, clients have more opportunities to identify both performance problems and solutions on their own.

Enabling Principles

There are several principles that need to be included when using the CO-OP Approach™. The first is to make it fun. Therapy sessions should be enjoyable to clients to keep them engaged and interested. The surest way to accomplish this is through the use of meaningful and client-centered goals. The second principle is to promote learning. The CO-OP Approach™ should be driven by self-discovery in which practitioners guide clients through the process of actively identifying

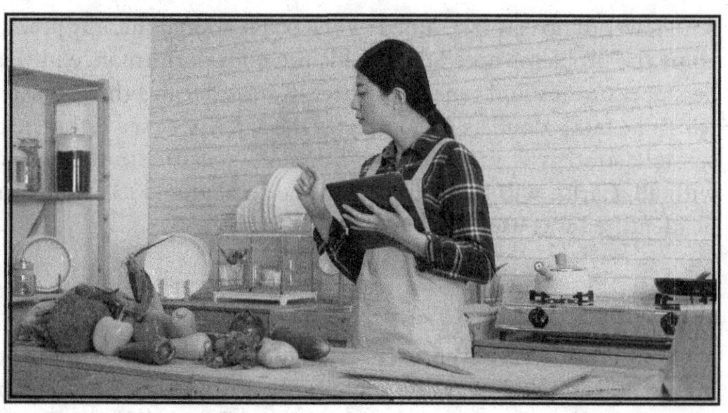

Figure 10-17. Using a metacognitive strategy, such as Goal-Plan-Do-Check from the CO-OP Approach™, can improve performance with occupation by having people set clear goals, make plans, execute plans, and check their progress to see if corrections need to be made. This woman is pausing in her meal preparation task to make sure she is on track with making a recipe accurately. (PRPicturesProduction/shutterstock.com)

strategies that can support their occupational performance. The third enabling principle is to work toward independence. Through the CO-OP Approach™, clients develop the skills to problem solve independently using the global strategy (Polatajko et al., 2011; Skidmore et al., 2017; Figure 10-17). The final enabling principle is to promote generalization and transfer. An important part of the CO-OP Approach™ consists of having clients use the global strategy outside of therapy sessions with occupations other than those that have been identified as specific goals. Clients are assigned homework and work with clinicians to problem solve how Goal-Plan-Do-Check can be used outside of therapy. Clients will make notes about their successes and difficulties in notebooks between sessions. Practitioners then follow up with clients to review the global strategy and to discuss how it worked for the client. Practicing the global strategy outside of therapy with different tasks and in different contexts is one of the ways that the CO-OP Approach™ is designed to promote generalization and transfer (McEwen & Houldin, 2017; Polatajko et al., 2011; Skidmore et al., 2017).

Caregiver Support

The first of the seven CO-OP Approach™ features that can be modified is the use of caregivers. As stated earlier, the CO-OP Approach™ was originally designed to be used with pediatric populations. When the approach was studied with adults, researchers realized that not all adult clients have caregivers who are available for training. As a result, caregivers may not be a part of treatment for adult clients. However, when caregivers are present, they should be trained with the global strategy to support its use outside of therapy. This can help increase the likelihood of generalization and transfer (McEwen et al., 2017; Skidmore et al., 2017).

Intervention Format

This is the final CO-OP Approach™ feature and includes session sequence, format, and materials that are used in intervention. This feature is modifiable depending on the client's needs. Typically, the CO-OP Approach™ is administered over the course of 10 to 12 weekly sessions, with sessions being approximately 50 minutes long (Polatajko et al., 2011; Skidmore et al., 2017). Studies that have examined the use of the CO-OP Approach™ with adults have had some variability with this, with sessions occurring more than once per week or with changes in the length of sessions or the overall number of sessions (Dawson et al., 2017; McEwen et al., 2017). The general sequence remains roughly the same for clients, again with some variation reported for different people. Goals are created, and a baseline is established in the first one or two sessions. The practitioner will also teach the client the global strategy of Goal-Plan-Do-Check. The following sessions follow the same general format. The session begins with an introduction to the session, a review of the global strategy, and a discussion of the homework that was assigned in the previous session. The client will then complete one of the occupations identified as a goal. The practitioner and client will collaboratively complete dynamic performance analysis and work to apply the global strategy to the task, allowing the client to identify domain-specific strategies that will be used. At the end of the session, homework is assigned for the next session, with the practitioner guiding the client in brainstorming how the global strategy can be used outside of the therapy time (Dawson et al., 2017; McEwen et al., 2017; Polatajko et al., 2011; Skidmore et al., 2017).

A number of intervention studies looking at the efficacy of the CO-OP Approach™ for adults with ABI have been conducted, including some pilot randomized controlled trials. Populations that have been studied have included adults with stroke (Henshaw et al., 2011; Houldin et al., 2018; McEwen et al., 2010) and adults with TBI (Dawson et al., 2009, 2013; Houldin et al., 2018). One study also examined the impact of the CO-OP Approach™ with women with chemotherapy-induced cognitive dysfunction (Wolf et al., 2016). Most studies have been conducted in outpatient settings, but one case report looked at the use of the CO-OP Approach™ with a man with a stroke who was being treated in inpatient rehabilitation (Skidmore et al., 2011). The researchers of that study concluded that the CO-OP Approach™ was feasible to use on inpatient rehabilitation units but that it required careful coordination with the team so that the metacognitive strategy of Goal-Plan-Do-Check could be regularly reinforced (Skidmore et al., 2011).

The research that has been completed with adult populations has shown that the CO-OP Approach™ has a positive impact on occupational performance. Participants in these studies had improvement in their COPM scores on both perceived performance and satisfaction with their occupational performance (Dawson et al., 2009, 2013; McEwen et al., 2010; Wolf et al., 2016). Many studies have reported moderate to large effect sizes, reflecting the robustness of the treatment (Dawson et al., 2013, 2017; Wolf et al., 2016). In addition to examining the efficacy of the CO-OP Approach™ on improving occupational performance on goals that were targeted in therapy, researchers in most of these studies considered participants' performance on additional occupations not addressed in treatment. This was done to examine the impact of the CO-OP Approach™ on untrained tasks as a way to explore transfer and generalization (discussed in more detail later in this chapter). In these studies, participants showed improvement in their COPM scores on both performance and satisfaction with the untrained tasks, indicating that the effects of the CO-OP Approach™ may result in generalization and transfer (Dawson et al., 2013, 2017; Houldin et al., 2018; McEwen et al., 2010, 2017; McEwen & Houldin, 2017).

The CO-OP Approach™ is a comprehensive and more complex intervention that can be useful when working with people with ABI who have cognitive deficits. To ensure that it is administered correctly, the developers recommended that practitioners receive additional training before using this approach (Skidmore et al., 2017). Interested readers are encouraged to visit https://icancoop.org/ for more details.

Generalization and Transfer

The terms *generalization* and *transfer* are often used interchangeably and do not have agreed-upon definitions in the literature (Geusgens et al., 2007). Some have argued that they are two different, but related, constructs and have given definitions that differentiate one from the other. These authors have defined generalization as a situation in which a person uses the same skill that was taught in therapy in another context (McEwen & Houldin, 2017; Polatajko et al., 2011). An example of generalization would be teaching a person to use a one-handed dressing strategy to don a button-down shirt in therapy. The person then uses the same dressing strategy to don a coat at home. In this case, the skill (using a one-handed dressing strategy for upper body dressing) is the same but is used in different contexts (with different articles of clothing and in different settings). Transfer occurs when a person uses one skill to learn something new that was untrained and is different from the specific task that was used for the training (McEwen & Houldin, 2017; Polatajko et al., 2011). An example of transfer is when a clinician teaches a client to use a kitchen timer to take oatmeal off of the stove during a cooking task in a therapy session. The person later sets a reminder on a smartphone to cue them to call to set up a doctor's appointment. There is some similarity between the two tasks in that an external device is giving a signal to the person to remember something. However, there are a lot of differences as well, including the task itself (cooking vs. medical management), the device (kitchen timer vs. an application on a smartphone), and the setting (the therapy kitchen vs. the home community).

In reality, generalization and transfer can be difficult to distinguish from one another and are often examined together. More importantly, they have also repeatedly been demonstrated as difficult to achieve. Historically, clinicians assumed that people used what they learned in treatment when they returned to their homes and communities (Toglia, 1991). However, numerous studies conducted with a variety of treatment techniques have shown that people will often improve in the training session (e.g., a lab or clinic) on the specific tasks or skills that were trained but that those improvements are less likely to carry over to other, untrained tasks in other areas of life (Houldin et al., 2018; Mogensen & Wulf-Andersen, 2017; Sohlberg & Turkstra, 2011). Without being able to achieve generalization and transfer, people will be less independent. They will not be able to use the skills they are learning in the clinic in their homes and communities to overcome challenges they face when they encounter tasks that are different from those they practiced in therapy. It is impossible for clinicians to specifically prepare clients for every possible issue they may face in the community, which is dynamic and increasingly complex. As a result, achieving transfer and generalization are of vital importance to enable clients to find solutions to untrained problems and to reach their full occupational potential (Geusgens et al., 2007; Houldin et al., 2018; Radomski & Giles, 2021).

Researchers have described factors that can increase the likelihood of transfer. One of the most cited articles was published by Geusgens and colleagues in 2007. The authors conducted a literature review of 39 articles (describing 41 studies) to examine how often transfer was achieved in rehabilitation and how researchers measured it. They found that transfer was reported in the majority of studies (36 of the 41 included in the review) but that almost half of those did not achieve significance. The studies in the review measured transfer in one of three ways. The first, and preferred, method was to measure the performance of nontrained tasks in the home and community. The second was to assess the performance of tasks in laboratory environments. The third was to administer self-report measures in which participants, caregivers, and/or staff assessed occupational performance. After conducting the review, the authors concluded that there were six prerequisites that needed to be present to increase the likelihood of transfer (Geusgens et al., 2007).

1. People need to be taught explicitly about transfer in their treatment. They need to understand what transfer is and how it works. Included in that discussion is defining transfer for people and telling them what they will need to do, both in therapy sessions and outside of therapy, to increase the chances of becoming more independent in a wider variety of tasks (Geusgens et al., 2007; McEwen et al., 2018; McEwen & Houldin, 2017).

2. People need to have a good understanding of their abilities and the areas in which they have performance breakdown (Geusgens et al., 2007; McEwen & Houldin, 2017; Toglia, 2018; Toglia et al., 2010). Working on improving awareness during therapy is essential if a person does not have an accurate picture of their abilities and deficits. (See the discussion of treating awareness deficits earlier.) People also need to be taught to analyze their own work, both the outcomes and the performance itself. Asking them whether the outcomes were what they expected and the strategies they used to achieve results can help with this (Haskins, 2012; Radomski & Giles, 2021; Toglia, 2018; Toglia & Maeir, 2018).

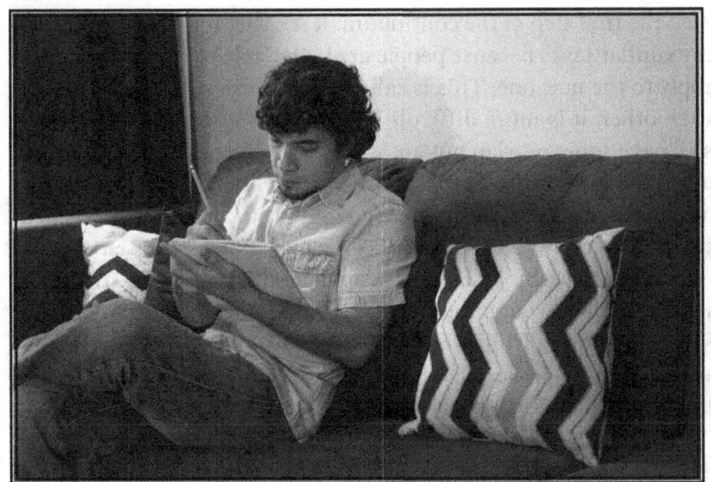

Figure 10-18. In order to increase the likelihood of transfer with metacognitive strategy use, therapists can instruct clients to utilize strategies outside of therapy sessions. Journaling about outside activities (the goals that were set, the process that was followed, and the outcomes that were achieved) and reviewing the entries with the therapist can help clients recognize how strategies can be used in a variety of situations. (Antonio Tanaka/shutterstock.com)

3. People need to know when and where the learned skills can be applied (Geusgens et al., 2007; McEwen & Houldin, 2017; Toglia, 2018). One way to work on this is by discussing what people will do outside of therapy time and how the skills they are learning can be used with those activities. Journaling can also assist with this because people can make notes about what they are doing outside of therapy time and discuss their observations with the clinician at follow-up sessions (McEwen & Houldin, 2017; Figure 10-18).
4. General strategies should be taught rather than teaching strategies that are too specific. A general strategy or framework (e.g., a metacognitive strategy) can be used in multiple situations and can give people guidance when they need to problem solve solutions to issues that arise. If clients are too rigid in their thinking by using only very specific strategies, they will be less able to adjust plans and accomplish a variety of activities in a variety of situations (Geusgens et al., 2007; McEwen & Houldin, 2017; Toglia, 1991; Toglia et al., 2010).
5. Varied practice is important. People need to have a lot of practice in applying strategies. This practice needs to occur at a variety of times, with a variety of tasks, and in a variety of environments. This can partly be accomplished in therapy sessions by having people practice at different times (e.g., early in the session vs. late) and with different occupations. To truly accomplish varied practice, however, people need to use strategies outside of therapy sessions as well (Geusgens et al., 2007; McEwen & Houldin, 2017; Sohlberg & Turkstra, 2011; Toglia, 1991, 2018). This requires communication with team members, including the client and caregivers.
6. Transfer needs to be addressed directly and deliberately in therapy. It is unlikely to happen automatically, so practitioners need to have an explicit plan for increasing the likelihood of transfer. Building in the previously described suggestions, in addition to gradually shifting the responsibility for analyzing activities and providing feedback from the clinician to the client, is essential when transfer is the goal (Geusgens et al., 2007; McEwen & Houldin, 2017; Sohlberg & Turkstra, 2011; Toglia, 1991, 2018; Toglia et al., 2010).

As stated earlier, a lack of transferability is an issue for many different disciplines, including occupational therapy. The multicontext approach, first described by Joan Toglia in 1991, was designed to help improve the likelihood of transfer with occupational therapy treatment. Practitioners who use the multicontext approach utilize several of the principles described previously, including self-awareness, understanding the value of using cognitive strategies, and varied practice (Toglia, 1991, 2018). A point that is emphasized with the multicontext approach is that transfer needs to be gradual. Toglia (1991, 2018) described a continuum with transfer. Tasks that are very similar to each other are on the first step of the continuum. It is easier for people to transfer learned skills between two very similar tasks because people are better able to recognize how a skill learned with one task can apply to the new one. This is called *near transfer*. As tasks become more and more different from each other, it is more difficult for transfer to occur. *Intermediate transfer* is required when tasks still have some overlap but are starting to diverge in several ways. *Far transfer* and *very far transfer* are the most difficult to achieve because the tasks are quite different from the original one, and people are less likely to recognize that the skills they learned and used with the original task will also apply to the new tasks (Toglia, 1991, 2018). Dr. Toglia theorized that making changes to tasks gradually by having people practice the same strategies with increasingly different tasks and moving through the stages of near to intermediate to far and very far transfer could improve the likelihood of transfer occurring. This gradual change could enable people to recognize the utility of strategies learned in treatment with a variety of different tasks occurring in a variety of different contexts (Toglia, 1991, 2018).

The multicontext approach should be used with functional and meaningful tasks that are at a just-right challenge to improve clients' motivation in therapy. Clients are taught to use cognitive strategies by using them in the context of activity. Ideally, the clients self-generate the cognitive strategies as they complete their activities in therapy (Toglia, 1991, 2018). Occupational therapy practitioners conduct an in-depth activity analysis of the first task that clients complete, which is the one that is used to first practice the cognitive strategy. The process of transfer is then initiated by having clients practice using the same cognitive strategy with a different but very similar task. This is done by changing one or two of the task characteristics while keeping the others constant to encourage clients to complete a near transfer. This can allow clients to see the benefits of using the cognitive strategy in a new situation that is similar to the original training task. The similarities between the two tasks can help people to recognize that the same strategy can still be helpful. Over time, more of the task characteristics are changed to allow clients to practice using the same strategy with intermediate transfer; far transfer; and, ultimately, very far transfer tasks. The gradual change can assist clients in seeing the relevance of strategy use with increasingly different activities (Toglia, 1991, 2018). In 2017, Dr. Toglia produced intervention kits with activities that are designed to assist clients in using cognitive strategies in a structured way. At the time of this writing, there were scheduling and menu modules with a business card module in development. For more details, readers can visit https://multicontext.net/

To illustrate the use of the multicontext approach, imagine Damien, a 45-year-old man who sustained a right cerebrovascular accident. He has issues with hemi-inattention and struggles to fully visually search his environment. His occupational therapy practitioner, Vivian, is working with him on using an organized search pattern to search for items. Vivian knows that transfer is difficult to achieve with clients and is addressing transfer deliberately in her treatment by using the multicontext approach. She starts the process by having Damien use his organized search pattern to find a carton of milk in a refrigerator door that has 10 items (Figure 10-19). This task deals with food in the kitchen. It also has Damien working on searching in a horizontal pattern on a vertical surface. The next task Vivian has Damien complete is to look for cake mix in a cupboard with 10 items. This activity also deals with food in the kitchen and has Damien searching in a horizontal pattern on a vertical surface. The changed characteristics of the task are the specific item he is looking for (milk vs. cake mix) and the specific location (refrigerator vs. cupboard). The next task has Damien searching for a picture of a butterfly on a wall with 10 pictures. This is an intermediate transfer task because more of the task characteristics have changed. Damien is continuing to use the same strategy and is still working on searching a vertical surface with 10 items, but many of the other aspects of the task are different. Vivian then chooses to have Damien look for a tennis shoe in a closet with 10 pairs of shoes, an intermediate to far transfer task, depending on how the items are arranged. Damien could then search for a wastebasket in a room with 10 pieces of furniture, which is a far transfer task. To achieve very far transfer, Damien would use the same strategy (i.e., organized searching) in numerous environments during his daily routines.

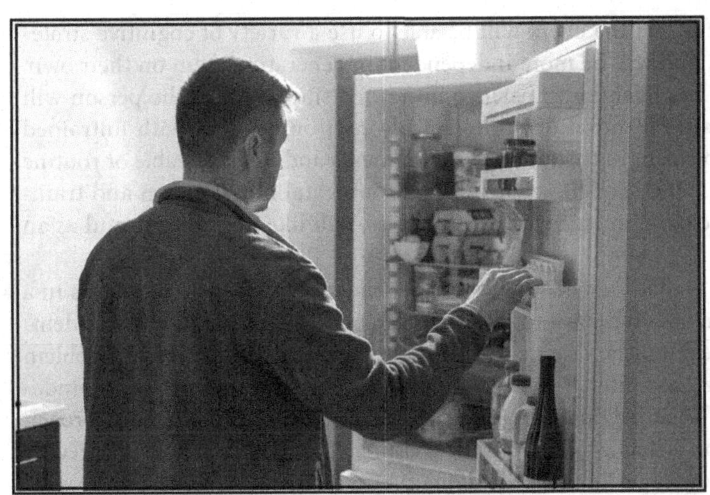

Figure 10-19. A man using an organized visual search pattern to locate milk in a refrigerator. (Aliaksandra Post/shutterstock.com)

Some intervention research has been performed with the multicontext approach. One was a case series conducted with four people with TBI (Toglia et al., 2010). The researchers found that the four participants improved with their occupational performance and self-regulation skills after being treated with the multicontext approach. They also had some improvements in awareness about their performance breakdowns but not about their awareness of their deficits in a more general way, indicating that occupational performance can be improved even if there is not an improvement in the impairments themselves (Toglia et al., 2010). Two other case studies with people with TBI have been reported in the literature. Both demonstrated improvement in occupational performance, including some transfer of skills after treatment with the multicontext approach. Both also showed improvement in awareness of occupational performance deficits (Landa-Gonzalez, 2001; Toglia et al., 2011). The carryover of learned skills was not consistent with the two individuals, with one showing continued use of learned strategies and independence 8 weeks after intervention had stopped (Landa-Gonzalez, 2011) and the other demonstrating deterioration of skills, although still better than the original baseline, after 4 weeks (Toglia et al., 2011).

Conclusion

In general, for people who undergo cognitive rehabilitation because of deficits from ABI, there are four possible outcomes (Haskins, 2012). For those with more severe deficits for whom the ability to learn is limited and/or the lack of awareness interferes with the independent use of cognitive strategies, independence will be less likely. In this case, people will probably need continuing assistance with many occupations, although their performance can be improved with routine and unvarying tasks (Haskins, 2012). For people who fall into this category, procedural learning and environmental modification will likely be the most useful intervention approaches for occupational therapy practitioners to use.

The second possible outcome is that a person will be able to use external aids independently, such as alarms or memory aids, but will need assistance setting them up. They will also need more assistance completing activities that are less predictable or amenable to routine. People at this level of recovery will benefit from consistency and routine but may be able to use some cognitive strategies with sufficient practice or some supervision (Haskins, 2012). Environmental modification will be a useful treatment technique for these clients. Whether procedural learning or more trial-and-error learning is best will be decided through clinical reasoning and will depend on factors such as the person's learning capacity, living environment, social support, and occupational goals.

The third possible outcome is that the client will be able to use a variety of cognitive strategies, both internal and external, and will be more independent in generating them on their own. However, these abilities will be less likely to transfer to untrained situations, so the person will probably need continued assistance in novel or unpredictable environments or with untrained tasks. These clients can be independent in their home environments and in predictable or routine community activities (Haskins, 2012). For these clients, environmental modification and training with cognitive strategies, including metacognitive strategies, will likely be most useful as an intervention approach.

The final possible outcome is that the client will be independent with a variety of tasks in a wide range of situations. This client will be able to self-generate cognitive strategies and will demonstrate the use of a variety of techniques. Clients with this outcome will also be able to problem solve solutions to issues that are encountered in untrained or novel situations and will be independent with most, if not all, of their occupations (Haskins, 2012)..The best treatment approach for clients in this category will be metacognitive strategy training. Through that training, people will likely develop their own knowledge about which domain-specific external or internal cognitive strategies and environmental modifications are most useful to them (Polatajko et al., 2011; Skidmore et al., 2017).

In reality, it is not always easy to predict how independent clients will be after a brain injury. Clinicians will need to be flexible in using different cognitive treatment approaches, making adjustments based on how clients respond to intervention (Ehlhardt et al., 2008). As stated previously, a major factor in determining which treatment approach to use is the client's learning potential. Another factor can be the timing of rehabilitation. Recall that there are different stages that clients go through when learning skills in rehabilitation (i.e., acquisition, application, and adaptation). Different treatment techniques can be useful in different ways at these stages of learning. For example, practitioners may find errorless learning techniques most useful in the acquisition phase as people are first learning new skills (Haskins, 2012; Sohlberg & Turkstra, 2011).

Ultimately, there is evidence to support a variety of treatment techniques for people with cognitive impairment after a brain injury (Ehlhardt et al., 2008). Which ones to use will depend on multiple factors, including the severity of the cognitive deficits and the person's learning potential. Taking into account clients' goals and types of tasks they need to complete are also important. If the person will be conducting more routine tasks in specific environments, errorless learning may be more useful. If generalization or transfer is the goal, allowing the person to make errors and learn to use a metacognitive strategy may be warranted. No matter what treatment technique is used, it is important to provide clients with plenty of practice with meaningful tasks as they learn to improve their occupational performance and to monitor how they respond to therapy using clinical reasoning about whether or not treatment is improving occupational performance and what changes, if any, may be needed.

References

American Occupational Therapy Association. (2020). Occupational therapy practice framework: Domain and process (4th ed.). *American Journal of Occupational Therapy, 74*(Suppl. 2), 7412410010. https://doi.org/10.5014/ajot.2020.74S2001

Below, C. P., & Lewis, K. (2021). Visual function intervention. In D. P. Dirette & S. A. Gutman (Eds.), *Occupational therapy for physical dysfunction* (8th ed., pp. 100-116). Wolters Kluwer.

Bertens, D., Kessels, R. P. C., Boelen, D. H. E., & Fasotti, L. (2016). Transfer effects of errorless Goal Management Training on cognitive function and quality of life in brain-injured persons. *NeuroRehabilitation, 38*, 79-84. https://doi.org/10.3233/NRE-151298

Bertens, D., Kessels, R. P. C., Fiorenzato, E., Boelen, D. H. E., & Fasotti, L. (2015). Do old errors always lead to new truths? A randomized controlled trial of errorless Goal Management Training in brain-injured patients. *Journal of the International Neuropsychological Society, 21*, 639-649. https://doi.org/10.1017/S1355617715000764

Campbell, L., Wilson, F. C., McCann, J., Kernahan, G., & Rogers, R. G. (2007). Single case experimental design study of carer facilitated errorless learning in a patient with severe memory impairment following TBI. *NeuroRehabilitation, 22*, 325-333. https://doi.org/10.3233/NRE-2007-22411

Cicerone, K. D., Goldin, Y., Ganci, K., Rosenbaum, A., Wethe, J. V., Langenbahn, D. M., Malec, J. F., Bergquist, T. F., Kingsley K., Nagele, D., Trexler, L., Fraas, M., Bogdanova, Y., & Harley, J. P. (2019). Evidence-based cognitive rehabilitation: Systematic review of the literature from 2009 through 2014. *Archives of Physical Medicine and Rehabilitation, 100*, 1515-1533. https://doi.org/10.1016/j.apmr.2019.02.011

Cohen, M., Ylvisaker, M., Hamilton, J., Kemp, L., & Claiman, B. (2010). Errorless learning of functional life skills in an individual with three aetiologies of severe memory and executive function impairment. *Neuropsychological Rehabilitation, 20*, 355-376. https://doi.org/10.1080/09602010903309401

Cohn, E. S., & Lew, C. (2015). Occupational therapy's perspective on the use of environments and contexts to facilitate health, well-being, and participation in occupations. *American Journal of Occupational Therapy, 69*, 1-13. https://doi.org/10.5014/ajot.2015.696S05

Dawson, D. R., Binns, M. A., Hunt, A., Lemsky, C., & Polatajko, H. J. (2013). Occupation-based strategy training for adults with traumatic brain injury: A pilot study. *Archives of Physical Medicine and Rehabilitation, 94*, 1959-63. https://doi.org/10.1016/j.apmr.2013.05.021

Dawson, D. R., Gaya, A., Hunt, A., Levine, B., Lemsky, C., & Polatajko, H. J. (2009). Using the Cognitive Orientation to Occupational Performance (CO-OP) with adults with executive dysfunction following traumatic brain injury. *Canadian Journal of Occupational Therapy, 76*, 115-127. https://doi.org/10.1177/000841740907600209

Dawson, D. R., Hunt, A. W., & Polatajko, H. J. (2017). Using the CO-OP Approach: Traumatic brain injury. In D. Dawson, S. E. McEwen, & H. J. Polatajko (Eds.), *Cognitive Orientation to Daily Occupational Performance in occupational therapy: Using the CO-OP approach to enable participation across the lifespan* (pp. 135-160). AOTA Press.

Ehlhardt, L. A., Sohlberg, M. M., Kennedy, M., Coelho, C., Ylvisaker, M., Turkstra, L., & Yorkston, K. (2008). Evidence-based practice guidelines for instructing individuals with neurogenic memory impairments: What have we learned in the past 20 years? *Neuropsychological Rehabilitation, 18*, 300-342. https://doi.org/10.1080/09602010701733190

Engel, L., Chui, A., Goverover, Y., & Dawson, D. R. (2017). Optimising activity and participation outcomes for people with self-awareness impairments related to acquired brain injury: An interventions systematic review. *Neuropsychological Rehabilitation, 29*(2), 163-198. https://doi.org/10.1080/09602011.2017.1292923

Evans, J. J., Wilson, B. A., Schuri, U., Andrade, J., Baddeley, A., Bruna, O., Canavan, T., Sala, S. D., Green, R., Laaksonen, R., Lorenzi, L., & Taussik, I. (2000). A comparison of "errorless" and "trial-and-error" learning methods for teaching individuals with acquired memory deficits. *Neuropsychological Rehabilitation, 10*, 67-101. https://doi.org/10.1080/096020100389309

Ferland, M. B., Laurente, J., Rowland, J., & Davidson, P. S. R. (2013). Errorless (re)learning of daily living routines by a woman with impaired memory and initiation: Transferrable to a new home? *Brain Injury, 27*, 1461-1469. https://doi.org/10.3109/02699052.2013.823661

Fleming, R., Bennett, K., Preece, T., & Phillipson, L. (2017). The development and testing of the dementia friendly communities environment assessment tool (DFC EAT). *International Psychogeriatrics, 29*, 303-311. https://doi.org/10.1017/S1041610216001678

Fong., K. N. K., & Howie, D. R. (2009). Effects of an explicit problem-solving skills training program using a metacomponential approach for outpatients with acquired brain injury. *American Journal of Occupational Therapy, 63*, 525-534. https://doi.org/10.5014/ajot.63.5.525

Gazzaniga, M. S., Ivry, R. B., & Mangun, G. R. (2019). *Cognitive neuroscience: The biology of the mind* (5th ed.). W. W. Norton & Company.

Geusgens, C. A. V., Winkens, I., van Heugten, C. M., Josses, J., & van den Heuvel, W. J. A. (2007). Occurrence and measurement of transfer in cognitive rehabilitation: A critical review. *Journal of Rehabilitation Medicine, 39*, 425-439. https://doi.org/10.2340/16501977-0092

Giles, G. M. (2018). Neurofunctional approach to rehabilitation after brain injury. In N. Katz & J. Toglia (Eds.), *Cognition, occupation, and participation across the lifespan* (4th ed., pp. 419-442). AOTA Press.

Gillen, G. (2018). Evaluation and treatment of limited occupational performance secondary to cognitive dysfunction. In H. M. Pendleton & W. Schultz-Krohn (Eds.), *Pedretti's occupational therapy: Practice skills for physical dysfunction* (8th ed., pp. 645-668). Elsevier.

Gillen, G. (2021). Treatment of cognitive-perceptual deficits: a function-based approach. In G. Gillen & D. M. Nilsen (Eds.), *Stroke rehabilitation: a function-based approach* (5th ed., pp. 593-626). Elsevier.

Gillen, G., Nilsen, D. M., Attridge, J., Banakos, E., Morgan, M., Winterbottom, L., & York, W. (2015). Effectiveness of interventions to improve occupational performance of people with cognitive impairments after stroke: An evidence-based review. *American Journal of Occupational Therapy, 69*, 6901180040. https://doi.org/10.5014/ajot.2015.012138

Gitlin, L. N., Corcoran, M., Winter, L., Boyce, A., & Hauck, W. W. (2001). A randomized, controlled trial of a home environmental intervention: Effect on efficacy and upset in caregivers and on daily function of persons with dementia. *The Gerontologist, 41*, 4-14. https://doi.org/10.1093/geront/41.1.4

Glogoski, C., Milligan, N. V., & Wheatley, C. J. (2006). Evaluation and treatment of cognitive dysfunction. In H. M. Pendleton & W. Schultz-Krohn (Eds.), *Pedretti's occupational therapy: Practice skills for physical dysfunction* (6th ed., pp. 589-608). Elsevier.

Goverover, Y., Johnston, M. V., Toglia, J., & Deluca, J. (2007). Treatment to improve self-awareness in persons with acquired brain injury. *Brain Injury, 21*, 913-923. https://doi.org/10.1080/02699050701553205

Haskins, E. C. (2012). *Cognitive rehabilitation manual: Translating evidence-based recommendations into practice.* American Congress of Rehabilitation Medicine.

Henshaw, E., Polatajko, H., McEwen, S., Ryan, J. D., & Baum, C. M. (2011). Cognitive approach to improving participation after stroke: Two case studies. *American Journal of Occupational Therapy, 65*, 55-63. https://doi.org/10.5014/ajot.2011.09010

Houldin, A., McEwen, S. E., Howell, M. W., & Polatajko, H. J. (2018). The Cognitive Orientation to Daily Occupational Performance approach and transfer: A scoping review. *OTJR: Occupation, Participation and Health, 38*, 157-172. https://doi.org/10.1177/1539449217736059

Johansson, K., Lundberg, S., & Borell, L. (2011). "The cognitive kitchen"—key principles and suggestions for design that includes older adults with cognitive impairments as kitchen users. *Technology and Disability, 23*, 29-40. https://doi.org/10.3233/TAD-2011-0310

Kelly, F., & Nikopoulos, C. K. (2010). Facilitating independence in personal activities of daily living after a severe traumatic brain injury. *International Journal of Therapy and Rehabilitation, 17*, 474-482. https://doi.org/10.12968/ijtr.2010.17.9.78037

Kennedy, M. R. T., Coelho, C., Turkstra, L., Ylvisaker, M., Sohlberg, M. M., Yorkston, K., Chiou, H.-H., & Kan, P.-F. (2008). Intervention for executive functions after traumatic brain injury: A systematic review, meta-analysis and clinical recommendations. *Neuropsychological Rehabilitation, 18*, 257-299. https://doi.org/10.1080/09602010701748644

Kessels, R. P. C., & de Haan, E. H. F. (2003). Implicit learning in memory rehabilitation: A meta-analysis on errorless learning and vanishing cues methods. *Journal of Clinical and Experimental Neuropsychology, 25*, 805-814. https://doi.org/10.1076/jcen.25.6.805.16474

Landa-Gonzalez, B. (2001). Multicontextual occupational therapy intervention: A case study of traumatic brain injury. *Occupational Therapy International, 8*, 49-62. https://doi.org/10.1002/oti.131

Lidsten-McQueen, K., Weiner, N. W., Wang, H.-Y., Josman, N., & Connor, L. T. (2014). Systematic review of apraxia treatments to improve occupational performance outcomes. *OTJR: Occupation, Participation and Health, 34*, 183-192. https://doi.org/10.3928/15394492-20141006-02

Lin, K., & Wroten, M. (2022). *Ranchos Los Amigos.* StatPearls Publishing. https://www.ncbi.nlm.nih.gov/books/NBK448151/

Manly, T., Hawkins, K., Evans, J., Woldt, K., & Robertson, I. H. (2002). Rehabilitation of executive function: Facilitation of effective goal management on complex tasks using periodic auditory alerts. *Neuropsychologia, 40*, 271-281. https://doi.org/10.1016/S0028-3932(01)00094-X

Matérne, M., Lundqvist, L.-O., & Strandberg, T. (2017). Opportunities and barriers for successful return to work after acquired brain injury: A patient perspective. *Work, 56*, 125-134. https://doi.org/10.3233/WOR-162468

McEwen, S. E., & Houldin, A. (2017). Generalization and transfer in the CO-OP Approach. In D. Dawson, S. E. McEwen, & H. J. Polatajko (Eds.), *Cognitive Orientation to Daily Occupational Performance in occupational therapy: Using the CO-OP Approach to enable participation across the lifespan* (pp. 31-42). AOTA Press.

McEwen, S. E., Mandich, A., & Polatajko, H. J. (2018). CO-OP Approach: A cognitive-based intervention for children and adults. In N. Katz & J. Toglia (Eds.), *Cognition, occupation, and participation across the lifespan* (4th ed., pp. 315-334). AOTA Press.

McEwen, S. E., Polatajko, H. J., Huijbregts, M. P. J., & Ryan, J. D. (2010). Inter-task transfer of meaningful, functional skills following a cognitive-based treatment: Results of three multiple baseline design experiments in adults with chronic stroke. *Neuropsychological Rehabilitation, 20*, 541-561. https://doi.org/10.1080/09602011003638194

McEwen, S. E., Poulin, V., Skidmore, E. R., & Wolf, T. J. (2017). Using the CO-OP Approach: Stroke. In D. Dawson, S. E. McEwen, & H. J. Polatajko (Eds.), *Cognitive Orientation to Daily Occupational Performance in occupational.* AOTA Press.

Medley, A. R., & Powell, T. (2010). Motivational interviewing to promote self-awareness and engagement in rehabilitation following acquired brain injury: A conceptual review. *Neuropsychological Rehabilitation, 20*, 481-508. https://doi.org/10.1080/09602010903529610

Middleton, E. L., & Schwartz, M. F. (2012). Errorless learning in cognitive rehabilitation: A critical review. *Neuropsychological Rehabilitation, 22*, 138-168. https://doi.org/10.1080/09602011.2011.639619

Mogensen, J., & Wulf-Andersen, C. (2017). Home and family in cognitive rehabilitation after brain injury: Implementation of social reserves. *NeuroRehabilitation, 41*, 513-518. https://doi.org/10.3233/NRE-160007

Morton, N., & Barker, L. (2010). The contribution of injury severity, executive and implicit functions to awareness of deficits after traumatic brain injury (TBI). *Journal of the International Neuropsychological Society, 16*, 1089-1098. https://doi.org/10.1017/S1355617710000925

Mount, J., Pierce, S. R., Parker, J., DiEgidio, R., Woessner, R., & Spiegel, L. (2007). Trial and error versus errorless learning of functional skills in patients with acute stroke. *NeuroRehabilitation, 22*, 123-132. https://doi.org/10.3233/NRE-2007-22208

Ownsworth, T., Fleming, J., Tate, R., Beadle, E., Griffin, J., Kendall, M., Schmidt, J., Lane-Brown, A., Chevignard, M., & Shum, D. H. K. (2017). Do people with severe traumatic brain injury benefit from making errors? A randomized controlled trial of error-based and errorless learning. *Neurorehabilitation and Neural Repair, 31*, 1072-1082. https://doi.org/10.1177/1545968317740635

Padilla, R. (2011). Effectiveness of interventions designed to modify the activity demands of the occupations of self-care and leisure for people with Alzheimer's disease and related dementias. *American Journal of Occupational Therapy, 65*, 523-531. https://doi.org/10.5014/ajot.2011.002618

Parish, L., & Oddy, M. (2007). Efficacy of rehabilitation for functional skills more than 10 years after extremely severe brain injury. *Neuropsychological Rehabilitation, 17*, 230-243. https://doi.org/10.1080/09602010600750675

Pitel, A. L., Beaunieux, H., Lebaron, N., Joyeux, F., Desgranges, B., & Eustache, F. (2006). Two case studies in the application of errorless learning techniques in memory impaired patients with additional executive deficits. *Brain Injury, 20*, 1099-1110. https://doi.org/10.1080/02699050600909961

Polatajko, H. J. (2017). History of the CO-OP Approach. In D. Dawson, S. E. McEwen, & H. J. Polatajko (Eds.), *Cognitive Orientation to Daily Occupational Performance in occupational therapy: Using the CO-OP Approach to enable participation across the lifespan* (pp. 5-10). AOTA Press.

Polatajko, H. J., Mandich, A., & McEwen, S. E. (2011). Cognitive Orientation to Daily Occupational Performance (CO-OP): A cognitive-based intervention for children and adults. In N. Katz (Ed.), *Cognition, occupation, and participation across the life span: Neuroscience, neurorehabilitation, and models of intervention in occupational therapy* (3rd ed., pp. 299-322). AOTA Press.

Radomski, M. V., & Giles, G. M. (2021). Cognitive intervention. In D. P. Dirette & S. A. Gutman (Eds.), *Occupational therapy for physical dysfunction* (8th ed., pp. 161-175). Wolters Kluwer.

Skidmore, E. R., Holm, M. B., Whyte, E. M., Dew, M. A., Dawson, D., & Becker, J. T. (2011). The feasibility of meta-cognitive strategy training in acute inpatient stroke rehabilitation: Case report. *Neuropsychological Rehabilitation, 21*, 208-223. https://doi.org/10.1080/09602011.2011.552559

Skidmore, E. R., McEwen, S. E., Green, D., van den Houten, J., Dawson, D. R., & Polatajko, H. J. (2017). Essential elements and key features of the CO-OP Approach. In D. Dawson, S. E. McEwen, & H. J. Polatajko (Eds.), *Cognitive Orientation to Daily Occupational Performance in occupational therapy: Using the CO-OP Approach to enable participation across the lifespan* (pp. 11-20). AOTA Press.

Sohlberg, M. M., & Turkstra, L. S. (2011). *Optimizing cognitive rehabilitation: Effective instructional methods.* The Guilford Press.

Stergiou-Kita, M., Dawson, D., & Rappolt, S. (2012). Inter-professional clinical practice guidelines for vocational evaluation following traumatic brain injury: A systematic and evidence-based approach. *Journal of Occupational Rehabilitation, 22*, 166-181. https://doi.org/10.1007/s10926-011-9332-2

Tate, R., Kennedy, M., Ponsford, J., Douglas, J., Velikonja, D., Bayley, M., & Stergiou-Kita, M. (2014). INCOG recommendations for management of cognition following traumatic brain injury, part III: Executive function and self-awareness. *Journal of Head Trauma Rehabilitation, 29*, 338-352. https://doi.org/10.1097/HTR.0000000000000068

Toglia, J. P. (1991). Generalization of treatment: A multicontext approach to cognitive perceptual impairment in adults with brain injury. *American Journal of Occupational Therapy, 45*, 505-516. https://doi.org/10.5014/ajot.45.6.505

Toglia, J. (2018). The Dynamic Interactional Model and the Multicontext Approach. In N. Katz & J. Toglia (Eds.), *Cognition, occupation, and participation across the lifespan* (4th ed., pp. 355-385). AOTA Press.

Toglia, J., Goverover, Y., Johnston, M. V., & Dain, B. (2011). Application of the multicontextual approach in promoting learning and transfer of strategy use in an individual with TBI and executive dysfunction. *OTJR: Occupation, Participation and Health, 31*, S53-S60. https://doi.org/10.3928/15394492-20101108-09

Toglia, J., Johnston, M. V., Goverover, Y., & Dain, B. (2010). A multicontext approach to promoting transfer of strategy use and self regulation after brain injury: An exploratory study. *Brain Injury, 24*, 664-677. https://doi.org/10.3109/02699051003610474

Toglia, J., & Kirk, U. (2000). Understanding awareness deficits following brain injury. *NeuroRehabilitation, 15*, 57-70. https://doi.org/10.3233/NRE-2000-15104

Toglia, J., & Maeir, A. (2018). Self-awareness and metacognition: Effect on occupational performance and outcome across the life span. In N. Katz & J. Toglia (Eds.), *Cognition, occupation, and participation across the lifespan* (4th ed., pp. 143-163). AOTA Press.

Toglia, J. P., Rodger, S. A., & Polatajko, H. J. (2012). Anatomy of cognitive strategies: A therapist's primer for enabling occupational performance. *Canadian Journal of Occupational Therapy, 79*, 225-236. https://doi.org/10.2182/cjot.2012.79.4.4

Trevena-Peters, J., McKay, A., Spitz, G., Suda, R., Renison, B., & Ponsford, J. (2018). Efficacy of activities of daily living retraining during posttraumatic amnesia: A randomized controlled trial. *Archives of Physical Medicine and Rehabilitation, 99*, 329-337. https://doi.org/10.1016/j.apmr.2017.08.486

van Hoof, J., Kort, H. S. M., van Waarde, H., & Blom, M. M. (2010). Environmental interventions and the design of homes for older adults with dementia: An overview. *American Journal of Alzheimer's Disease and Other Dementias, 25*, 202-232. https://doi.org/10.1177/1533317509358885

Vanderploeg, R. D., Schwab, K., Walker, W. C., Fraser, J. A., Sigford, B. J., Date, E. S., Scott, S. G., Curtiss, G., Salazar, A. M., & Warden, D. L. (2008). Rehabilitation of traumatic brain injury in active duty military personnel and veterans: Defense and Veterans Brain Injury Center randomized controlled trial of two rehabilitation approaches. *Archives of Physical Medicine and Rehabilitation, 89*, 2227-2238. https://doi.org/10.1016/j.apmr.2008.06.015

Warren, M. (2018). Evaluation and treatment of visual deficits after brain injury. In H. M. Pendleton & W. Schultz-Krohn (Eds.), *Pedretti's occupational therapy: Practice skills for physical dysfunction* (8th ed., pp. 594-630). Elsevier.

Wolf, T. J., Doherty, M., Kallogjeri, D., Coalson, R. S., Nicklaus, J., Ma, C. X., Schlaggar, B. L., & Piccirillo, J. (2016). The feasibility of using metacognitive strategy training to improve cognitive performance and neural connectivity in women with chemotherapy-induced cognitive impairment. *Oncology, 91*, 143-152. https://doi.org/10.1159/000447744

Wong, A. W. K., Ng, S., Dashner, J., Baum, M. C., Hammel, J., Magasi, S., Lai., J.-S., Carlozzi, N. E., Tulsky, D. S., Miskovic, A., Goldsmith, A., & Heinemann, A. W. (2017). Relationships between environmental factors and participation in adults with traumatic brain injury, stroke, and spinal cord injury: A cross-sectional multi-center study. *Quality of Life Research, 26*, 2633-2645. https://doi.org/10.1007/s11136-017-1586-5

World Health Organization. (2001). *International classification of functioning, disability and health (ICF)*. World Health Organization.

Wortzel, H. S., & Arciniegas, D. B. (2012). Treatment of post-traumatic cognitive impairments. *Current Treatment Options Neurology, 14*, 493-508. https://doi.org/10.1007/s11940-012-0193-6

CHAPTER 11

Use of Everyday Technology

At its core, occupational therapy focuses on occupational performance and people's ability to engage in meaningful occupations in their homes and communities (American Occupational Therapy Association [AOTA], 2020). Occupations that are often addressed for adults include activities of daily living (ADLs), instrumental activities of daily living (IADLs), work, including both paid employment and volunteering, education, social participation, leisure, and rest or sleep (AOTA, 2020). These occupations change throughout the lifespan as interests, demands, and roles evolve over time. Occupations are also influenced by the environment, including social trends (AOTA, 2020). The use and availability of technology are one such trend.

Technology has become an integral part of modern life in many places around the globe and is used by a wide variety of people, both with and without disabilities. One type of technology, called *assistive technology* (AT), is used specifically by people with disabilities. AT is defined in the Assistive Technology Act of 2004 as "any item, piece of equipment, or product system, whether acquired commercially off the shelf, modified, or customized, that is used to increase, maintain, or improve functional capabilities of individuals with disabilities" (Brain Injury Association of America, 2022). The technology that is available and used by the general public is called *everyday technology* (ET). ET may be used as AT by people with disabilities, but it is used by millions of people without disabilities as well. ET includes everything from low-tech devices (e.g., washing machines, microwaves) to high-tech devices (e.g., smartphones, computers; Malinowsky et al., 2011). The primary focus of this chapter is high-tech ET devices.

Trends With Technology Use

The use of ET is increasingly widespread, and its impact on the way in which people complete many of their occupations is substantial (Baker-Sparr et al., 2018; Brunner et al., 2017; Chu et al., 2014; de Joode et al., 2012; Fallahpour et al., 2014; Goverover & DeLuca, 2015; Gustavsson et al.,

Kaminsky, T. A., & Powell, J. M.
Zoltan's Vision, Perception, and Cognition: Evaluation and Treatment of the Adult With Acquired Brain Injury, Fifth Edition (pp. 303-327).

2018; Kassberg, Malinowsky et al., 2013; Kassberg et al., 2016; Lindén et al., 2010, 2011; Lund et al., 2012, 2014; Malinowsky et al., 2012; Malinowsky & Lund, 2014, 2016; Nygård & Rosenberg, 2016). Technology use can be observed in IADLs (e.g., online bill paying), leisure (e.g., virtual reality games), social participation (e.g., texting, using social media), education (e.g., using the internet to do research for a paper), and work (e.g., using spreadsheets to track inventory). High-tech ET devices are commonly used in the United States. In 2021, the Pew Research Center reported that approximately 93% of adults in the United States use the internet, 97% own a cellphone (85% have smartphones), 77% own a computer, and 53% own a tablet. To be fully engaged in all areas of occupation, it is increasingly necessary for people to be able to use ET successfully, which is supported by research that found that difficulties with using ET are linked to limitations in occupational performance, including ADLs (Fallahpour et al., 2015) and work (Kassberg, Prellwitz et al., 2013; Lund et al., 2014).

People with disabilities have been shown to use technology at lower rates than people without disabilities. In 2021, the Pew Research Center reported that compared with people without disabilities, those with disabilities were less likely to own a computer (62% of people with disabilities vs. 81% of people without), smartphone (72% vs. 88%), and tablet (47% vs. 54%) and were slightly less likely to have internet at home (72% vs. 78%), although this gap has narrowed in recent years. People with disabilities are also less likely to use the internet daily, with approximately 75% of people with disabilities making daily use of the internet compared with 87% of people without disabilities (Perrin & Atske, 2021). The populations with disabilities least likely to use technology tended to be older, have a lower socioeconomic status, and live in rural locations (Baker-Sparr et al., 2018).

At the time of this writing, we are still in the midst of the COVID-19 pandemic, which could have a lasting impact on how technology is used by numerous groups, including those with disabilities. One qualitative study looking at the impact of the pandemic on technology use was conducted with 20 dyads of participants made up of people with mild to moderate cognitive impairment and their caregivers. The researchers found that technology use by all participants increased during quarantine and was used to overcome isolation, reduce boredom, and assist caregivers (e.g., through telehealth appointments, eliminating the need to transport care recipients). The limitations of the technology for people with cognitive impairment in this study were similar to other research that was conducted before the pandemic, results of which are described later in this chapter (Albers et al., 2022). Whether or not the increased use of technology will continue after the pandemic has ended is unknown at this time.

Influences on Effective Technology Use

Numerous factors can interfere with a person's ability to use ET, including the person's skills, the environment, and the demands of the technology (Scherer & Craddock, 2002; Scherer & Federici, 2015). Physical, sensory, and cognitive deficits all have the potential to negatively impact technology use. These types of deficits can all be present, to different degrees, for people with acquired brain injury (ABI) with a subsequent impact on their ability to use technology (Scherer & Federici, 2015). For example, individuals with fine motor control deficits can have difficulty accessing inputs, such as controlling touch screens or pushing buttons. Individuals with sensory deficits, specifically vision loss, can have difficulty seeing print or icons on screens (Hakobyan et al., 2013) or get overwhelmed by cluttered web pages (Dixon & Lazar, 2020). Using touch screens can be especially difficult for people with vision impairment because they must rely on vision to use them, and touch screens do not provide tactile feedback. Some applications that enable hands-free use of devices (e.g., voice control) can help to minimize this difficulty (Hakobyan et al., 2013).

People with cognitive impairments have many deficits that can make ET use difficult. These deficits can include memory loss, poor attention, and executive dysfunction (e.g., poor planning, decision making, and/or problem solving; Chu et al., 2014). Research performed with people with cognitive deficits after ABI reported that this population often struggles with a variety of aspects of ET, including finding functions on the devices (Engström et al., 2010; Evald, 2015; Goverover & DeLuca, 2015; Lindén et al., 2010; Lund et al., 2012; Malinowsky & Lund, 2016), remembering passwords (Engström et al., 2010; Kassberg et al., 2016; Lindén et al., 2010; Lund et al., 2012; Malinowsky & Lund, 2016), properly sequencing steps (Engström et al., 2010; Goverover & DeLuca, 2015; Kassberg, Malinowsky, et al., 2013; Lund et al., 2012), and keeping track of information (Chu et al., 2014; Engström et al., 2010). People with cognitive impairment may also forget or lose their devices and/or forget how the devices work (Adolfsson et al., 2015; Engström et al., 2010; Evald, 2015; Lund et al., 2011; Wong et al., 2017). These issues are often worse for people with more severe cognitive deficits after ABI (Fallahpour et al., 2014; Kassberg, Malinowsky, et al., 2013; Lund et al., 2014). Finally, fatigue is frequently an issue that many people with ABI, with or without cognitive deficits, report. Fatigue can have an impact on technology use because it can exacerbate other deficits (Engström et al., 2010; Kassberg et al., 2016; Kassberg, Malinowsky, et al., 2013; Kassberg, Prellwitz, et al., 2013; Lund et al., 2012).

In addition to factors within the person, there are influences outside the person that can impact their ability to use technology. Cost is the biggest barrier reported by people with ABI and their families because it can limit what types of devices and how many devices people are able to acquire (Brown et al., 2017; Charters et al., 2015; Chu et al., 2014; Crossland et al., 2014; de Joode et al., 2012; Hart et al., 2003; Kassberg et al., 2016; Wang et al., 2016; Wild, 2013; Wong et al., 2017). Other barriers to ET use that have been reported include issues with reliability (Chu et al., 2014; Lindqvist & Borell, 2012), usability (Chu et al., 2014), accessibility (Brunner et al., 2015; Chu et al., 2014), and ease of use (Brown et al., 2017; Brunner et al., 2017; Chu et al., 2014; Lund et al., 2011; Wang et al., 2016; Wong et al., 2017). Safety, including the risk of people becoming victims of fraud or oversharing personal information, has been mentioned by those with ABI, caregivers, and health care professionals (Baker-Sparr et al., 2018; Brown et al., 2017; Brunner et al., 2017; Charters et al., 2015; Chu et al., 2014; Evald, 2015; Lund et al., 2011; Oliver, 2019; Wang et al., 2016; Wong et al., 2017). Keeping up with rapidly changing technology and issues such as short battery lives are other concerns that have been identified (Engström et al., 2010; Evald, 2015; Kassberg, Prellwitz, et al., 2013; Wang et al., 2016).

In addition to personal characteristics and abilities and device features, people with ABI report that the environment that surrounds them while they use ET can also impact their performance. In some cases, this external environment can facilitate ET use. For example, because of the widespread use of high-tech ET, people with disabilities may be open to using ET to assist functioning because it is socially acceptable; even people without cognitive deficits will often use ET to assist their functioning, as outlined previously (Brunner et al., 2017; Charters et al., 2015; Chu et al., 2014; Ferguson et al., 2015; Gustavsson et al., 2018; Hakobyan et al., 2013; Hendricks et al., 2015; Livingstone-Lee et al., 2014; Lund et al., 2011; Wild, 2013; Wong et al., 2017). In other cases, the environment can create a barrier. Noisy spaces and the presence of other people have been reported as distractions that interfere with ET use, with the latter resulting in users feeling pressured to speed up (e.g., when using an ATM) or feeling judged when making mistakes (Chu et al., 2014; Engström et al., 2010; Kassberg et al., 2016; Kassberg, Malinowsky, et al., 2013; Kassberg, Prellwitz, et al., 2013). Another barrier is that caregivers are often the people who need to set up and manage ET for care recipients (Bartfai & Bowman, 2014; Dixon & Lazar, 2020; Lindqvist & Borell, 2012). If the caregiver does not think that the ET is appropriate for the care recipient or does not have the required knowledge or skills, it is more likely that the person with ABI will not use technology (de Joode et al., 2012).

Despite difficulties with ET, many people with ABI have a desire to use it and will often seek it out with or without the assistance of health care professionals (Gustavsson et al., 2018). Smartphones or other mobile devices are the most commonly reported type of high-tech ET that is used among people with ABI, although people report using other devices, including tablets and computers (Baker-Sparr et al., 2018; Brunner et al., 2017; Wong et al., 2017). Often people return to using the technology they utilized before their injuries, although many report having more difficulty with their devices after their injuries (Engström et al., 2010). Most people with ABI report not getting official training with technology during the rehabilitation process (Bartfai & Boman, 2014; Brunner et al., 2017; Chu et al., 2014; Ferguson et al., 2015; Lindqvist & Borell, 2012; Lund et al., 2011; Oliver, 2019). Because of clients' difficulties in using ET on their own and a lack of formal training, caregivers are usually the people setting up technology for those with ABI. Although caregiver assistance is invaluable, many caregivers do not know what technology options are available and how technology can assist people with ABI in fully participating in occupation. As a result, it is important for occupational therapy practitioners to evaluate technology use by adult clients with ABI and to incorporate it as part of their treatment.

Assessment of Technology Use

As stated earlier, adept use of technology is becoming an increasingly important skill for people to be able to fully engage in their occupations in their homes and communities. As a result, it is essential that occupational therapy practitioners consider clients' technology use during the assessment process. As of the writing of this chapter, there were a few standardized assessments that have been or are being developed for people with ABI. One assessment is designed to evaluate ET use by people with neurovisual deficits in addition to cognitive deficits; this assessment, which utilizes the Performance Assessment of Self-Care Skills (PASS), is being developed for use within the United States. In addition, two subtests of the Executive Function Performance Test (EFPT; described in detail in Chapter 8) now have the option of using ET. Two additional standardized assessments, the Management of Everyday Technology Assessment (META) and the Everyday Technology Use Questionnaire (ETUQ), are available in Sweden. The ETUQ is undergoing development for use by therapists in other countries. Both specifically consider the use of ET by people with cognitive deficits.

Performance Assessment of Self-Care Skills (Rogers et al., 2016)

Description

The Performance Assessment of Self-Care Skills (PASS) is described in detail in Chapter 8. The PASS is a standardized, occupation-based assessment tool with a variety of tasks that can be used to assess a person's performance during activity. The tasks can be used to assess both physical and cognitive skills. The authors of the PASS encourage community clinicians to develop test items that use the format of the assessment tool, and they provide instructions on how to create new test items (Rogers et al., 2016). One group of researchers is creating PASS assessment tasks, called the Functionally Simulated Technology Tasks, that examine performance with computerized activities (Cardell et al., 2013). These researchers have created two simulated technology tasks, one that allows clients to complete online bill paying and one that enables them to complete online shopping. The tools are free and available for general use. Practitioners who would like to use the tools with clients can download materials that are needed, including instructions, simulated credit cards, and simulated bills, at https://health.utah.edu/occupational-recreational-therapies/colleagues-clinicians

As a result of ongoing psychometric testing, at the time of this writing the authors of the Functionally Simulated Technology Tasks recommended that the subtests not be used for standardized testing. However, they suggested that they could be used as interventions to practice online bill paying and shopping (University of Utah College of Health, 2022). In the future, these tools may help provide valuable information about ET use by clients with ABI.

Procedure

Both the online bill paying and online shopping tasks have standardized instructions that describe the materials needed, how the task should be set up, the directions that are given to the client, and the scoring criteria. These can be found at https://health.utah.edu/occupational-recreational-therapies/colleagues-clinicians

Scoring

As stated previously, the developers of these tasks recommend that these assessments not be used as standardized tests due to ongoing psychometric testing, although they do include scoring criteria that are consistent with PASS scoring (described in Chapter 8). With this method, clients are scored in three areas (i.e., independence, safety, and outcome) using an ordinal scale. Independence is assessed using both the level of assistance and the type of assistance that is given on each subtask in the test item. To determine the assistance that is needed, a dynamic process is used where the evaluating clinician gives the client assistance in a graded fashion. There is a hierarchy of assistances levels examiners are to use, ranging from a general verbal assist (e.g., encouragement) through total physical assistance (i.e., when the examiner completes the task for the client). Safety is assessed by making observations of unsafe behaviors exhibited by the client during the task. Finally, outcome is assessed by considering both the person's efficiency as well as the quality of the performance. To assign the adequacy score, the client's performance as a whole is considered.

Psychometric Properties

Both the online bill paying and online shopping activities have been developed as PASS subtests and are currently undergoing research to establish inter-rater reliability and content validity (University of Utah College of Health, 2022). Preliminary content validity testing demonstrated that these tools were able to discriminate between people with and without cognitive deficits. There was also a good to excellent relationship between the Functionally Simulated Technology Tasks and the Montreal Cognitive Assessment, a screening tool for cognition (Cardell et al., 2013).

Executive Function Performance Test Subtests (Rand et al., 2018)

Description

In 2018, a research group from Israel described internet-based tasks that can be used with the Executive Function Performance Test (EFPT) subtests (described in detail in Chapter 8; Rand et al., 2018). These researchers had study participants complete the telephone subtest using Google rather than a telephone book. Participants also completed the bill-paying subtest using a specially designed computer program. The software for this program can be downloaded for free from http://www.tau.ac.il/~portnoys/Internet-based_Bill_Paying_Task.html. These subtests provide a standardized way to assess two tasks in which people often use ET.

Procedure

Clients complete the EFPT as described in Chapter 8 with two exceptions. Clients use a Google search rather than a telephone book in the telephone subtest and use the online bill-paying module instead of the checkbook and paper bills. For further information about how to administer the EFPT, see Chapter 8 and the EFPT test manual.

Scoring

Clients are scored on each subtest separately with the scoring the same for clients who use the technology options (Google and online bill paying) as those who use the original versions of these tasks. The examiner scores the client's performance using a 6-point scale as follows: 0 = independent, 1 = verbal guidance, 2 = gestural guidance, 3 = verbal direct instruction, 4 = physical assistance, and 5 = done for the participant. Clients also receive scores for several behaviors including (a) initiation or beginning the task; (b) execution, which includes organization, sequencing, and judgment/safety; and (c) completion. In addition, the examiner notes the time it takes participants to complete the activity. Scores for each subtest are then summarized and the client's actual performance is compared to the client's prediction of how well they will do. For additional details about scoring, see the EFPT test manual.

Psychometric Properties

These researchers found that the online options of the subtests correlated well with the original paper-based tasks from the EFPT. They were also correlated with the Trail Making Task, a neuropsychological assessment of executive functions. In addition, the online-based subtests were able to distinguish between people with a CVA and those without (Rand et al., 2018).

Management of Everyday Technology Assessment (Karolinska Institutet, 2022b)

Description

Two assessment tools looking at ET use by people with cognitive deficits have been developed in Sweden and have undergone some psychometric testing in that country. One of the assessments, the Management of Everyday Technology Assessment (META), is a standardized tool that allows a clinician to assess a client using ET. At the time of this writing, the META was only available for clinicians in Sweden, although its use may be extended to practitioners in other countries in the future (Karolinska Institutet, 2022b).

Procedure

The client is observed while using two to three technologies of their choice. The ET must belong to the client, be relevant and currently used, and be somewhat challenging as reported by the client. The test manual, which can be ordered from Sweden, provides additional details (https://www.arbetsterapeuterna.se/foerbundet/english/ot-instruments/management-of-everyday-technology-assessment-meta/).

Scoring

The META allows clinicians to rate 11 different performance-related skills for the client, the environment's impact on ET use, the client's personal capacities for using the ET, and the client's opinions about how relevant the technology is for them (Karolinska Institutet, 2022b). The performance on each skill is scored on a three-category rating scale: no difficulty, minor difficulty, or major difficulty (Malinowsky et al., 2016).

Psychometric Properties

Psychometric testing on the META has shown fair to good test–retest reliability (Malinowsky et al., 2016) and acceptable intra-rater reliability (Malinowsky et al., 2011). It also was able to distinguish among those with different levels of ability with using technology (Malinowsky et al., 2011).

Everyday Technology Use Questionnaire (Karolinska Institutet, 2022a)

Description

The Everyday Technology Use Questionnaire (ETUQ) is the second assessment of ET use by people who have cognitive deficits that has been developed recently in Sweden. The ETUQ is a semi-structured standardized interview tool that asks about 93 technological devices or services grouped into 8 activity areas. The results of the ETUQ provide the clinician with information about which ET the client finds useful or relevant in addition to the person's perceived ability when using the ET. It takes approximately 30 to 45 minutes to complete the interview.

At the time of this writing, the ETUQ was available for use by clinicians in Sweden. Research into the applicability of the ETUQ to people in other countries has been started. In 2020, Wallcook and colleagues reported on a study of the ETUQ that had been completed in three countries: Sweden, the United States, and England. In total, 315 people, both with and without cognitive impairment, participated in the study. The researchers found that of the items in the questionnaire, only five showed a statistically significant difference by country. All of the five items involved technology that is found in public spaces (e.g., ATM, automatic ticket gate, self-check-in kiosk, baggage drop-off, and gas pump). The researchers stated that, because the majority of items were not impacted by the country in which participants lived and the overall scores were comparable, the study supported the ETUQ being used in other countries (Wallcook et al., 2020). However, they stressed that practitioners should be aware of the technology that is commonly used in their geographic areas and consider familiarity of ET for their clients. In order to support the use of the ETUQ in other countries, online training in English was being developed so that English-speaking practitioners could access the tool and be trained with its use. Additional information on the on-line training is available at https://akademin.arbetsterapeuterna.se/LuvitPortal/activities/activitydetails_ext.aspx?inapp=1&id=56

A shorter version of the ETUQ (S-ETUQ) has been developed and tested for use with people with mild cognitive impairment and Alzheimer's disease. The S-ETUQ has 32 items and can be administered in 10 to 20 minutes.

Procedure

For each of the 32 items on the assessment, the clinician determines if that ET item is relevant to the client. ET is considered relevant if the client is using it or intends to start using it. If an item is relevant, the client is asked about perceived difficulty with using the device (Malinowsky et al., 2020).

Scoring

Perceived difficulty for each relevant item is rated on a six-level scale (Malinowsky et al., 2020).

Psychometric Properties

Psychometric testing done on the ETUQ has found that it has acceptable scale validity and is able to distinguish between people with and without cognitive impairment (Rosenberg et al., 2009). Researchers found that the S-ETUQ was also able to distinguish between people with and without cognitive impairment, although it may not be as sensitive as the longer version of the ETUQ (Kottorp & Nygård, 2011). The S-ETUQ was also found to have good test–retest reliability (Malinowsky et al., 2020).

Matching Person and Technology Assessment Tool (Scherer & Federici, 2015)

Description

The Matching Person and Technology assessment tool is another assessment that could be useful to clinicians who are considering technology use by their clients. This is a general tool for considering AT use, not one specifically geared toward ET use by people with cognitive and/or visual impairment. It is based on the Matching Person and Technology Model, which is designed to maximize the fit among the person's abilities, the characteristics of the desired AT, and the demands of the environment. The tool considers the needs, preferences, and characteristics of the person, including their goals for technology use and their abilities. The AT under consideration is also assessed, including the device's features and functions and whether or not the device can help the person achieve their goals. Finally, the environment surrounding the person when the technology will be used is considered.

Procedure

The Matching Person and Technology assessment tool has several forms that can be completed with clients, depending upon their needs. All of the forms can be downloaded, along with user manuals, from https://sites.google.com/view/matchingpersontechnology/menu/products. The first form can help with goal creation and consideration of possible devices that may help the person achieve goals. A second form considers prior use of devices and what features of those devices are desired. Additional forms consider specific features of the devices that are being considered for the client (Institute for Matching Person and Technology, 2021).

Scoring

The assessment tool is scored differently based upon which form is used. For details, readers should refer to the user manuals.

Psychometric Properties

Psychometric testing has found internal consistency ratings of $\alpha = 0.73$ to 0.89 for the different forms (Scherer et al., 2005). Another study found that the tool had good inter-rater reliability, but the researchers did not report the relevant statistics (Scherer & Craddock, 2002). These researchers also reported that the tool was useful in predicting which clients would adopt versus abandon ET (Scherer & Craddock, 2002; Scherer et al., 2005).

Non-Standardized Assessment

Because of the lack of available standardized assessments looking specifically at ET use by people with cognitive and/or visual impairment, most practitioners will need to assess this area of occupational performance through non-standardized methods. When considering ET use, researchers in this area recommend that practitioners use a combination of observation and interview to gather a more complete picture of ET use for clients, including the types of technology that are relevant and the factors that both support and hinder its use (Goverover & DeLuca, 2015; Kassberg et al., 2016; Kassberg, Prellwitz, et al., 2013; Malinowsky & Lund, 2014). Observation can enable practitioners to see where breakdown occurs and the types of errors that are made. An interview can provide information about the types of ET that are used currently, the types of ET that were used before injury, and the perceived ability related to ET use. It is not uncommon for the interview and the observation to not match up exactly. People may perceive that they are struggling even though they may be able to complete tasks, demonstrating that their performance may not be as efficient as it was before injury even if it is functional (Malinowsky & Lund, 2014). People may also overestimate their abilities, demonstrating impaired awareness of their deficits related to technology use (Goverover & DeLuca, 2015; Malinowsky & Lund, 2014).

Interviews will be similar to those completed to create the occupational profile, but questions about ET use should be specifically asked. The person should be asked about what ET was used before ABI and how ET was used for a variety of occupations, including IADLs, work, leisure, and social participation. The person's goals regarding technology should also be ascertained, and it can be helpful to ask about motivation for using technology (Leopold et al., 2015; Scherer & Federici, 2015). Some types of technology to consider are high-tech ET, including smartphones, computers, and tablets, in addition to low-tech ET, such as microwave ovens, washing machines, and stoves (Malinowsky et al., 2011; Figure 11-1). In addition to the interview, skilled observation of the client using ET should be completed. Ideally, the person's own ET would be used. The tasks with which the person is successful, tasks in which they are not, and deficits that are likely contributing to problems should be noted. Deficits may include some combination of motor, sensory, and cognitive skills (Bartfai & Bowman, 2014; Chu et al., 2014; Hart et al., 2003; Leopold et al., 2015; Lindén et al., 2010; Oliver, 2019; Scherer & Federici, 2015). Observation of the person using ET in multiple environments is recommended because the context surrounding the person will likely impact their success with using ET (Malinowski et al., 2012; Figures 11-2 and 11-3).

Intervention With Technology

When using ET in treatment with people with ABI, there are two general approaches a clinician may use. The first is to use ET as a compensatory strategy, focusing on increasing occupational performance despite deficits that are present after the brain injury. The second is to use ET as remediation, aiming to improve the deficits themselves. Little has been written about how ET can benefit people with visual impairments after ABI, but the literature that has been published reports several ways that ET can be used by those with vision loss as a compensatory tool. More research has been published about the use of ET by people with cognitive impairment after ABI. This research has explored the use of ET as both compensation and as remediation.

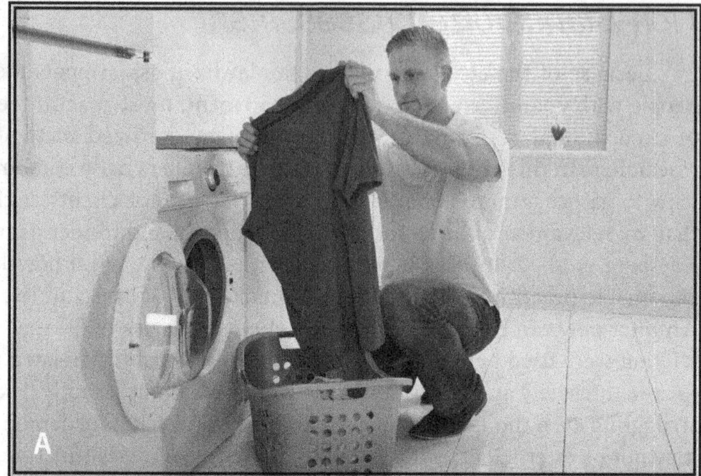

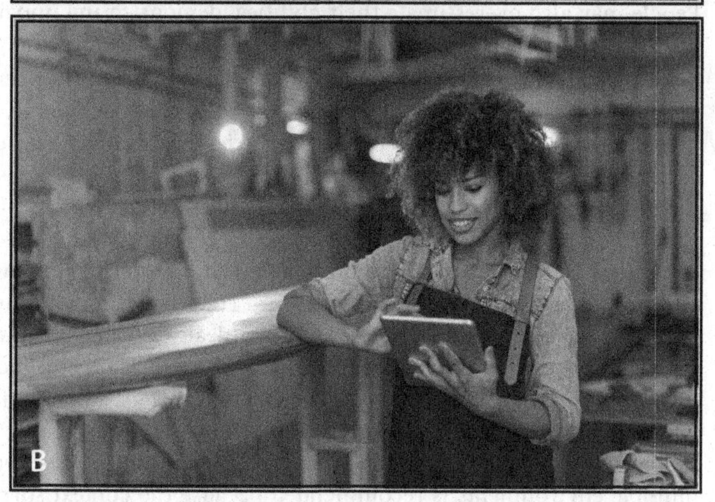

Figure 11-1. Non-standardized observation of people using technology, both (A) low-tech devices such as washing machines and (B) high-tech devices such as tablets, can provide information about skills and needs clients have with completing tasks that require the use of technology. (A: Andrey_Popov/shutterstock.com; B: pikselstock/shutterstock.com)

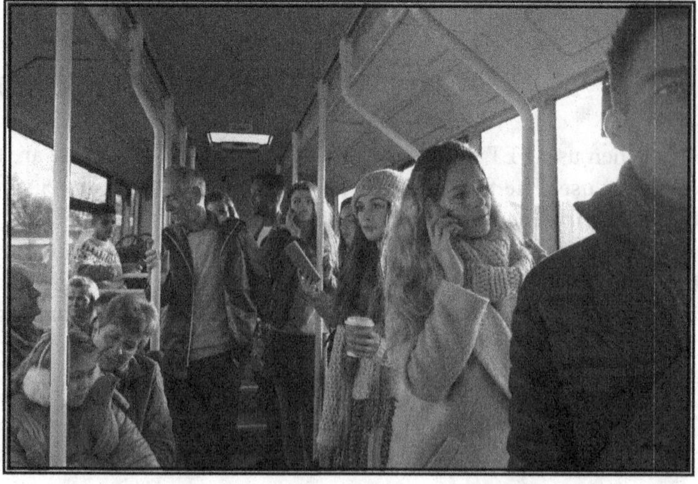

Figure 11-2. Considering technology use in multiple environments is important. Using a phone while standing on a crowded and moving bus is a challenging task that requires advanced cognitive and physical skills. (DGLimages/shutterstock.com)

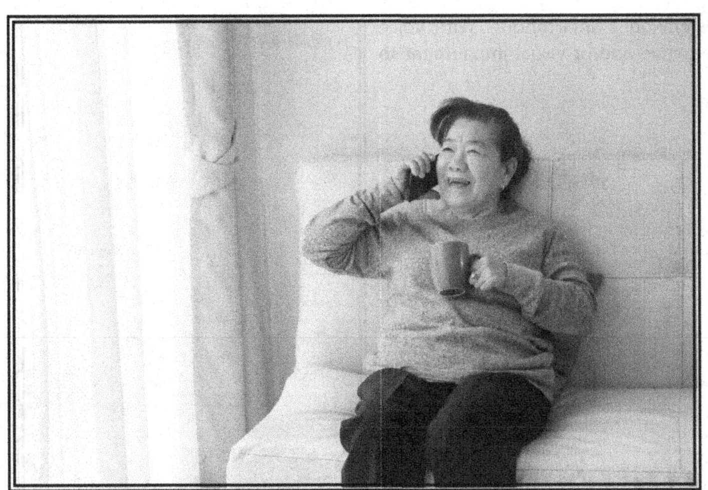

Figure 11-3. Sitting at home in a nondistracting environment while using the phone will prove to be an easier task for people who may have cognitive deficits, such as impairments in selective attention. (StudioByTheSea/shutterstock.com)

Compensatory Everyday Technology for Neurovisual Impairment

One of the most prevalent uses of ET by those with visual impairment is for assistance with navigation or pathfinding, with applications such as global positioning devices with voice output being especially helpful (Figure 11-4; Copolillo & Dahlin-Ivanoff, 2011; Hakobyan et al., 2013). Other ways that ET can be used to support this population include identifying objects in a grocery store using a specialized application that scans labels and barcodes (Figure 11-5; Hakobyan et al., 2013), taking pictures and enlarging the images to allow magnification (Figure 11-6; Crossland et al., 2014), determining colors through specialized applications (Crossland et al., 2014), and tracking public transportation (Hakobyan et al., 2013).

To better enable the use of devices, the same principles for those with vision deficits that were outlined in Chapter 4 for environmental modification can be used, specifically the consideration of lighting, magnification, and contrast (Copolillo & Dahlin-Ivanoff, 2011). Lighting can be considered with devices themselves, including their screen brightness, because this can greatly impact the visibility of information on screens. Environmental lighting will also need to be considered, especially if it creates a glare on the screens of devices people are trying to use. Teaching people to enlarge information on their devices, including font size, is important because the magnification of information can make it easier for many people to decipher (Figure 11-7). The contrast of information on screens can also be adjusted to find the level of contrast that is most effective for people as well as reducing clutter on the screen by deleting un-needed icons (Figure 11-8). There are an increasing number of accessibility features that are included on ET (e.g., ones that enable changes to font and contrast), and it is essential for practitioners working with people with ABI to familiarize themselves with these features (Copolillo & Dahlin-Ivanoff, 2011).

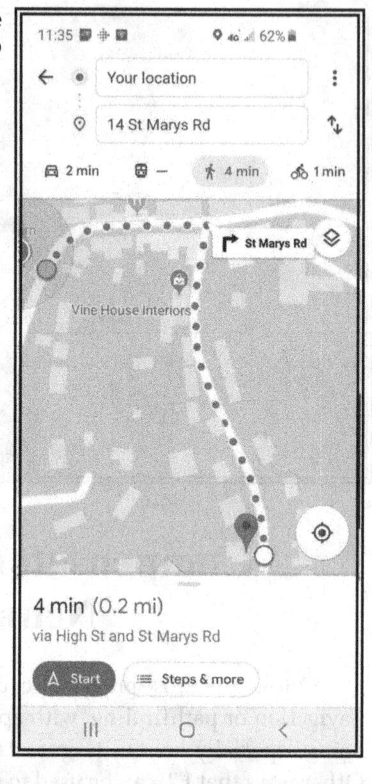

Figure 11-4. A global positioning system on a smartphone. With voice output, this can assist people with cognitive and/or visual impairment to navigate in the community.

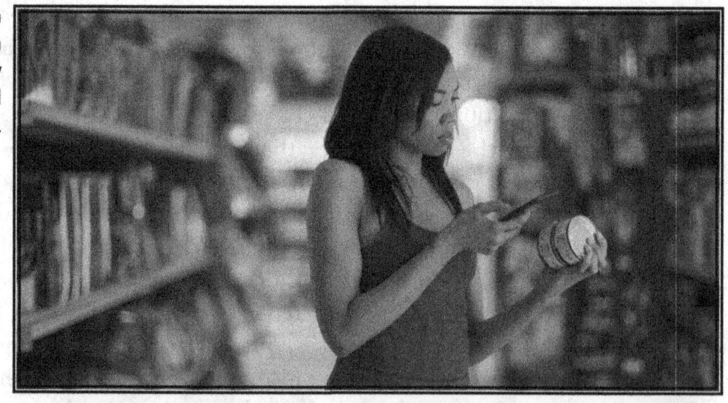

Figure 11-5. Applications on smartphones can be used to scan barcodes of items in the grocery store to assist people with visual impairment in object identification. (Rocketclips, Inc./shutterstock.com)

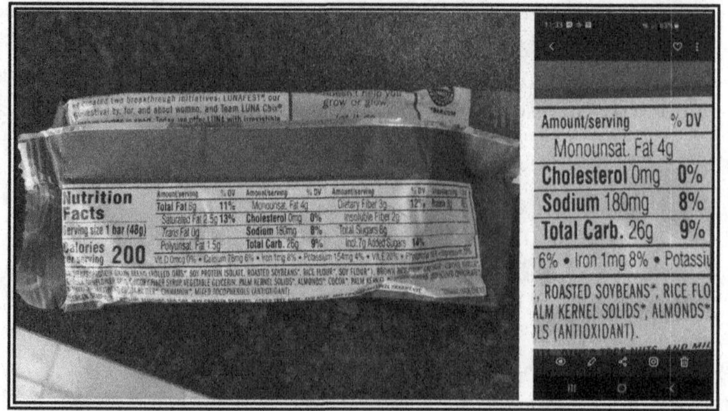

Figure 11-6. Using the camera to magnify. The original photo taken with the smartphone is on the left. The magnified image through the zoom function is on the right. This would assist someone with visual impairment who needed to monitor sodium intake with reading nutrition labels.

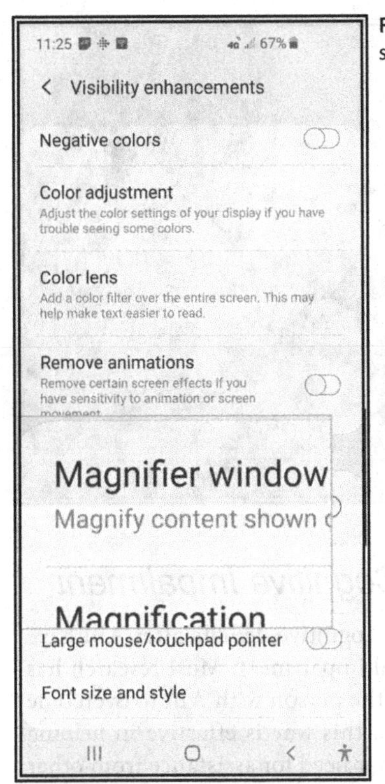

Figure 11-7. The magnification function from the accessibility features of a smartphone.

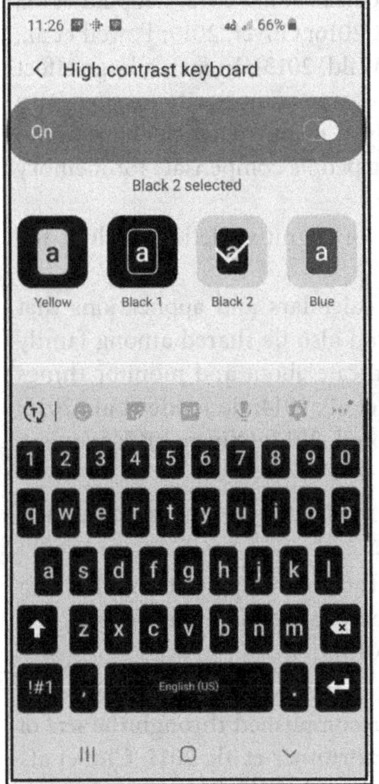

Figure 11-8. A high-contrast on-screen keyboard from the accessibility features of a smartphone.

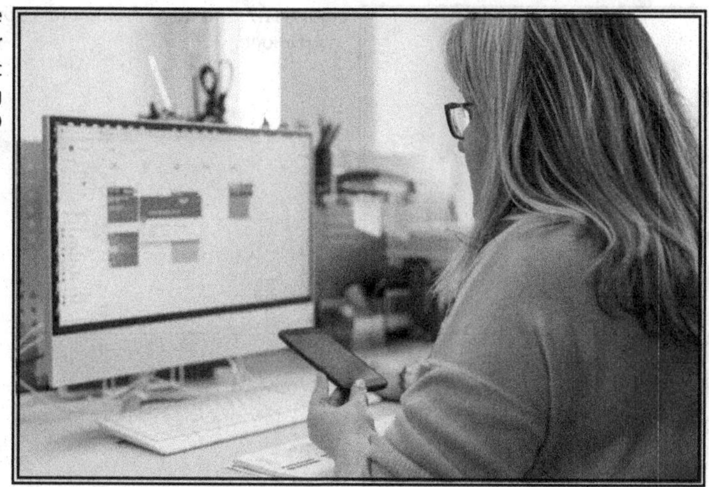

Figure 11-9. Online schedules can be shared among family members or with other caregivers. This can assist in the coordination and monitoring of appointments or other tasks. (ABO PHOTOGRAPHY/shutterstock.com)

Compensatory Everyday Technology for Cognitive Impairment

The ways in which ET can be used to support people with cognitive deficits after ABI have been studied more extensively than for people with neurovisual impairment. Most research has focused on the use of ET as a compensatory tool that can assist the person with ABI to overcome cognitive deficits. There is increasing evidence that ET used in this way is effective in helping people increase their occupational performance and decrease their need for assistance from other people (Adolfsson et al., 2015; Bartfai & Bowman, 2014; Chu et al., 2014; de Joode et al., 2010, 2012; Ferguson et al., 2015; Gentry, 2018; Gustavsson et al., 2018; Hendricks et al., 2015; Leopold et al., 2015; Lindén et al., 2011; Lund et al., 2011; Nygård & Rosenberg, 2016; Oliver, 2019; Powell et al., 2015; Veterans Health Administration, 2010; Wang et al., 2016; Wild, 2013). In fact, a large effect size was found in a meta-analysis looking at the use of technology to compensate for cognitive deficits (Jamieson et al., 2014). Other studies looking specifically at memory deficits have found medium to large effect sizes with the use of technology in helping people compensate for memory deficits (Charters et al., 2015; Evald, 2015; Wong et al., 2017).

Specific ways that technology has been used to compensate for cognitive deficits include the following:

- Planning and maintenance of schedules, including using calendars and applications that can help with the prioritization of tasks. These schedules can also be shared among family members or other caregivers so that it is easier to communicate about and monitor things such as appointments (Figure 11-9; Brown et al., 2017; Chu et al., 2014; de Joode et al., 2012; Gustavsson et al., 2018; Leopold et al., 2015; Lindqvist & Borell, 2012; Oliver, 2019; Wang et al., 2016; Wild, 2013; Wong et al., 2017).
- Sequencing tasks with multiple steps through the use of applications, such as checklists (Gentry, 2018; Lund et al., 2012).
- Navigating and pathfinding in the community, including the use of applications that can assist with public transportation use (Chu et al., 2014; Gillespie et al., 2012; Lindén et al., 2011; Livingstone-Lee et al., 2014; Stock et al., 2011; Wang et al., 2016).
- Helping people remember to perform tasks, especially those that need to be accomplished at specific times (e.g., medication management). This can be accomplished through the use of alarms or other reminders (Figure 11-10; Brown et al., 2017; Brunner et al., 2017; Chu et al., 2014; Evald, 2015; Ferguson et al., 2015; Gentry, 2018; Gillespie et al., 2012; Lindén et al., 2011; Lindqvist & Borell, 2012; Oliver, 2019; Wang et al., 2016; Wong et al., 2017).

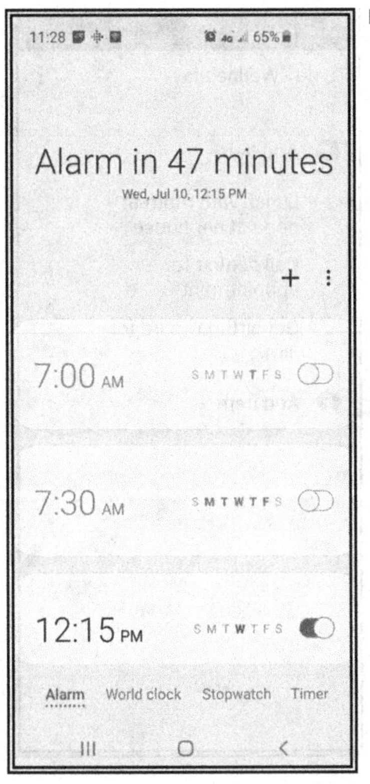

Figure 11-10. The timer/alarm function on a smartphone.

- Recalling events through the use of cameras built in to devices to create photo journals or through the use of note-taking applications (Chu et al., 2014; Evald, 2015; Gustavson et al., 2018); this would take the place of paper memory logs (Figure 11-11).
- Regulating emotions through applications that support guided meditation or biofeedback to monitor agitation (Chu et al., 2014; Gentry, 2018; Gillespie et al., 2012; Wild, 2013).
- Maintaining safety though the use of reminders to check that stoves have been turned off (Lindqvist & Borell, 2012) or device tracking to enable caregivers to monitor the location of the ABI survivor (Figure 11-12; Chu et al., 2014; Livingstone-Lee et al., 2014; Oliver, 2019; Stock et al., 2011). Mobile phones also enable people to call for assistance when needed (Gustavsson et al., 2018).
- Accessing information through the internet (Baker-Sparr et al., 2018; Gustavsson et al., 2018; Lindén et al., 2011; Oliver, 2019).

Many of these compensatory strategies can be set up using the applications and functions that are built in to a variety of ET devices, including smartphones, tablets, and computers. Table 11-1 provides examples of built-in functions that may be used to support people with deficits after ABI. The reader should note that Table 11-1 does not include all possible functions that can be used to help people compensate for deficits. Instead, it lists common applications that are available on most ET high-tech devices that people commonly use. It also does not include specialized applications, which may be available to address the compensatory strategies listed previously and more. Because of the rapidly changing nature of technology, specific applications and functions are not listed in this chapter. Practitioners are encouraged to explore options that become available on a regular basis.

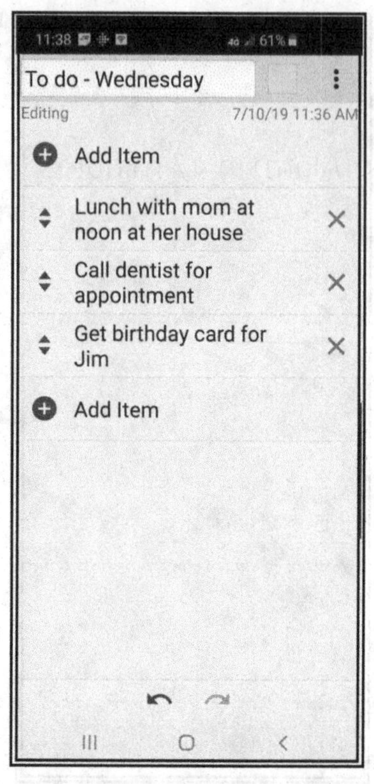

Figure 11-11. A note-taking application on a smartphone. This application can be used to create checklists and/or to log activities throughout the day to serve as a memory log.

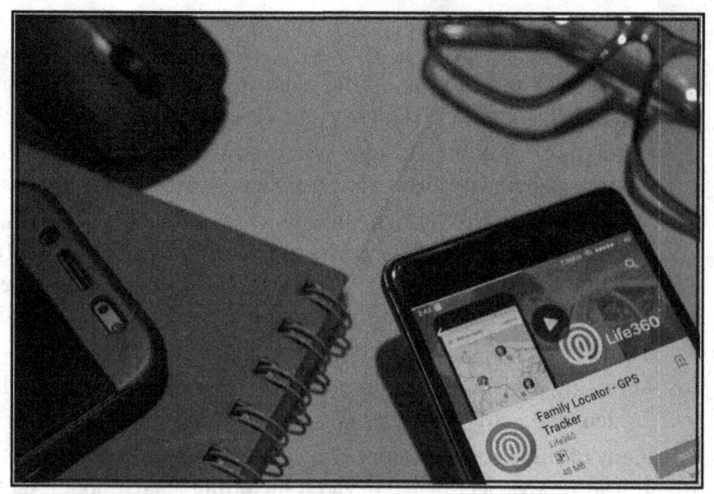

Figure 11-12. Features such as device tracking can assist caregivers in monitoring the status of the person with ABI. (bangoland/shutterstock.com)

Remedial Everyday Technology for Cognitive Impairment

As a reminder, remediation focuses on improving the deficits directly. The theory is that improving impairments will result in improvements in function (Maskill & Tempest, 2017). There are increasing numbers of studies examining the impact of computer-based treatments for the remediation of cognitive deficits. A systematic review by Cicerone and colleagues (2019) that included studies published between 2009 and 2014 examined a variety of treatment options for people with cognitive impairment after traumatic brain injury, including computer-based

Table 11-1

Built-In Functions and Applications That Can Be Used to Compensate for Deficits After Acquired Brain Injury

APPLICATION/ FUNCTION	COMPENSATORY STRATEGY
Accessibility settings	All high-tech ET devices, including smartphones, tablets, and computers, have accessibility settings that can be customized for individual users. Some common settings include changing the contrast or color of screens, changing font size, changing screen brightness, and activating voice output. Deleting unused applications and reducing visual clutter can also help people after ABI, with both visual and cognitive impairment.
Alarms and timers	Timers may be set to help people remember appointments or tasks, such as medication management. Recurring reminders may also be set for appointments or tasks that are regularly occurring.
Calendar	Calendars can be used for tracking schedules and remembering appointments. A calendar can also be shared among users, enabling caregivers to set up appointments on the care recipient's devices.
Camera	For people with visual impairment, cameras may be used to help magnify information. For example, they can take a picture of a sign and then zoom in to enlarge the print. For people with cognitive impairment, cameras may be used to help remember activities and information. For example, people can take pictures intermittently during the day to create a photo journal/ memory log.
Global positioning systems	Can be used by both people with visual impairment and those with cognitive impairment for route following and pathfinding. Voice output may be used for both populations to supplement or replace visual instruction.
Note-taking	Can be used to create notes to remember a variety of things, including codes, to-do lists, and sequences of activities.

treatment. The authors found that computer-based treatment did have a positive impact on cognitive functioning, especially with attention, and that there was some evidence that this improvement carried over to self-reported functioning in everyday activities. Based on these findings, the authors recommended that computer-based remedial treatment be used as one component of cognitive rehabilitation in post-acute care. The impact of computer-based treatment in acute care was inconclusive. Not all studies have found that computer-based remedial treatment improves performance with everyday tasks. Some studies, including some that were completed after the studies included in the previously discussed review, showed improvements on neuropsychological testing but did not show significant gains in everyday functioning and real-life contexts (Li et al., 2015; van de Ven et al., 2016, 2017).

Even without a clear impact of computer-based remediation on functional activities, there are aspects of this treatment modality that may be valuable for meeting therapeutic goals. Participants in studies that examined computer-based cognitive rehabilitation found the training to be motivating. They also reported that they appreciated that it provided another way in which they could participate in the rehabilitation process (Erikkson & Dahlin-Ivanoff, 2002; Li et al., 2015; van de Ven et al., 2016). Because many of the training programs are available on portable devices, they could be used outside of therapy time, which enabled people to get more opportunities to practice skills (Erikkson & Dahlin-Ivanoff, 2002; van de Ven et al., 2017). Remediation programs also sometimes helped people understand some of their cognitive deficits, including their increased fatigue and how it affected performance. Participants in one study stated that the use of the computer training enabled them to see that they needed to take breaks more frequently than they did before their ABI (Erikkson & Dahlin-Ivanoff, 2002). In the studies that have been conducted with computer-based remediation programs, participants and researchers stated that they thought that computer training should be a complement to, not a replacement of, in-person cognitive rehabilitation. The skills taught by the occupational therapy practitioner, in addition to other members of the rehabilitation team, and practiced during therapy sessions were considered essential for improving occupational performance (Cicerone et al., 2019; Erikkson & Dahlin-Ivanoff, 2002; van de Ven et al., 2017).

Everyday Technology and Occupational Therapy Intervention

Occupational therapy intervention can help people with ABI understand how ET can assist them and how the technology can be better matched to their changed abilities after ABI. Without professional intervention, the benefits of ET may be underutilized (Evald, 2015; Kassberg, Prellwitz, et al., 2013; Wang et al., 2016). People with ABI who have received technology training from a professional have reported that it is helpful in allowing them to be more successful with using ET (Lund et al., 2011; Wang et al., 2016).

One of the ways in which occupational therapy practitioners can support people with ABI is by better enabling a match among the person's abilities, the features of the devices themselves, the demands of the environment, and the task components themselves. Through careful assessment of the person and the desired device, the occupational therapy practitioner can make decisions about how the device can be adapted to better allow the person to use it (de Joode et al., 2010; Engström et al., 2010; Fallahpour et al., 2014; Leopold et al., 2015). One outcome may include using accessibility features on the client's existing devices (i.e., the ones used before injury) to improve the client's access to the device and its features. Another outcome from the evaluation may be that the clinician has the information needed to guide the client and caregiver in choosing new devices that will best match the person's abilities and goals if existing technology is not usable (Oliver, 2019; Figure 11-13).

When considering which devices to use, it is best to start with the client's existing technology. Familiarity with devices can enable clients to be more proficient with their use and can also allow them to use the routines they had before their ABI (Brown et al., 2017; Brunner et al., 2017; Charters et al., 2015; Ferguson et al., 2015; Gustavsson et al., 2018; Hendricks et al., 2015; Kassberg et al., 2016; Lindén et al., 2011; Livingston-Lee et al., 2014; Lund et al., 2011, 2012; Oliver, 2019; Wong et al., 2017). If a different device is needed, it is essential that both the client and the caregivers be involved in the decision-making process. The client needs to be motivated to use the technology in occupation, and the caregiver will need to support the client's use of the device, including set-up and maintenance (Adolfsson et al., 2015; Albers et al., 2022; Bartfai & Boman, 2014; Brunner et al., 2017; Chu et al., 2014; Federici et al., 2014; Lindqvist & Borell, 2012; Oliver,

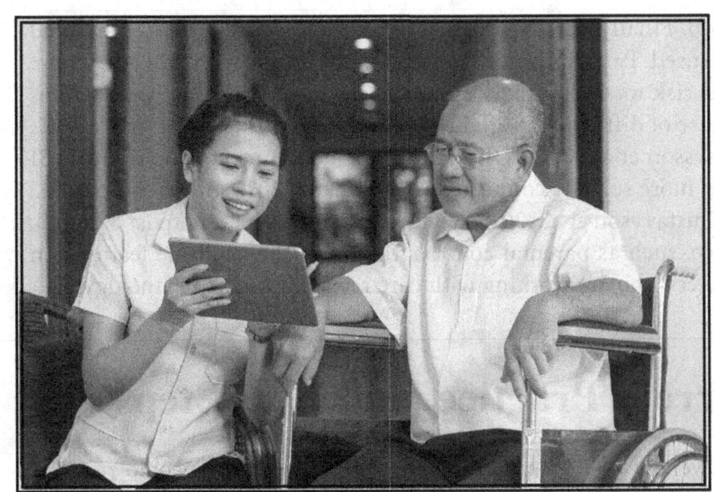

Figure 11-13. Caregivers are an important factor to consider in rehabilitation. In the case of technology, it is often the caregiver who needs to set up, monitor, and maintain devices for people with ABI. (xmee/shutterstock.com)

2019; Veterans Health Administration, 2010). If existing technology will no longer work for the client, the practitioner should first consider other commercially available ET before moving to more specialized AT (Oliver, 2019). This approach will help control costs (Oliver, 2019). In addition, commercially available ET is more socially acceptable to clients and more likely to be used rather than abandoned because it does not direct attention to their disability (Brunner et al., 2017; Charters et al., 2015; Chu et al., 2014; Ferguson et al., 2015; Gustavsson et al., 2018; Hakobyan et al., 2013; Hendricks et al., 2015; Lund et al., 2014; Wild, 2013; Wong et al., 2017).

Another essential piece of the occupational therapy intervention is training the client with the device, specifically in the context of occupation where the focus is on how ET can help improve occupational performance (Lindén et al., 2011). It is helpful to consider the technology as another compensatory strategy, similar to other strategies clients may use, such as checklists or memory logs. As a result, the training that happens with technology uses the same approaches as those used in cognitive rehabilitation in general (described in detail in Chapters 9 and 10). Research has found that errorless learning can be a useful technique when clients are in the acquisition phase of learning to use ET or if generalization is not expected (Bartfai & Bowman, 2014; Bertens et al., 2015; Cicerone et al., 2019; Lindén et al., 2011; Lund et al., 2011; Powell et al., 2015; Radomski & Giles, 2021). Metacognitive strategy training can be helpful when the goal is generalization of ET use (e.g., using the alarm for both medication management and to remember pet care; Lund et al., 2012; Polatajko, 2017; Skidmore et al., 2017). Similar to cognitive rehabilitation with other treatment modalities besides ET, training in context is important so that clients can have practice using devices during actual meaningful activities rather than in artificial environments. This also enables clients to problem solve solutions to situations that may arise in environments that are less controlled (Leopold et al., 2015; Lindén et al., 2010; Livingstone-Lee et al., 2014; Oliver, 2019; Powell et al., 2015; Scherer & Federici, 2015). Adequate time to work with devices through repetition and reinforcement, including time spent using ET outside of therapy sessions, is important for learning and generalization of tasks (de Joode et al., 2012; Federici et al., 2014; Geusgens et al., 2007; Kassberg et al., 2016; Lindén et al., 2011; Oliver, 2019).

Although there is a great deal of overlap between training a client to use a nontechnological compensatory strategy and one that uses ET, there are some factors that are unique to technology as a treatment modality. First, time needs to be spent with clients and caregivers problem solving solutions for scenarios for when the technology fails, such as when the battery runs out, the device is lost, or it malfunctions in another way (Wild, 2013). Second, clients and caregivers also need to know how to maintain devices and keep them fully updated (Oliver, 2019; Veterans Health

Administration, 2010; Wild, 2013). Finally, there are safety concerns that need to be considered depending on how the ET will be used. Passwords need to be secured. People with ABI are a more vulnerable population and are at risk for becoming victims of fraud. Interpersonal interactions online may also be an issue because of difficulties with behavior management (Baker-Sparr et al., 2018; Brunner et al., 2015; Gustavsson et al., 2018; Oliver, 2019), although most people with ABI report that ET can help them feel more socially connected (Albers et al., 2022; Baker-Sparr et al., 2018; Brunner et al., 2015, 2017; Gustavvson et al., 2018; Hendricks et al., 2015; Lindqvist & Borell, 2012). Having safeguards in place, such as parental controls that limit the available features on devices, may be useful for caregivers who are working with care recipients using technology.

Barriers, Current Practice, and Next Steps

The evidence on the effectiveness of ET as a compensatory strategy for people recovering from ABI is strong. The inclusion of technology training in the rehabilitation process has been named as a practice standard for people with cognitive impairment after brain injury by both the American Congress of Rehabilitation Medicine (Wild, 2013) and the Veterans Health Administration (2010). Despite the evidence and the implementation of practice standards regarding technology inclusion in rehabilitation, most occupational therapy practitioners, along with other rehabilitation professionals, have not been training clients with ET in therapy (Bartfai & Boman, 2014; de Joode et al., 2012; Hart et al., 2003). In 2012, de Joode and colleagues described a survey of 147 rehabilitation professionals, approximately 25% of whom were occupational therapy practitioners. These researchers found that only about 28% of these practitioners had used technology in their treatment with clients with ABI. This finding was similar to another study that was completed with practitioners in 2004 with approximately 30% of professionals using technology in rehabilitation. Despite increasing personal use of technology by the general public, the use of technology in rehabilitation was essentially unchanged between these two surveys (de Joode et al., 2012). A third survey that was completed in 2015 showed that only 20% of occupational therapists ($n = 40$) consistently used ET in treatment with clients with ABI, although an additional 45% did occasionally use it (Ladner & Davis, 2015).

There are several reasons that many clinicians have not used technology with their clients. The most commonly cited issue was the cost and availability of the technology (de Joode et al., 2012; Hart et al., 2003; Ladner & Davis, 2015). This may become less of an issue with time because the cost of many types of ET has been decreasing as it becomes more common (Hakobyan et al., 2013; Hendricks et al., 2015). In addition, it is increasingly likely that clients with ABI will have their own devices that may be used in rehabilitation, especially because clients are likely to return to using ET whether or not they receive training, albeit less effectively (Gustavsson et al., 2018).

Another major issue relates to clinician knowledge and confidence in their ability to train people with ABI to use ET (Bartfai & Boman, 2014; de Joode et al., 2012; Hart et al., 2003; Ladner & Davis, 2015; Nygård & Rosenberg, 2016; Wild, 2013). In a survey of 81 rehabilitation professionals, 21% of whom were occupational therapy practitioners, Hart and colleagues (2003) found that more than two-thirds of respondents were either not at all confident or only slightly confident in their ability to use technology in treatment with clients with ABI.

Researchers have made several recommendations to clinicians about how to build knowledge and confidence about ET. The first recommendation is to seek out continuing education opportunities for increasing knowledge about how ET can be used with people with ABI. Identifying peers who can provide mentoring is another way to improve both knowledge and confidence (Bartfai & Boman, 2014; de Joode et al., 2012). A second recommendation is to attend to and reflect on personal ET use. Many of the ways in which the general public, including clinicians themselves, use

ET can also help to support people with ABI (Hart et al., 2003). Finally, researchers recommend that clinicians focus on the ultimate goal of occupational performance and view the technology as a tool that can enable people to better engage in occupation. By approaching technology use as another activity to analyze versus something that is wholly unique, occupational therapy practitioners can make use of existing skills to approach technology as a treatment modality (Covington & Kim, 2014; Lindén et al., 2011).

Conclusion

Technology is increasingly prevalent in today's societies. Being skilled with using a variety of forms of technology is essential for many to be able to fully engage in numerous occupations, both in the home and in the community. To enable people with ABI to maximize their occupational performance, occupational therapy practitioners need to consider how well their clients are using technology. Exploring technology use needs to be a part of occupational therapy evaluation through both interview and observation. Systematic and individualized intervention that incorporates technology as a compensatory strategy will enable people with brain injury to better use the resources they have available to them and to identify new options and opportunities.

References

Adolfsson, P., Lindstedt, H., & Janeslätt, G. (2015). How people with cognitive disabilities experience electronic planning devices. *NeuroRehabilitation, 37*, 379-392. https://doi.org/10.3233/NRE-151268

Albers, E. A., Mikal, J., Millenbah, A., Finlay, J., Jutkowitz, E., Mitchell, L., Horn, B., & Gaugler, J. E. (2022). The use of technology among persons with memory concerns and their caregivers in the United States during the COVID-19 pandemic: Qualitative study. *JMIR Aging, 5*(1), e31552. https://doi.org/10.2196/31552

American Occupational Therapy Association. (2020). Occupational therapy practice framework: Domain and process (4th ed.). *American Journal of Occupational Therapy, 74*(Suppl. 2), 7412410010. https://doi.org/10.5014/ajot.2020.74S2001

Baker-Sparr, C., Hart, T., Bergquist, T., Bogner, J., Dreer, L., Juengst, S., Mellick, D., O'Neil-Pirozzi, T. M., Sander, A. M., & Whiteneck, G. G. (2018). Internet and social media use after traumatic brain injury: A traumatic brain injury model systems study. *Journal of Head Trauma Rehabilitation, 33*, E9-E17. https://doi.org/10.1097/HTR.0000000000000305

Bartfai, A., & Boman, I.-L. (2014). A multiprofessional client-centred guide to implementing assistive technology for clients with cognitive impairments. *Technology and Disability, 26*, 11-21. https://doi.org/10.3233/TAD-140400

Bertens, D., Kessels, R. P. C., Fiorenzato, E., Boelen, D. H. E., & Fasotti, L. (2015). Do old errors always lead to new truths? A randomized controlled trial of errorless goal management training in brain-injured patients. *Journal of the International Neuropsychological Society, 21*, 639-649. https://doi.org/10.1017/S1355617715000764

Brain Injury Association of America. (2022). Assistive technology acts. https://www.biausa.org/public-affairs/public-policy/assistive-technology-act

Brown, J., Hux, K., Hey, M., & Murphy, M. (2017). Exploring cognitive support use and preference by college students with TBI: A mixed-methods study. *NeuroRehabilitation, 41*, 483-499. https://doi.org/10.3233/NRE-162065

Brunner, M., Hemsley, B., Palmer, S., Dann, S., & Togher, L. (2015). Review of the literature on the use of social media by people with traumatic brain injury (TBI). *Disability and Rehabilitation, 37*, 1511-1521. https://doi.org/10.3109/09638288.2015.1045992

Brunner, M., Hemsley, B., Togher, L., & Palmer, S. (2017). Technology and its role in rehabilitation for people with cognitive-communication disability following a traumatic brain injury (TBI). *Brain Injury, 31*, 1028-1043. https://doi.org/10.1080/02699052.2017.1292429

Cardell, B., Swain, L., & Burnett, A. (2013). Construct validity of the Functionally Simulated Technology Task: An exploratory study. *Occupational Therapy in Health Care, 27*, 345-354. https://doi.org/10.3109/07380577.2013.845928

Charters, E., Gillett, L., & Simpson, G. K. (2015). Efficacy of electronic portable assistive devices for people with acquired brain injury: A systematic review. *Neuropsychological Rehabilitation, 25*, 82-121. https://doi.org/10.1080/09602011.2014.942672

Chu, Y., Brown, P., Harniss, M., Kautz, H., & Johnson, K. (2014). Cognitive support technologies for people with TBI: Current usage and challenges experienced. *Disability and Rehabilitation: Assistive Technology, 9*, 279-285. https://doi.org/10.3109/17483107.2013.823631

Cicerone, K. D., Goldin, Y., Ganci, K., Rosenbaum, A., Wethe, J. V., Langenbahn, D. M., Malec, J. F., Bergquist, T. F., Kingsley K., Nagele, D., Trexler, L., Fraas, M., Bogdanova, Y., & Harley, J. P. (2019). Evidence-based cognitive rehabilitation: Systematic review of the literature from 2009 through 2014. *Archives of Physical Medicine and Rehabilitation, 100*, 1515-1533. https://doi.org/10.1016/j.apmr.2019.02.011

Copolillo, A., & Dahlin-Ivanoff, S. (2011). Assistive technology and home modification for people with neurovisual deficits. *NeuroRehabiltation, 28*, 211-220. https://doi.org/10.3233/NRE-2011-0650

Covington, R., & Kim, G. (2014). *Occupational therapists' evaluation and treatment of everyday technology with adult patients with traumatic brain injury* [Unpublished master's thesis]. University of Puget Sound.

Crossland, M. D., Silva, R. S., & Macedo, A. F. (2014). Smartphone, tablet computer and e-reader use by people with vision impairment. *Ophthalmic & Physiological Optics, 34*, 552-557. https://doi.org/10.1111/opo.12136

de Joode, E. A., van Boxtel, M. P. J., Verhey, F. R., & van Heugten, C. M. (2012). Use of assistive technology in cognitive rehabilitation: Exploratory studies of the opinions and expectations of healthcare professionals and potential users. *Brain Injury, 26*, 1257-1266. https://doi.org/10.3109/02699052.2012.667590

de Joode, E., van Heugten, C., Vergey, F., & van Boxtel, M. (2010). Efficacy and usability of assistive technology for patients with cognitive deficits: A systematic review. *Clinical Rehabilitation, 24*, 701-714. https://doi.org/10.1177/0269215510367551

Dixon, E., & Lazar, A. (2020). The role of sensory changes in everyday technology use by people with mild to moderate dementia. *ASSETS, 41*. https://doi.org/10.1145/3373625.3417000

Engström, A-L. L., Lexell, J., & Lund, M. L. (2010). Difficulties in using everyday technology after acquired brain injury: A qualitative analysis. *Scandinavian Journal of Occupational Therapy, 17*, 233-243. https://doi.org/10.3109/11038120903191806

Erikkson, M., & Dahlin-Ivanoff, S. (2002). How adults with acquired brain damage perceive computer training as a rehabilitation tool: A focus-group study. *Scandinavian Journal of Occupational Therapy, 9*, 119-129. https://doi.org/10.1080/11038120260246950

Evald, L. (2015). Prospective memory rehabilitation using smartphones in patients with TBI: What do participants report? *Neuropsychological Rehabilitation, 25*, 283-297. https://doi.org/10.1080/09602011.2014.970557

Fallahpour, M., Kottorp, A., Nygård, L., & Lund, M. L. (2014). Perceived difficulty in use of everyday technology in persons with acquired brain injury of different severity: A comparison with controls. *Journal of Rehabilitative Medicine, 46*, 635-641. https://doi.org/10.2340/16501977-1818

Fallahpour, M., Kottorp, A., Nygård, L., & Lund, M. L. (2015). Participation after acquired brain injury: Associations with everyday technology and activities in daily life. *Scandinavian Journal of Occupational Therapy, 22*, 366-376. https://doi.org/10.3109/11038128.2015.1011229

Federici, S., Scherer, M. J., & Borsci, S. (2014). An ideal model of an assistive technology assessment and delivery process. *Technology and Disability, 26*, 27-38. https://doi.org/10.3233/TAD-140402

Ferguson, S., Friedland, D., & Woodberry, E. (2015). Smartphone technology: Gentle reminders of everyday tasks for those with prospective memory difficulties post-brain injury. *Brain Injury, 29*, 583-591. https://doi.org/10.3109/02699052.2014.1002109

Gentry, T. (2018). Consumer technologies as cognitive aids. In N. Katz & J. Toglia (Eds.), *Cognition, occupation, and participation across the lifespan* (4th ed., pp. 219-230). AOTA Press.

Geusgens, C. A. V., Winkens, I., van Heugten, C. M., Josses, J., & van den Heuvel, W. J. A. (2007). Occurrence and measurement of transfer in cognitive rehabilitation: A critical review. *Journal of Rehabilitation Medicine, 39*, 425-439. https://doi.org/10.2340/16501977-0092

Gillespie, A., Best, C., & O'Neill, B. (2012). Cognitive function and assistive technology for cognition: A systematic review. *Journal of the International Neuropsychological Society, 18*, 1-19. https://doi.org/10.1017/S1355617711001548

Goverover, Y., & DeLuca, J. (2015). Actual reality: Using the internet to assess everyday functioning after traumatic brain injury. *Brain Injury, 29*, 715-721. https://doi.org/10.3109/02699052.2015.1004744

Gustavsson, M., Ytterberg, C., Marwaa, M. N., Tham, K., & Guidetti, S. (2018). Experiences of using information and communication technology within the first year after stroke—A grounded theory study. *Disability and Rehabilitation, 40*, 561-568. https://doi.org/10.1080/09638288.2016.1264012

Hakobyan, L., Lumsden, J., O'Sullivan, D., & Barlett, H. (2013). Mobile assistive technologies for the visually impaired. *Survey of Ophthalmology, 58*, 513-528. https://doi.org/10.1016/j.survophthal.2012.10.004

Hart, T., O'Neill-Pirozzi, T. O., & Morita, C. (2003). Clinician expectations for portable electronic devices as cognitive-behavioural orthoses in traumatic brain injury rehabilitation. *Brain Injury, 17*, 401-411. https://doi.org/10.1080/0269905021000038438

Hendricks, D. J., Sampson, E., Rumrill, P., Leopold, A., Elias, E., Jacobs, K., Nardone, A., Sherer, M., & Stauffer, C. (2015). Activities and interim outcomes of a multi-site development project to promote cognitive support technology use and employment success among postsecondary students with traumatic brain injuries. *NeuroRehabilitation, 37*, 449-458. https://doi.org/10.3233/NRE-151273

Institute for Matching Person and Technology, Inc. (2021). Matching person and technology. https://sites.google.com/view/matchingpersontechnology/home

Jamieson, M., Cullen, B., McGee-Lennon, M., Brewster, S., & Evans, J. J. (2014). The efficacy of cognitive prosthetic technology for people with memory impairments: A systematic review and meta-analysis. *Neuropsychological Rehabilitation, 24*, 419-444. https://doi.org/10.1080/09602011.2013.825632

Karolinska Institutet. (2022a). Everyday Technology Use Questionnaire, ETUQ. https://ki.se/en/nvs/everyday-technology-use-questionnaire-etuq

Karolinska Institutet. (2022b). Management of Everyday Technology Assessment, META. https://ki.se/en/nvs/management-of-everyday-technology-assessment-meta

Kassberg, A.-C., Malinowsky, C., Jacobsson, L., & Lund, M. L. (2013). Ability to manage everyday technology after acquired brain injury. *Brain Injury, 27*, 1583-1588. https://doi.org/10.3109/02699052.2013.837196

Kassberg, A.-C., Prellwitz, M., & Lund, M. L. (2013). The challenges of everyday technology in the workplace for persons with acquired brain injury. *Scandinavian Journal of Occupational Therapy, 20*, 272-281. https://doi.org/10.3109/11038128.2012.734330

Kassberg, A.-C., Prellwitz, M., Malinowsky, C., & Larsson-Lund, M. (2016). Interventions aimed at improving the ability to use everyday technology in work after brain injury. *Scandinavian Journal of Occupational Therapy, 23*, 147-157. https://doi.org/10.3109/11038128.2015.1122835

Kottorp, A., & Nygård, L. (2011). Development of a short-form assessment for detection of subtle activity limitations: Can use of everyday technology distinguish between MCI and Alzheimer's disease? *Expert Review of Neurotherapeutics, 11*, 647-655. https://doi.org/10.1586/ern.11.55

Ladner, J., & Davis, A. (2015). *The use of everyday technology in occupational therapy practice for clients with acquired brain injury* [Unpublished master's thesis]. University of Puget Sound.

Leopold, A., Lourie, A., Petras, H., & Elias, E. (2015). The use of assistive technology for cognition to support the performance of daily activities for individuals with cognitive disabilities due to traumatic brain injury: The current state of the research. *NeuroRehabilitation, 37*, 359-378. https://doi.org/10.3233/NRE-151267

Li, K., Alonso, J., Chadha, N., & Pulido, J. (2015). Does generalization occur following computer-based cognitive retraining?—An exploratory study. *Occupational Therapy in Health Care, 29*, 283-296. https://doi.org/10.3109/07380577.2015.1010246

Lindén, A., Lexell, J., & Lund, M. L. (2010). Perceived difficulties using everyday technology after acquired brain injury: Influence on activity and participation. *Scandinavian Journal of Occupational Therapy, 17*, 267-275. https://doi.org/10.3109/11038120903265022

Lindén, A., Lexell, J., & Lund, M. L. (2011). Improvements of task performance in daily life after acquired brain injury using commonly available everyday technology. *Disability and Rehabilitation: Assistive Technology, 6*, 214-224. https://doi.org/10.3109/17483107.2010.528142

Lindqvist, E., & Borell, L. (2012). Computer-based assistive technology and changes in daily living after stroke. *Disability and Rehabilitation: Assistive Technology, 7*, 364-371. https://doi.org/10.3109/17483107.2011.638036

Livingstone-Lee, S. A., Skelton, R. W., & Livingston, N. (2014). Transit apps for people with brain injury and other cognitive disabilities: The state of the art. *Assistive Technology, 26*, 209-218. https://doi.org/10.1080/10400435.2014.930076

Lund, M. L., Engström, A.-L. L., & Lexell, J. (2012). Response actions to difficulties in using everyday technology after acquired brain injury. *Scandinavian Journal of Occupational Therapy, 19*, 164-175. https://doi.org/10.3109/11038128.2011.582651

Lund, M. L., Lövgren-Engström, A.-L., & Lexell, J. (2011). Using everyday technology to compensate for difficulties in task performance in daily life: Experiences in persons with acquired brain injury and their significant others. *Disability and Rehabilitation: Assistive Technology, 6*, 402-411. https://doi.org/10.3109/17483107.2011.574309

Lund, M. L., Nygård, L., & Kottorp, A. (2014). Perceived difficulty in the use of everyday technology: Relationships with everyday functioning in people with acquired brain injury with a special focus on returning to work. *Disability and Rehabilitation, 36*, 1618-1625. https://doi.org/10.3109/09638288.2013.863388

Malinowsky, C., Almkvist, O., Nygård, L., & Kottorp, A. (2012). Individual variability and environmental characteristics influence older adults' abilities to manage everyday technology. *International Psychogeriatrics, 24*, 484-495. https://doi.org/10.1017/S1041610211002092

Malinowsky, C., Kassberg, A.-C., Larsson-Lund, M., & Kottorp, A. (2016). Stability of person ability measures in people with acquired brain injury in the use of everyday technology: The test-retest reliability of the Management of Everyday Technology Assessment (META). *Disability and Rehabilitation: Assistive Technology, 11*, 395-399. https://doi.org/10.3109/17483107.2014.968812

Malinowsky, C., & Lund, M. L. (2014). The association between perceived and observed ability to use everyday technology in people of working age with ABI. *Scandinavian Journal of Occupational Therapy, 21*, 465-472. https://doi.org/10.3109/11038128.2014.919020

Malinowsky, C., & Lund, M. L. (2016). The match between everyday technology in public space and the ability of working-age people with acquired brain injury to use it. *British Journal of Occupational Therapy, 79*, 26-34. https://doi.org/10.1177/0308022614563943

Malinowsky, C., Nygård, L., & Kottorp, A. (2011). Psychometric evaluation of a new assessment of the ability to manage technology in everyday life. *Scandinavian Journal of Occupational Therapy, 18*, 26-35. https://doi.org/10.3109/11038120903420606

Malinowsky, C., Nygård, L., Pantzar, M., & Kottorp, A. (2020). Test-retest reliability of the short version of the everyday technology use questionnaire (S-ETUQ). *Scandinavian Journal of Occupational Therapy, 27*, 567-576. https://doi.org/10.1080/11038128.2020.1744715

Maskill, L., & Tempest, S. (2017). Intervention for cognitive impairments and evaluating outcomes. In L. Maskill & S. Tempest (Eds.), *Neuropsychology for occupational therapists: Cognition in occupational performance* (4th ed., pp. 33-49). Wiley Blackwell.

Nygård, L., & Rosenberg, L. (2016). How attention to everyday technology could contribute to modern occupational therapy: A focus group study. *British Journal of Occupational Therapy, 79*, 467-474. https://doi.org/10.1177/0308022615613354

Oliver, M. (2019). Assistive technology in polytrauma rehabilitation. *Physical Medicine and Rehabilitation Clinics of North America, 30*, 217-259. https://doi.org/10.1016/j.pmr.2018.08.002

Perrin, A., & Atske, S. (2021). Americans with disabilities less likely than those without to own some digital devices. Pew Research Center. https://www.pewresearch.org/fact-tank/2021/09/10/americans-with-disabilities-less-likely-than-those-without-to-own-some-digital-devices/

Pew Research Center. (2021). Fact sheets. https://www.pewresearch.org/publications/?formats=fact-sheet&research-teams=internet-tech

Polatajko, H. J. (2017). History of the CO-OP Approach. In D. Dawson, S. E. McEwen, & H. J. Polatajko (Eds.), *Cognitive Orientation to daily Occupational Performance in occupational therapy: Using the CO-OP Approach to enable participation across the lifespan* (pp. 5-10). AOTA Press.

Powell, L. E., Gland, A., Pinkelman, S., Albin, R., Harwick, R., Ettel, D., & Wild, M. R. (2015). Systematic instruction of assistive technology for cognition (ATC) in an employment setting following acquired brain injury: A single case, experimental study. *NeuroRehabilitation, 37*, 437-447.

Radomski, M. V., & Giles, G. M. (2021). Cognitive intervention. In D. P. Dirette & S. A. Gutman (Eds.), *Occupational therapy for physical dysfunction* (8th ed., pp. 161-175). Wolters Kluwer.

Rand, D., Lee Ben-Haim, K., Malka, R., & Portnoy, S. (2018). Development of internet-based tasks for the Executive Function Performance Test. *American Journal of Occupational Therapy, 72*, 7202205060. http://doi.org/10.5014/ajot.2018.023598

Rogers, J. C., Holm, M. B., & Chisholm, D. (2016). *Performance Assessment of Self-Care Skills: Scoring guidelines.* University of Pittsburgh.

Rosenberg, L., Nygård, L., & Kottorp, A. (2009). Everyday Technology Use Questionnaire: Psychometric evaluation of a new assessment of competence in technology use. *OTJR: Occupation, Participation and Health, 29*, 52-62. https://doi.org/10.3928/15394492-20090301-05

Scherer, M. J., & Craddock, G. (2002). Matching Person & Technology (MPT) assessment process. *Technology and Disability, 14*, 125-131. https://doi.org/10.3233/TAD-2002-14308

Scherer, M. J., & Federici, S. (2015). Why people use and don't use technologies: Introduction to the special issue on assistive technologies for cognition/cognitive support technologies. *NeuroRehabilitation, 37*, 315-319. https://doi.org/10.3233/NRE-151264

Scherer, M. J., Sax, C., Vanbiervliet, A., Cushman, L. A., & Scherer, J. V. (2005). Predictors of assistive technology use: the importance of personal and psychosocial factors. *Disability and Rehabilitation, 27*, 1321-1331. https://doi.org/10.1080/09638280500164800

Skidmore, E. R., McEwen, S. E., Green, D., van den Houten, J., Dawson, D. R., & Polatajko, H. J. (2017). Essential elements and key features of the CO-OP Approach. In D. Dawson, S. E. McEwen, & H. J. Polatajko (Eds.), *Cognitive Orientation to daily Occupational Performance in occupational therapy: Using the CO-OP Approach to enable participation across the lifespan* (pp. 11-20). AOTA Press.

Stock, S. E., Davies, D. K., Wehmeyer, M. L., & Lachapelle, Y. (2011). Emerging new practices in technology to support independent community access for people with intellectual and cognitive disabilities. *NeuroRehabilitation, 28*, 261-269. https://doi.org/10.3233/NRE-2011-0654

University of Utah College of Health. (2022). OT therapeutic activities. https://health.utah.edu/occupational-recreational-therapies/colleagues-clinicians/

van de Ven, R. M., Buitenweg, J. I. V., Schmand, B., Veltman, D. J., Aaronson, J. A., Nijboer, T. C. W., Kruiper-Doesborgh, S. J. C., van Bennekom, C. A. M., Rasquin, S. M. C., Ridderinkhof, K. R., & Murre, J. M. J. (2017). Brain training improves recovery after stroke but waiting list improves equally: A multicenter randomized controlled trial of a computer-based cognitive flexibility training. *PLoS ONE, 12*(3), e0172993. https://doi.org/10.1371/journal.pone.0172993

van de Ven, R. M., Murre, J. M. J., Veltman, D. J., & Schmand, B. A. (2016). Computer-based cognitive training for executive functions after stroke: A systematic review. *Frontiers in Human Neuroscience, 10*, 150. https://doi.org/10.3389/fnhum.2016.00150

Veterans Health Administration. (2010). Veterans Health Administration Prosthetic Clinical Management Program (PCMP) clinical practice recommendations electronic cognitive devices. https://www.prosthetics.va.gov/Docs/CPR_ElectronicCognitiveDevices.pdf

Wallcook, S., Malinowsky, C., Nygård, L., Charlesworth, G., Lee, J., Walsh, R., Gaber, S., & Kottorp, A. (2020). The perceived challenge of everyday technologies in Sweden, the United States and England: Exploring differential item functioning in the everyday technology use questionnaire. *Scandinavian Journal of Occupational Therapy, 27*, 554-566. https://doi.org/10.1080/11038128.2020.1723685

Wang, J., Ding, D., Teodorski, E. E., Mahajan, H. P., & Cooper, R. A. (2016). Use of assistive technology for cognition among people with traumatic brain injury: A survey study. *Military Medicine, 181*, 560-566. https://doi.org/10.7205/MILMED-D-14-00704

Wild, M. R. (2013). Assistive technology for cognition following brain injury: Guidelines for device and app selection. *Perspectives on Neurophysiology and Neurogenic Speech and Language Disorders, 23*, 49-58. https://doi.org/10.1044/nnsld23.2.49

Wong, D., Sinclair, K., Seabrook, E., McKay, A., & Ponsford, J. (2017). Smartphones as assistive technology following traumatic brain injury: A preliminary study of what helps and what hinders. *Disability and Rehabilitation, 39*, 2387-2394. https://doi.org/10.1080/09638288.2016.1226434

Index

Printed in the United States
by Baker & Taylor Publisher Services

Printed in the United States
by Baker & Taylor Publisher Services